LINCOLN CHRISTIAN COLLEGE AN

HOMOSEXUALITY, SCIENCE, AND THE "PLAIN SENSE" OF SCRIPTURE

Homosexuality, Science, *and the* "Plain Sense" of Scripture

Edited by

DAVID L. BALCH

WILLIAM B. EERDMANS PUBLISHING COMPANY
GRAND RAPIDS, MICHIGAN / CAMBRIDGE, U.K.

© 2000 Wm. B. Eerdmans Publishing Co.
255 Jefferson Ave. S.E., Grand Rapids, Michigan 49503 /
P.O. Box 163, Cambridge CB3 9PU U.K.
All rights reserved

Printed in the United States of America

05 04 03 02 01 00 7 6 5 4 3 2 1

Library of Congress Cataloging-in-Publication Data

Homosexuality, science, and the "plain sense" of scripture /
edited by David L. Balch.
p. cm.
Includes bibliographical references.
ISBN 0-8028-4698-X (pbk.)
1. Homosexuality — Religious aspects —Christianity — Congresses.
I. Balch, David L.

BR115.H6 P58 2000
261.8′35766 —dc21

99-055787

For Prof. Stephen V. Sprinkle,
valued friend and colleague,
director of field education and supervised ministry,
instructor in practical theology at Brite Divinity School/TCU,
and a founder and co-pastor of Angel of Hope Christian Church
(Disciples of Christ) (www. angelofhope.org.)

Contents

Contributors ix

Abbreviations xi

Introduction 1
David L. Balch

1. Muddling Through: The Church and Sexuality/Homosexuality 6
Mark G. Toulouse

2. Same-Sex Eros: Paul and the Greco-Roman Tradition 43
William R. Schoedel

3. The Use, Misuse, and Abuse of Science in the Ecclesiastical Homosexuality Debates 73
Stanton L. Jones and Mark A. Yarhouse

4. The Bible and Science on Sexuality 121
Christine E. Gudorf

5. The Bible in Christian Ethical Deliberation concerning Homosexuality: Old Testament Contributions 142
Phyllis A. Bird

6. Sexuality and Scripture's Plain Sense: The Christian Community and the Law of God 177
Christopher Seitz

7. Natural and Unnatural Use in Romans 1:24-27: Paul and the Philosophic Critique of Eros 197
David E. Fredrickson

8. The Social Context and Implications of Homoerotic References in Romans 1:24-27 223
Robert Jewett

9. The Logic of the Interpretation of Scripture and the Church's Debate over Sexual Ethics 242
Kathryn Greene-McCreight

10. Christian Vocation, Freedom of God, and Homosexuality 261
Nancy J. Duff

Concluding Observations by the Editor, Including a Comparison of Christian with Jewish Biblical Interpretation 278
David L. Balch

Index of Contemporary Authors 305

Scripture Index 313

Index of Other Ancient Authors 317

Contributors

David L. Balch is professor of New Testament at Brite Divinity School, Texas Christian University, Fort Worth, Texas.

Phyllis A. Bird is professor of Old Testament interpretation at Garrett-Evangelical Theological Seminary, Evanston, Illinois.

Nancy J. Duff is associate professor of Reformed theological ethics at Princeton Theological Seminary, Princeton, New Jersey.

David E. Fredrickson is associate professor of New Testament at Luther Seminary in St. Paul, Minnesota.

Kathryn Greene-McCreight is visiting lecturer in the religion department of Smith College, North Hampton, Massachusetts.

Christine E. Gudorf is professor of ethics at Florida International University, Miami, Florida.

Robert Jewett is professor emeritus at Garrett-Evangelical Theological Seminary and in 2000 will become a research professor at the University of Heidelberg, Germany.

Stanton L. Jones is provost of Wheaton College, Wheaton, Illinois.

William R. Schoedel is retired professor of classics and religious studies at the University of Illinois, Urbana, Illinois.

Christopher Seitz is chair of the department of Old Testament and theological studies, University of St. Andrews, Scotland.

Mark G. Toulouse is the dean of Brite Divinity School, Texas Christian University, Fort Worth, Texas.

Mark A. Yarhouse is assistant professor of psychology at Regent University in Virginia Beach, Virginia.

Abbreviations

Akk.	Akkadian
ABD	*Anchor Bible Dictionary*
AOAT	Alter Orient und Altes Testament
APA	American Psychiatric Association
BAGD	W. Bauer, *A Greek-English Lexicon of the New Testament,* trans. W. F. Arndt and F. W. Gingrich, 2nd ed. rev. and augmented by F. W. Gingrich and F. W. Danker (Chicago, 1979)
BCC	Beth Chayim Chadashim
BDB	Brown, Driver, and Briggs, *Hebrew and English Lexicon of the Old Testament* (1907)
BET	Beiträge zur biblischen Exegese und Theologie
BRM	Babylonian Records in the Library of J. Pierpont Morgan
BibS(N)	*Biblische Studien* (Neukirchen)
BThZ	*Berliner Theologische Zeitschrift*
CBQ	*Catholic Biblical Quarterly*
CCAR	Central Conference of American Rabbis
CRINT	Compendia rerum iudaicarum ad novum testamentum
CT	Cuneiform Texts from Babylonian Tablets in the British Museum, London
DSM	*Diagnostic and Statistical Manual*
EC	Evangelicals Concerned
EKK	Evangelisch-Katholischer Kommentar zum Neuen Testament
ELCA	Evangelical Lutheran Church in America
FC	The Fathers of the Church
HNT	Handbuch zum Neuen Testament
HSS	Harvard Semitic Studies

HTR	*Harvard Theological Review*
HWP	*Historisches Wörterbuch der Philosophie*
JAAR	*Journal of the American Academy of Religion*
JBL	*Journal of Biblical Literature*
JRE	*Journal of Religious Ethics*
JSOT	*Journal for the Study of the Old Testament*
KAI	H. Donner and W. Röllig, *Kanaanäische und aramäische Inschriften,* 3 vols. (Wiesbaden, 1962-64)
KAV	*Keilschrifttexte aus Assur verschieden Inhalts,* ed. O. Schroeder (Leipzig and Berlin, 1920)
LSJ	H. G. Liddell, R. Scott, and H. S. Jones, with the assistance of R. McKenzie, *Greek-English Lexicon* (revised 1968)
MCC	Metropolitan Community Church
NovT	*Novum Testamentum*
NRSV	New Revised Standard Version
NRTh	*Nouvelle Revue Théologique*
NTSupp	*Novum Testamentum* Supplements
OBO	Orbis biblicus et orientalis
PJC	Presbyterian Judicial Commission
PW	A. Pauly–G. Wissowa, *Real-Encyclopädie der klassichen Altertumswissenschaft*
RB	*Revue Biblique*
RSV	Revised Standard Version
SAA	State Archives of Assyria
SANT	Studien zum Alten und Neuen Testament
SBT	Studies in Biblical Theology
SNTS	Society for New Testament Studies
TDNT	*Theological Dictionary of the New Testament*
ThWAT	*Theologisches Wörterbuch zum Alten Testament*
TS	*Texts and Studies*
UAHC	Union of American Hebrew Congregations
UCC	United Church of Christ
UF	*Ugarit-Forschungen: Internationales Jahrbuch für die Altertumskunde Syrien-Palästinas*
UMC	United Methodist Church
USQR	*Union Seminary Quarterly Review*
VC	*Vigiliae Christianae*
VTSup	Vetus Testamentum Supplements
WUNT	Wissenschaftliche Untersuchungen zum Neuen Testament
ZAW	*Zeitschrift für die alttestamentliche Wissenschaft*
ZEE	*Zeitschrift für evangelische Ethik*
ZNW	*Zeitschrift für die neutestamentliche Wissenschaft*

Introduction

DAVID L. BALCH

This book arises out of current discussions in our churches concerning the interpretation of the Bible in relation to the morality of homosexual acts and relationships. At a meeting in Washington, D.C., in 1993 of persons who are both ordained pastors and professors, we had a vigorous discussion of a proposed social statement of human sexuality by a church body. I emphasize that this debate arose among persons concerned for the church, not primarily in the academy. The group asked Karl Donfried and me to help generate more discussion. The Louisville Institute first gave a planning grant, then a conference grant that supported further, balanced debate. In the proposal to the Louisville Institute and at the conference, I arranged the discussions so that persons who represent both poles of the discussion presented their interpretations of evangelical and mainline church understandings of science, Old and New Testaments, and theology. I am grateful to the Louisville Institute and Wm. B. Eerdmans Publishing Company for making these discussions and their publication possible, but neither institution is responsible for any of the particular writers' opinions.

1. Mark Toulouse, a Disciples of Christ minister, surveys the current state of the discussion among both evangelicals and mainstream churches. There has been change over the past forty years in both these groups' discussion of sexuality, as reflected in their widely read church journals. He concludes that language of "culture wars" is inappropriate to describe our present conflicts over sexuality, but that the majority of Christians leaning left and those leaning right can be described as belonging to a "muddled middle." Several recent denominational social statements belong to this muddled middle.

2. Planners for the conference insisted that science must be a central aspect of the discussions, since somehow what is (nature) is related to what ought to be (ethics). Bill Schoedel, a member of the Lutheran Church–Missouri Synod, writes on the subject of his doctoral dissertation for Robert Grant at Chicago, Greco-Roman anthropology, on which he has had an entire academic career to reflect. He shows that Greco-Roman biology, medicine, and embryology in the first and second centuries C.E. may well have informed the ethics of Hellenistic Jews like Philo and Christians like Paul, Barnabas, and Clement of Alexandria. Schoedel also documents ancient debates about whether sexuality is a continuum between male and female, with some males and females being intersexual, a possibility rejected by most Jews and Christians like Philo and Clement of Alexandria, who also appeal to binary conceptions of purity/impurity.

3. Stanton Jones, now a member of the Evangelical Presbyterian Church, and Mark A. Yarhouse, an Episcopalian, write on contemporary psychology. Jones and Yarhouse object to the way scientific research has been used to caricature the traditionalist view. As psychologists, they survey contemporary scientific research into both the prevalence and the causes of homosexual orientation. They conclude that "the traditionalist argument is essentially that God has revealed that heterosexual union in marriage or chastity are the two desired outcomes with regard to genital sexual experience for which God created humans, and that God commands us to refrain from all noncommended sexual behaviors, including homosexual ones, regardless of the sources of our urges to do otherwise."

4. Christine Gudorf, a Roman Catholic, disputes Jones's and Yarhouse's claim that "God's standard for . . . all persons [is] chastity in marriage or celibacy outside of marriage." Like Phyllis Bird below, she begins by stating her understanding of the Bible as a resource for Christian ethics. It is a, not the, primary resource; to see the Bible as the sole source of Christian ethics is idolatry. Science, too, needs interpretation. The most fundamental recent scientific insight, especially Kinsey's research in the late forties and early fifties, is the discovery of sexual orientation that for most persons is fixed relatively early in life. Catholicism teaches that the discoveries of science contribute to understandings of God's original intention and ongoing will, a contrast to classical Protestantism, which rejected nature as corrupted by sin. Given the traditionally anti-intellectual ethos of conservative Protestantism, recognizing science as uncovering divine intention within creation will not be easy.

5. From science, our discussions moved to the Old Testament. Phyllis Bird, a Methodist professor, presents sexuality in Old Testament legal, narrative, and wisdom literature, noting Egyptian, Mesopotamian, and Canaanite

parallels or the lack of them. She begins with her understanding of Scripture, which supplies governing principles, the starting point for the church's conversation, not the end. These principles demand love of God and neighbor that finds expression in concrete acts. She differs from Christopher Seitz, writer of the following paper in this volume, in insisting on the historical character of the biblical witness. Then she deals with the narrative texts Genesis 19:1-29 and Judges 19:22-24 and the legal texts Leviticus 18:22 and 20:13. Her conclusion section is as extensive as her exegesis. We may not absolutize even the creation stories, which assume the common pattern of sexual relations between male and female as the basis for reproduction of the species but do not prescribe any behavior or institution.

6. The Episcopalian Old Testament scholar Christopher Seitz writes concerning "Sexuality and Scripture's Plain Sense." He also interprets the New Testament and carries on a debate with the Episcopalian bishop John Spong. In contrast to Gudorf and Bird, Seitz sees Scripture alone as the authority that guides the church's reflection on sexual behavior. He focuses on the law of God as revealed to Israel in the Old Testament and radically reconsidered by Jesus Christ. He characterizes the Christian before God's law by interpreting Romans 3:31; 7:13-25; Matthew 5:17-48; Galatians 5:16-24; John 8:1-11; 19:30; Deuteronomy 22:23-24; Leviticus 20:13; Hebrews 10:1-31; and Mark 7:1-23. To historical-critical interpretation, which tries to uncover the novel and is not connected to church life, Seitz opposes the text's plain literal sense. Old Testament ritual law was only the shadow of reality. Responding to other essays in the third section of this book, Seitz questions appealing to Greco-Roman sources to interpret Paul, since Israel's Scriptures are the single, epistemologically privileged witness of God's revelation.

7. Then we moved to the New Testament. David Fredrickson, a Lutheran (ELCA) professor, asks how ways of conceptualizing sexual matters in Paul's philosophic and literary environment help make sense of his argument. He concludes that Paul points to the problem of insatiable "passion" without introducing the modern dichotomy of homo/heterosexual. Further, in 1 Corinthians 6:9 Paul's term "soft" refers to the problem of self-control, not to the boy prostitute, and the Greek term *arsenokoites* refers to the pederast whose vice is not misplaced desire but injustice. Greeks thought of sexual activity as "use" *(chresis)*, a term Paul employs in Romans 1:26, 27 that is often mistranslated "intercourse" or by the modern term "relation," which implies mutuality. When the terms "nature" and "use" are combined, the question concerns controlling excessive "passion." "Romans 1:24-27 is not an attack on homosexuality as a violation of divine law but a description of the human condition informed by the philosophic rejection of passionate love."

Fredrickson concludes: "it is anachronistic and inappropriate to think that Paul condemns homosexuality as unnatural and praises heterosexuality as a reflection of the God-given order of things. Sexual activity between males is not portrayed as the violation of a male-female norm given with creation but as an example of passion into which God has handed over persons who have dishonored him. The immediate problem is passion, not the gender of the persons having sex."

8. In utter contrast Robert Jewett, also a Methodist, writes in his first sentence of "the denunciation of homoerotic relations in Romans 1:24-27," then gives a detailed exegesis of these verses. An aggressive campaign against God reverses the proper relationship between creation and Creator (v. 25); assault on the right relationship to God means deliverance to dishonest relationships, "to dishonorable passions." In verse 26b Paul introduces the example of homoerotic intercourse, an example used as a rhetorical proof, and he employs the most effective example first, that of lesbian relations as sexual perversity, which would generate revulsion in his audience. His aim is not to prove the evil of homoerotic behavior; rather he simply assumes it. On this point Schoedel, Fredrickson, and Jewett agree. Next follows Paul's weaker example, male homoeroticism, because more pagan writers approved this. For Paul all same-sex relations are a proof of divine wrath. Finally, slavery was the social background of most of Paul's audience in Rome, and sexual servicing of owners was a necessity for a slave in a culture marked by aggressive bisexuality.

9. Finally, we asked constructive theologians to interpret these Scriptures. Kathryn Greene-McCreight, a United Church of Christ scholar, suggests that the argument is really about hermeneutics, the interpretation and use of Scripture. Traditional biblical hermeneutics includes approaching Scripture expecting to be taught, waiting to be transformed, to be built up in the love of God and neighbor. Valid interpretation would at least not contradict the faith of the church and would be based on a publicly accessible sense of a passage interpreted according to the rules of faith and charity, the "plain sense" of Scripture, the *sensus literalis* (see her n. 11 for bibliography), which is what the Reformers meant by *sola Scriptura.* It excludes random proof texting and reads parts of Scripture according to the whole. Finally, she insists, traditional hermeneutics did not make Enlightenment notions of equity and tolerance basic, but rather the righteousness of God and of God's grace toward fallen humanity. We cannot appeal to our experience over against Scripture and tradition.

10. Nancy Duff, who is Presbyterian, writes concerning "Christian Vocation, Freedom of God, and Homosexuality." She contends that while some are called by God into heterosexual relationships and some into the celibate life,

others are called into homosexual relationships. The starting point for theological reflection on moral issues is not human freedom but divine freedom. The second part of her essay applies the theology of God's calling to the dispute about the ethics of homosexual relationships. Same-sex unions are no more idolatrous, self-centered, or devoid of the ability to give life than heterosexual unions are. Some homosexual unions are enhanced by mutual love, give children homes, and teach the gospel. The goodness of human sexual intercourse has two purposes: the unitive and procreative. These are affirmations, not prescriptions, a statement true for both heterosexual and homosexual couples.

11. I make concluding comments,[1] which attempt to clarify aspects of the modern discussion of biblical hermeneutics, especially the way of reading the Bible shared by Brevard Childs, George Lindbeck, and Hans Frei, all of Yale Divinity School. They insist on a "plain," literal reading for the church in light of the ancient rules of faith and charity that outline the story of the gospel. These authors all suggest that a "plain" reading of Scripture would benefit from paying attention to the way Jews have read the Bible. I discovered that the debates among and between Jewish communities about the morality of homosexual relationships are quite similar to our Christian ones. Since contemporary Jews are reading (portions of) the same Scriptures, I outline their arguments, hoping that viewing the subject from a different perspective might shed new light on the issues. Strikingly, contemporary rabbis are also debating the relative importance of Leviticus 19:18 (love your neighbor as yourself) and Leviticus 20:13 (one who commits homosexual acts shall be put to death), which sounds amazingly like ancient Jewish Christian hermeneutical debates reflected in Matthew and Romans.

All the authors in this book offer their observations and arguments to the church, hoping that they contribute to our hearing the word of God.

1. This book is intentionally balanced, with arguments at both poles of the debate. I draw my own conclusions from the conference elsewhere: see "Romans 1:24-27, Science, and Homosexuality," *Currents in Theology and Mission* 25, no. 6, an issue dedicated to Edgar Krentz, of the Lutheran School of Theology at Chicago (December 1998): 433-40. I find this research compatible with study of the early Christian family: see Carolyn Osiek and David L. Balch, *Families in the New Testament World: Households and House Churches* (Louisville: Westminster/John Knox, 1997).

CHAPTER 1

Muddling Through: The Church and Sexuality/Homosexuality

MARK G. TOULOUSE

An examination of Christian struggles dealing with the issue of human sexuality indicates the emergence of some clear trends over the last forty years that should be taken seriously. Of course, taking trends too seriously can be dangerous. Trends are not hard-and-fast realities. By their very nature, trends are simply trends. They have not completely materialized and reached their final resting place. They point in a particular direction, but pointing does not mean absolutely that things are ultimately going to end up the way they are heading. Trends can be depressing or hopeful. But the people who make these responses to trends need to recognize that things can change; trends do not define future reality. People and events do that by the way they interact between now and then, just as the trends to be discussed here have emerged from the way people and events have interacted over the past forty years.

A word about the context for these emerging trends needs to be said as well. If you, the reader, could get into a time machine; set the date back to about forty years ago, perhaps around November 1956; turn the dial for a traveling destination to any city in America; and push the start button, when the machine stopped and the door opened you would find yourself in a very strange place indeed. Dwight D. Eisenhower would have just won his second term as president. You might pick up a newspaper and read editorials about the Soviet crushing of Hungarian freedom fighters the month before, or about the yearlong Montgomery bus boycott led by twenty-eight-year-old

Martin Luther King. If you landed in Los Angeles, you might want to visit two-year-old Disneyland, where you could plunk down $2.72 for admission and rides, and another 18¢ for souvenirs, things like Disneyland pennants, maps, and Donald Duck caps.

What would you see around you relating to the topic of homosexuality in the fall of 1956? Not much. It simply was not a topic of conversation. There weren't any trends because it was mostly invisible. It was present, and in about the same percentages as now. But people lived hidden lives with their own forms of hidden pain. For purposes of this discussion, in a time when many members of most churches are weary of extended discussions about homosexuality because it seems the discussion has lasted forever, it is important to recall that meaningful discussion has really been relatively short-lived in the context of the church's history, even if one limits that history to a consideration of the church in America.

As soon as you stepped out of your time machine, you could, however, get a sense of the uptight way most Christians dealt with sexuality by reading magazines describing the cultural phenomenon known as "rock 'n' roll." White leadership in Birmingham condemned it as part of a "Negro plot" against whites. Roman Catholic leaders in Boston wanted all Catholics to boycott the music. *Time* magazine, representing the older generation, listed among the characteristics of the music the fact that it usually contains "a choleric saxophone honking mating-call sounds."[1]

Christianity Today, in some ways the voice of what we commonly describe as American evangelicalism in the early 1960s, mourned the passing of the days when Pat Boone could be trusted. His involvement with rock 'n' roll and white shoes had transformed his character. During his film *State Fair* (1962), the journal editorialized, a "sideshow girl" danced with "seductive abandon" and captured Boone in "as torrent and violent love-making as is possible to depict on a screen."[2] Few would describe that scene that way today. By the standards of 1962, most American Christians today would be liberals.

Liberal Protestants, represented by the pages of the *Christian Century,* waited until 1960 to respond to Elvis Presley, but their response was no less uncomplimentary than evangelical concern about Pat Boone. When Presley appeared on *The Ed Sullivan Show,* his "revolting exhibitionism," with its "two wiggles and . . . two songs," underscored "the depth of decadence" soci-

1. See "Yeh-Heh-Heh-Hes, Baby," *Time,* 18 June 1956, p. 54.

2. See "Hollywood Seduces a Teen-Age Idol . . . and the Kids Love It," *Christianity Today,* 11 May 1962, p. 794. Boone is experiencing conservative disapproval again these days due to his recently released, with tongue in cheek, album of heavy-metal music.

ety had reached, as well as the damage the "new media of communication" could wreak on family values.[3] No less a liberal authority than the *New York Times* described his "one specialty" in 1956 as "an accented movement of the body that hitherto has been primarily identified with the repertoire of the blond bombshells of the burlesque runway."[4] I suppose, as part of the context for the church's discussion of human sexuality, it would be good to remember that liberal positions tend to look increasingly conservative as time passes.

"Liberal" and "conservative" are, of course, relative terms. Some of my relatives think I am conservative; other relatives think I am liberal. This little piece of anecdotal evidence is mentioned to illustrate just how relative such terms are. Though the terms are problematic, they are shorthand for differences between individuals and groups of Christians. My use of the terms carries with it the recognition that, though they are not totally useless, they are often foggy and ambiguous.

The terms "evangelical" and "mainline" (or "mainstream") are themselves troublesome in many respects. By using the term "evangelical," I mean to denote those church groups who traditionally have not been active in the National Council of Churches. Evangelicals generally stress biblical authority and emphasize the need for individuals to experience personally the grace of God leading to salvation, usually described by such terms as "new birth" or "conversion," or being "born again." They place high value on an individual's relation to God and promote evangelism as probably the most effective tool in the church's fight against the sins of society. There are, however, vast differences between and among evangelicals on many issues. Evangelicals themselves cannot agree precisely about what it means to be an evangelical.[5]

The term "mainline" is difficult to get a hold on as well. If one means by it to describe those churches possessing large memberships and powerful identities, the groups described by the term have certainly changed since the 1950s. By this definition many of the evangelical churches would definitely qualify as mainline. My use of the term follows the one suggested by Richard G. Hutcheson, Jr., in 1981: "large historical denominations having membership reflecting great diversity, but leadership and official positions putting

3. See "Beware Elvis Presley," *America,* 23 June 1956, pp. 294-95; the *New York Times* was quoted in this editorial. See also "What a Twisted Scale of Values," *Christian Century,* 25 May 1960, p. 630.

4. Quoted in "Beware Elvis Presley," pp. 294-95.

5. See, for example, Donald Dayton, ed., *The Variety of American Evangelicalism* (Knoxville: University of Tennessee Press, 1991).

them generally in the liberal, ecumenically included and socially concerned wing of Christians."[6]

Today's postdenominational context has made such lines harder to draw. Many traditional mainline churches today contain individuals who would define themselves as evangelicals. Some individuals among evangelicals might define themselves as mainline, though this is more unlikely since the latter term has fallen into such disrepute in recent years. Some traditional mainline churches might today more accurately be described as "sideline" churches, since they have lost much of the cultural leadership they enjoyed in earlier decades. On the whole, clear lines of division and clear definitions do not work very well these days. With these caveats in place, I will still use these terms to distinguish between the "conservative"-leaning Christian groups and the more generally "liberal" ones.

Time machine travel would reveal the state of Christianity to be unbelievably good in 1956. The 1950s "revival" of "religion in general" was one of the dominating features of the domestic situation in America at this time. Church membership rose steadily (five percentage points) during the early part of the decade. Two years before your time machine landed, Congress added the words "under God" to the Pledge of Allegiance. The words "In God We Trust" were officially adopted as the national motto in 1956. Corporations and civic organizations decided that providing outlets for prayer made good business sense. Church building boomed. Religious book sales soared. Television, the propaganda potential of which people were only beginning to realize, spread religious images far and wide. Billy Graham's urban crusades were packed with people, and he became America's most well-known religious figure for the next several decades. By the end of the 1950s, nearly 69 percent of Americans were church members. The trend was very good for the church, and it looked like the whole population would be attending church by the 1970s. What happened?

Martin E. Marty suggested that, by the end of the 1950s, the revival, rather than benefiting Protestantism, actually served as the agent to usher in the "post-Protestant" years of American life. Rather than reviving Christianity, the revival actually took its place. It fostered "an attitude toward religion" which Marty claimed became "a religion itself." Whereas the "old shape" of American religion had been "basically Protestant," the "new shape" became something else. Protestantism's power "as virtual monopolist in penetrating and molding the religious aspect of national culture" had "disappeared." For

6. See Richard G. Hutcheson, Jr., *Mainline Churches and the Evangelicals* (Atlanta: John Knox, 1981), p. 39.

the most part, the cultural revival presented a God who was "understandable and manageable, . . . an American jolly good fellow."[7] Rather than thinking of God as the one who sent Jesus Christ to save all humanity, including the communists, Americans tended to think of God as an American, just like them. And this led many American Christians to confuse the trappings of their culture with God's will. For these Christians, women belonged in the kitchen and blacks belonged in menial jobs; certainly God never intended for blacks and whites to live in the same neighborhoods. For Protestants, culture reflected what they perceived to be their values.

But change was brewing in the land. Catholicism, as illustrated by Kennedy's victory in 1960, had finally made great strides toward the equal footing it deserved in American culture. By the mid-1960s, other religious expressions became both more common and more visible in America. Rapid urbanization, technology, mobility, an emerging drug culture, a rebellious generation of youth, a civil rights movement, a fledgling feminist movement, the beginnings of an Asian war — all contributed to an atmosphere where traditional Protestant values in America were seriously challenged.

The pluralism represented by these changes affected the Christian response to sexual issues as well. Developments within culture always affect the way the church thinks about important issues. The trends of the last forty years illustrate the fact that the church simply cannot avoid its cultural context when it theologizes about sexual ethics. A discussion of these trends will also bring more clarity to the concept of the muddled middle and what those situated there, regardless of significant theological differences, are coming to share in common.

I do not intend for the term "muddled middle" to carry with it a necessarily negative connotation. Some confusion is always a good thing in that it prevents individuals and groups from taking a self-righteous perspective of these issues. The muddle of the middle represents, as well, the diversity that exists within subgroups of Christianity, some of whom possess a fair degree of clarity in their thinking but without what might be described as consensus.

7. Martin E. Marty, *The New Shape of American Religion* (New York: Harper & Row, 1959), pp. 27-28 and 32. Sidney E. Mead challenges the post-Protestant concept in his essay entitled "The Post-Protestant Concept and America's Two Religions," in Mead, *The Nation with the Soul of a Church* (New York: Harper & Row, 1975), pp. 11-28. Mead's point is that the "constitutional and legal structure" of the United States had never been Protestant. This is certainly true; but prior to the 1950s, Protestants took that structure for granted and most Americans interpreted it in ways fully consistent with Protestant values and beliefs. After the late fifties, such interpretations were challenged. See also Marty, chap. 4, pp. 67-89, "America's Real Religion: An Attitude," esp. pp. 73f., and pp. 37-39.

Further, I am using the term "muddle" somewhat in the old English sense of "muddling through" by encouraging continued discussion and debate in order to advance public understanding and create the proper environment for a careful and deliberative process. Finally, part of the muddle of the middle may arise due to the development of a broad consensus on values (caring, response to people's needs, importance of human relationships, etc.), while complete consensus concerning the issues raising "values" kinds of questions remains, at present, unachievable.

Four Trends Related to Sexuality in General

1. *The first trend emerged from the sexual revolution. Though rejected in the main by most Christians, the sexual revolution has led many Christian theologians to shift from a rule-oriented ethic toward a more realistic assessment of the context of sexual activity.*

Most Christians, left and right, rejected Joseph Fletcher's *Situation Ethics,* one of the major books offering an ethical rationale for the sexual revolution of the 1960s. In 1964 Robert Fitch, dean at the Pacific School of Religion, spoke for many when he said trends associated with Fletcher scared him so much they almost made him want to become a Catholic.[8] But many Christians, as a result of the sexual revolution, did begin to ask contextual questions instead of merely referring to rules. They shifted from an emphasis on sex as an act to an emphasis on sexuality as involving a relationship. This trend has been more active among the moderate-to-liberal Christians than among the more conservative Christians.

The foundation for this new morality rested in the work of contextual ethicists like H. Richard Niebuhr and Paul Lehmann. Both published books in 1963 that captured the style of ethics they had long represented in their work. As James T. Laney put it:

> [T]hey insisted upon an appreciation of both the historical and the contemporary social contexts in discerning the will of God in a given situation. They allowed scriptural tradition to define their perspective, but not to delimit their horizon; they appreciated the novelty of God's demand, but insisted upon its being concordant with the life and teachings of Christ; and they emphasized the personal element, but set up means by

8. Robert Fitch, "The Sexplosion," *Christian Century,* 29 January 1964.

which it was to be informed by an equal sense of responsibility, both to others and to God.[9]

The work of Niebuhr and Lehmann is, however, barely recognizable in the more simplistic ethic of *Situation Ethics* (1966), by Joseph Fletcher, the theologian of the sexual revolution. Fletcher's ethic, in his words, "subordinates principles to circumstances and the general to the particular, as well as making the 'natural' and the biblical and the theoretical give way to the personal and the actual." For Fletcher, writing in 1966, all of Christian ethics is reduced to the act of love. What does love demand of the situation?[10] Fletcher's work provided after-the-fact legitimation for sexual changes already well practiced in the culture. It also paved the way for increasing family squabbles in the mainline.

In May 1967 the first sympathetic exploration of the "new morality" appeared in the pages of the *Christian Century.* Cyrus Pangborn, chair of the department of religion at Douglass College of Rutgers, stressed the "pervasive and creative nature of sexuality as a dimension of being." He challenged the view that sexuality can or should be regulated by the imposition of law:

> The immediate reply of the traditionalists is that this simply makes sex easy for everyone. But this misses the new moralists' point: sex as act is only the objective, the external, expression of our sexuality; sexuality is a 'dimension' rather than an addable or subtractable part of our being. . . . If this concept of sexuality were generally understood, some adult confusion about the changing roles of fathers and mothers, about youthful hairdos and clothing styles would be dispersed. The worry, so an endless stream of articles tells us, is that men can't feel masculine while changing diapers, that women can't feel feminine as chairmen of corporation boards, that boys aren't masculine if they wear their hair long, that girls can't be feminine if they wear shirts and levis. . . . It could be that today's dressed-to-look-alikes are mounting unconscious protest against the widespread belief that sex is external, are indirectly suggesting that the inner awareness of sexuality can be recovered only when limiting symbolic expressions of it are discarded. . . . What [new morality] does call for is an end to the isolation of sex as a set of external acts and an integration of

9. See the discussion of Niebuhr and Lehmann in James T. Laney, "The New Morality and the Religious Communities," *Annals of the American Academy of Political and Social Science* (January 1970): 16-18; the books published were H. Richard Niebuhr, *The Responsible Self* (New York: Harper & Row, 1963), and Paul Lehmann, *Ethics in a Christian Context* (New York: Harper & Row, 1963).

10. Fletcher, "Love Is the Only Measure," *Commonweal,* 14 January 1966, pp. 427-32.

enriched notions of sexuality into our view of what comprises wholeness, complete personhood.[11]

The new moralists hoped to redefine the meaning of sexual sin. In their view sexual sin was not so much the commission of a sexual act that violated a particular, and always consistent, Christian rule. Instead, sexual sin involved dehumanization of others, acting in ways that deny what it means to be human as defined by the loving God who became fully human.

Such thinking led some of these theologians to rethink the traditional Christian taboo regarding premarital sex.[12] Reinhold Niebuhr recognized certain distinctions one should make in premarital sex and called for "discriminating wisdom in young people and their guides," which in its own way left the ethical door open for the possibility of sexual intercourse before marriage for engaged couples.[13] Harvey Cox put it more bluntly: "[W]e must face the real question of whether avoidance of intercourse beforehand is always the best preparation." He urged that guidance be given to specific persons in specific contexts and toward the end that conduct will "serve to strengthen the chances of sexual success and fidelity in marriage." Cox set forth an evangelical sexual ethic he felt would provide a better way:

> [P]reaching the Gospel . . . means making clear the distorted images of sex from which the Gospel delivers us. . . . it entails protecting sex as a fully human activity against all the principalities and powers that seek to dehumanize it. In our day these include the forces, both within and without, that pervert sex into a merchandising technique, a means of self-aggrandizement, a weapon for rebelling against parents, a recreational pursuit. . . . Evangelical ethics cease to be Law and once again become Gospel when the Word liberates people from cultural conventions and social pressures, when persons discover their sexuality as a delightful gift of God that links them in freedom and concern to their fellows.[14]

11. Cyrus Pangborn, "Sex and the Single Standard," *Christian Century,* 17 May 1967, p. 649.

12. Societal leaders were rethinking this as well. In early 1964, for example, Dr. Warren Johnson, head of health education at the University of Maryland, published a new textbook advocating the acceptability of premarital sex. See "Sex Test Antidote," *Christian Century,* 11 April 1964, p. 501.

13. Reinhold Niebuhr, "Christian Attitudes toward Sex and Family," *Christianity and Crisis,* 27 April 1964, p. 74.

14. Harvey Cox, "Evangelical Ethics and the Ideal of Chastity," *Christianity and Crisis,* 27 April 1964, pp. 79-80.

As evidenced in *The Secular City* (1963), Cox represented an unqualified optimism about the ability of human beings to be problem solvers. Though he seemed to underestimate, for most theologians at the time and in retrospect, a failure to appreciate the power of sin generally, and some might argue especially so in matters related to sexuality, he did lift the popular discussion of sexual ethics to a new level.[15] And the trend since has generally affirmed the importance of the relational character of sexual activity.

2. *Second, in response to the birth control pill, the trend has been toward the development of a new sexual ethic stressing marriage, the positive place of sex within it, and the essential unity of body and spirit as a key component of human sexuality.*

If you picked up a newspaper when you stepped out of the time capsule in November 1956, you might read that G. D. Searle and Company was about to release a new pill that prevented conception during sexual intercourse. This little pill, when it became publicly available around 1960, changed the course of human sexuality. Besides being a major contributing factor in the sexual revolution, it led Christians to understand that they did not possess a good sexual ethic. In the age before the pill, the Christian sexual ethic was an abstinence based upon the fears of "infection, detection, [and] conception."[16] Parents warned their children not to fool around because they might get venereal disease, get caught, or get pregnant. In the age of the pill and the condom, Christians began to emphasize the role sex played in embodying "the mutual dependence, the utter need of one for the other," that is God's will for marriage.[17]

Within this more positive approach, Christians came to stress "the theological doctrines of creation, incarnation and resurrection" as they related to sex. Each of these three doctrines made clear the Christian affirmation of the "goodness of the physical dimension of life." Sex is a gift from God. Christians sounded a theme that has become important in Christian sexual ethics during the last three decades: the body and spirit are unified

15. Harvey Cox, *The Secular City* (New York: Macmillan, 1963); see esp. pp. 192-216 where the *Christianity and Crisis* article quoted throughout here forms the heart of this chapter.

16. Gordon Clanton, "Understanding Sex in the Age of the Pill," *Christian Century,* 8 January 1969, pp. 43-47.

17. For this material, see Hamilton, "Moralism and Sex Ethics: A Defense," *Christianity and Crisis,* 28 October 1957, pp. 140-42. See also Joseph Hough, "Rules and the Ethics of Sex," *Christian Century,* 29 January 1969, pp. 148-51, where he makes a strong ethical case for marriage as the only appropriate relationship for sexual relations by reconsidering the meaning of the Christian covenant with God.

and, together, are central to what it means to be human. Leaders among both right-leaning and left-leaning Christians helped to develop a Christian ethical approach to sex that renounced the "sexual dualism" of earlier tradition.[18] Most in the muddled middle continue to believe in the unity of body and spirit, though they still have not done a good job of reaching agreement (or even of accomplishing meaningful discussion) around the implications of this belief.

3. *Third, one of the great accomplishments of both the feminist and sexual revolutions during these forty years has rested in their ability to expose sexist attitudes. As a result, the trend in many Christian groups has been to remove such attitudes and to affirm more meaningfully the equality of women, both within the life of the church and within their role as sexual beings.*

Christians have had to reconsider presuppositions that had long supported the traditional standards of sexuality taught by the church, especially those dealing with gender roles. Walking out of your mythical time machine, you would discover most Americans believing that female sexuality found its ideal in devoted women who served their husband's needs and the needs of the household. Movies portrayed the dangers of aggressive women by showing that such characters ruined their marriages and found tragic ends before the final credits rolled across the silver screen.[19] Many connected sex in marriage with an inferior view of women, and the culture itself supported a double standard where women were concerned.

Theologians of the time addressed the double standard. In early 1964 Helmut Thielicke came close to providing a theological rationale for it. A chapter of his book *The Ethics of Sex* appeared in the *Christian Century.* "It is, so to speak," he wrote, "the 'vocation' of the woman to be lover, companion and mother." A woman is created to give her whole "'self' when she gives herself sexually, . . . whereas the husband brings in only a part, a very substantial part, but still only a part, of himself." The double standard of morality "does have some basis — which we would not wish to be understood as legitimation of it! — in the physiological structure of the sex organs . . . the woman receives something from the sexual encounter, . . . whereas the man discharges and thus rids himself of something." Though Thielicke had no intention of promoting the double standard, his theological explanation of the nature ("animal") of man being "polygamous" and that of woman being

18. James B. Nelson, "Reuniting Sexuality and Spirituality," *Christian Century,* 25 February 1987, p. 188. In this article, Nelson discusses several shifts in Christian sexual ethics that have occurred as a result of the sexual revolution.

19. Elaine Tyler May makes this point in her book *Homeward Bound* (New York: Basic Books, 1988), and provides an excellent discussion of family life in the 1950s.

"monogamous" provided an ontological excuse for men who were not particularly drawn to the Christian demands of agape.[20]

Reinhold Niebuhr echoed these calls for the recognition of the differences between male and female sexuality. Because "the woman is so intimately related to the family impulse, . . . she is frequently the reluctant partner in premarital intercourse. She submits herself for only one of two reasons: because she loves the man and regards her action as a proof of her love; or because she wants to bind the man to her in reciprocal love."[21] Here the woman is portrayed as either the hopeless romantic or the deceptive seductress. Neither is a great role for women to have to play in order to express their human sexuality.

Of course, more damaging still was the theological argument contrasting "the creative, redemptive initiative of God with the receptive, humble response of Israel," where "God calls Israel to be his wife." With this point Robert Osborn, associate professor of religion at Duke University, hoped for a return to the use of the sexual language from the Bible to discuss proper roles in marriage for men and women. These roles would help prevent the woman from filling "her need for a man by playing the male part herself" by "competing more openly for the male position in society." The dilemma Americans faced, according to Osborn, was in no small measure due to the theological work of people like Harvey Cox, Thomas J. J. Altizer, and the new feminist theologians. Their work "castrated theology." "I would say," he wrote, "that the knowledge of God is no longer a matter of intercourse but of masturbation."[22] Such quips marked the beginning of serious family conflicts in the mainline camp.

For many years fundamentalists and evangelicals had difficulty viewing passion, even within marriage, very positively. And when they finally did, they tended to connect it with an inferior view of women. Moderate evangelicals today have abandoned both their views on the inferiority of women and their emphasis on rules in favor of stressing the importance of "truthful relationships," the "personal responsibility for one another's larger lives" made possible only in marriage.[23]

20. Helmut Thielicke, "Realization of the Sex Nature," *Christian Century,* 15 January 1964, pp. 73-75.

21. Reinhold Niebuhr, pp. 73-75.

22. Robert T. Osborn, "Sex and the Single God," *Christian Century,* 7 September 1967, pp. 1078-80.

23. Richard Rohr, "An Appetite for Wholeness," *Sojourners,* 30 November 1982, p. 32; see also Richard J. Foster, "God's Gift of Sexuality," *Sojourners,* 16 July 1985, pp. 15-19, where he emphasizes the "mutuality, fidelity, and discipline" of the "faithful covenantal relationships" represented by marriage. See also "Really Good Sex," *Christianity Today,* 19 August 1991, p. 12.

Many mainline and evangelical theologians during the 1960s were actually trying to keep sexuality in its private sphere, with every dimension of it held in its so-called proper place. No longer are sexual issues purely individual or solely private, reserved for hushed conversations between lovers or between parent and child (if those conversations ever took place). Trends point to a sexuality that has found a very public voice. The church can no longer afford to ignore the full meaning of sexuality. The events of these years after the sexual revolution have exposed sexist attitudes for what they are. The church has had to face and reconsider presuppositions that have long undergirded the traditional standards of sexuality in the church, especially those dealing with gender roles and sexual orientation. Though there are continuing theological differences among those occupying the muddled middle, characteristic of all of them have been an increasing sophistication in articulating the importance of the role of women in the church and in sexual relationships and the desire to eliminate the double standard in human sexuality.

4. *Vatican II and other developments in American culture have led to a growing compatibility over the last four decades between Catholics and Protestants in America on the issue of sexuality.*

American Catholics in general responded more slowly to the claims of the sexual revolution than some Protestants did. Throughout the 1950s and much of the 1960s, birth control caused them great consternation as they struggled to hold the line against it, finally reconciling themselves to it by 1967, thereby joining the muddled middle on the issue.[24] Sections in chapter I of Schema 13, the Vatican II document on marriage in the modern world, likely had something to do with these more liberal views, as did the 1967 report of the papal commission on birth control that recommended acceptance of artificial birth control methods.[25] The conciliar document accepted the communion of conjugal love as an equal end in marriage alongside the procreation and education of children. Gone were any emphases on the "primary and secondary ends of marriage."[26] In this way the council gave sex in marriage an entirely new status in Catholic thought.

24. Earlier, see, for example, "Change the Natural Law?" *America,* 2 November 1957, p. 124, and "Birth Control and Policy," *America,* 11 May 1963, p. 662. Later, see "Powerful Voice Heard," *America,* 4 February 1967, p. 168, and "Contraception and the Synod of Bishops," *America,* 30 September 1967, p. 339.

25. Quoted in "The Symbol of Birth Control," *Commonweal,* 28 April 1967, pp. 163-64.

26. This quote is found in John T. Noonan, Jr., "Contraception and the Council," *Commonweal,* 11 March 1966, p. 658. The quote is from section 49 of Schema 13, *The Church in the Modern World.* Gregory Baum's essay is also a good description of the pro-

Ignoring the majority report of the papal study commission on the subject, Pope Paul VI issued an encyclical, *Humanae Vitae* (Human Life), in 1968 condemning all forms of artificial birth control. American church leaders expressed great disappointment. John Cogley, writing for *Catholic America*, emphasized that "the *Humanae Vitae* debacle marked a fundamental change in the character of American Catholicism. Reverential deference to the pronouncements of a reigning pontiff would probably never be the same again."[27] From this point on, Catholic leadership in America moved toward new expressions in the area of human sexuality. These tendencies brought American Catholics and the more moderate of American Protestants much closer together in their thinking about human sexuality.

Charles Curran's work challenging traditional Catholic notions of the natural law also contributed to this convergence between Catholics and Protestants. "Catholic theologians," he wrote in 1966, "have been afraid of the consequences that might come from any leak in the dike; but a realistic morality must come to grips with the ambiguity presented by the existence of sin in the world." In Curran's view, natural law theory did not take seriously enough the "disrupting influence of sin in the world." He accented "the incarnational character of Christian life." He reminded readers that Christian morality rests in Christ and calls Christians to live "out of the new life we have received, the existence that flows from our baptismal rebirth in Christ, the fruit of the Spirit Who dwells within us and transforms our beings." His emphasis for thinking about human sexuality was decidedly placed on the theological meaning of the new creation.

Curran urged Catholic moral theologians to take more seriously the reality of situations mature Christians face and to recognize the concept of compromise in human actions. "In the face of the sinful situation man must do the best he can."[28] This critique of Catholic natural theology coincided with Protestant expressions of the "new morality" during the 1960s, espe-

---

cess resulting in this kind of language: Baum, "Birth Control — What Happened?" *Commonweal,* 24 December 1965, pp. 369-71.

27. Cogley is quoted in Robert Handy, *A History of the Churches in the United States and Canada* (New York: Oxford University Press, 1977), p. 423; on this point of a crisis in authority, see also "Birth Control Crisis," *Commonweal,* 4 October 1968, p. 3. On disappointment of American church leaders, see "Dilemmas of Pope and President," *America,* 17 August 1968, p. 91; Gregory Baum, "The Right to Dissent," *Commonweal,* 23 August 1968, pp. 553-54; "Pope Denounces Birth Control as Millions Starve," *Commonweal,* 27 September 1968, p. 657 — this page is an ad signed by several notable Catholic laypeople.

28. Charles Curran, "To the Editors," *Commonweal,* 18 February 1966, p. 581.

cially in its emphasis on the importance of the situation in which moral decisions must be made.

On a more popular level, American Catholics knew they had to deal with the sexual revolution when a *Boston Globe* poll of Massachusetts youth in 1970 revealed that 79 percent of Catholic college students thought premarital sex was acceptable for people in love, and 64 percent said they had no problem with unmarried couples living together. Official church responses to these developments were continually ineffective in America. In 1975 the church issued *Declaration on Certain Questions concerning Sexual Ethics.* This document reiterated the standards of traditional morality, including complete condemnation of both masturbation and homosexuality.

In response, the Catholic Theological Society of America, the major professional association of American Catholic theologians, issued the results of its own study. A group of five Catholic theologians had been appointed in 1972 to study Christian sexual ethics and published its report in 1977. Titled *Human Sexuality: New Directions in American Catholic Thought,* this report revealed a significant and organized effort among American Catholics to integrate modern thought and Christian faith in this area.[29]

According to Rosemary Ruether's early assessment of the document, it represented "a major effort to shift the basis of sexual ethics from act-oriented to person-oriented principles." Resting on Scripture, tradition, and the empirical sciences as a sort of tripod of authority, the report criticized the outdated dimensions of the natural law and condemned its preoccupation with procreation. A Catholic ethic that "treated masturbation as a more serious sin than rape, since the former 'wasted the seed' while the latter preserved . . . procreation," had to be challenged. The document set the "person-oriented ethics of Jesus" over against "the patriarchalism of the Old Testament and the later Pauline tradition."[30]

Sounding like Harvey Cox, the Society described a "humanized sexuality" that is "self-liberating, other-affirming, honest, faithful, socially responsible, life-serving and joyous." (One critic jokingly foresaw "a questionnaire in every bedroom.")[31] Dehumanization occurs when sex consistently negates one or another of these humanizing principles. As Ruether put it,

29. For the full text, see Anthony Kosnik et al., *Human Sexuality: New Directions in American Catholic Thought* (New York: Paulist, 1977).

30. Rosemary Ruether, "Time Makes Ancient Good Uncouth: The Catholic Report on Sexuality," *Christian Century,* 3-10 August 1977, pp. 682-85.

31. Joe Cuneen, "Two Rousing Cheers," *Christianity and Crisis,* 31 October 1977, p. 248.

> The study also discards all double standards of sexual ethics that judge women differently from men, single persons (including celibates) differently from married persons, and homosexuals differently from heterosexuals. All persons, in whatever walk of life or sexual orientation, are sexual beings who must find self-development through sexual maturation. The standards of humanizing versus dehumanizing sexuality can be applied equally to all. . . .[32]

This document was a liberal cutting edge for American Catholicism (writers in *America* clearly opposed its conclusions), and for American Christianity, in its undifferentiated treatment of heterosexuality and homosexuality. This view allowed for sexuality among all singles, provided such conduct was clearly "creative and integrative of the human person."[33] The report also illustrates the growing compatibility between liberal Protestant and liberal Catholic theological understanding in America after Vatican II.[34] But the liberal views of both faced serious opposition from more moderate Christians, especially concerning homosexuality. Even so, Catholics and Protestants found more significant areas of agreement as both abandoned the rule- and act-oriented approaches to human sexuality, paid more attention to contexts and situations, and took more seriously the role of women.

Unifying Trends Emerging from the Homosexuality Debate

Several trends have emerged from the homosexuality debate during the last forty years. The details of the cultural and church events leading to these trends deserve an essay in their own right, but a brief listing is appropriate here: the influence of the British Wolfenden report of 1957 that called for homosexual civil rights in Britain; the 1963 Quaker study from London which called for complete equality in all respects, including sexual expression, between homosexuals and heterosexuals; the founding of the Metropolitan

32. Ruether, pp. 682-85.

33. See Kosnik, pp. 170-86.

34. Ruether, "Time Makes Ancient Good Uncouth: The Catholic Report on Sexuality," *Christian Century,* 3-10 August 1977, pp. 682-85; Tom F. Driver also praised the document, though he criticized its conspicuous silence on the topic of orgasm (Driver, "A Stride toward Sanity," *Commonweal,* 31 October 1977, pp. 243-46); see Francis X. Meehan, "Love and Sexuality in Catholic Tradition," *America,* 15 October 1977, pp. 231-34; see also the review of the document written by James Gaffney, "A Brace of Controversies: Sex and Authority," *America,* 9 July 1977, pp. 14-15.

Community Church (MCC) in Los Angeles in 1968; the police raid of the gay bar known as Stonewall Inn on 28 June 1969 that gave birth to the gay liberation movement in American culture; the first ordination of an openly gay man, William Reagan Johnson,[35] by a mainline denomination, the United Church of Christ, on 27 June 1972, which spawned a number of gay caucuses in the Protestant denominations, leading to increased activism in churches on behalf of the ordination of homosexuals and the advocacy of civil rights for homosexuals in society; the host of other heavily publicized events in the last ten to fifteen years associated with the increased visibility of homosexuality in American culture, including the formation of evangelical activist groups in Protestant circles and countless popular media stories about AIDS, military harassment of gays and lesbians, gay marriages, and the adoption of babies by gay couples — all these events have contributed content and issues around which the debate has swirled for forty years. Two significant trends point to the development of a "muddled middle" in the churches, rather than an all-out culture war, in relationship to this issue.

1. *First, there has been a shifting of theological ground over the last forty years among the leadership in both mainline and evangelical churches as those leaders have thought about the relationship between sin and homosexuality.*

This movement is primarily defined by a historical shift in thinking about homosexuality that has moved through three stages.

First Stage: Homosexuals as Degenerates

During the 1950s, nearly all Christians (Protestant and Catholic, liberal and conservative) viewed homosexuals as degenerates. In other words, homosexuality was sin, pure and simple. It constituted degenerate behavior in all of its aspects.

Conservatives, certain of the biblical prohibitions in Genesis 19, Leviticus 20, and Romans 1, the most often cited passages, remained convinced throughout the first portion of our period that homosexuality was against nature ("contrary to God's created order for the sexes") and a sin.[36] In the

35. The United Church of Christ announced in March 1997 that William R. Johnson had become the first national staff minister for lesbian and gay concerns. Since 1990 Johnson has been the HIV/AIDS ministries specialist for the United Church Board for Homeland Mission. See "UCC Appoints Minister to Address Gay Issues," *Christian Century*, 9 April 1997, pp. 359-60.

36. On the biblical argument, see Kenneth Kantzer, "Homosexuals in the Church," *Christianity Today*, 22 April 1983, pp. 8-9; "The Laws against Homosexuals," *Christianity*

mid-1970s, for example, Anita Bryant quipped that if God had wanted homosexuals, God would have created "Adam and Bruce."[37] In the 1960s' conservative view, the fact that some homosexuals seemed proud of their orientation only demonstrated the severity of the nation's moral decay.

Because they understood homosexuality as a sin, it was treated primarily as an individual failing. The more conservative one is, the more likely one has been to place the emphasis upon sexual sin as an individual act. Evangelicals and fundamentalists, during this period, stressed that homosexuals had no hope of reaching heaven unless they repented and changed. "The Bible condemns homosexual behavior," wrote Harold Lindsell, "and [it] says that homosexuals cannot inherit the kingdom of God" (1 Cor. 6:9-11).[38] In general, because conservatives during the 1950s and 1960s felt so strongly about homosexuality as sin, they were frightened by the trend of increasing activism among homosexuals in American culture. FBI director J. Edgar Hoover, writing for the conservative *Christianity Today* during this period, surely without intending any pun in the matter, argued that "hope for a reversal of [this] immoral trend [tolerating homosexuality] lies with an aroused public."[39]

Liberals, prior to the 1960s, also generally emphasized homosexuality as

---

Today, 7 November 1969, p. 33: "Romans 1:18-32 shows that homosexuality is contrary to nature, and that it is part of the degeneration of man that guarantees ultimate disaster in this life and in the life to come. Homosexuality was one of the leading sins that brought about God's final judgment on Sodom and Gomorrah." See "Confusion over Criteria a Sign That Morality Is Declining," *Christianity Today,* 14 September 1962, p. 25; "Giving Away What You Don't Own," *Christianity Today,* 25 November 1966, pp. 26-27; "The Debilitating Revolt," *Christianity Today,* 21 July 1967, pp. 24-25; B. L. Smith, "Homosexuality in the Bible and the Law," *Christianity Today,* 18 July 1969, pp. 7-10.

37. This is a favorite quip of the antigay conservative Christians. How could these homosexuals actually think they could "find the same fulfillment as the heterosexual"? an editorial in *Christianity Today* asked. The answer: "A San Francisco graffiti writer knew better. He wrote: 'If God had wanted homosexuals, he would have created Adam and Freddy.'" Anita Bryant repeated this idea seven years later in Dade County, only her version included "Adam and Bruce." "Adam and Freddy" comment in "'Gays' Go Radical," *Christianity Today,* 4 December 1970, pp. 40-41; "Adam and Bruce" comment is covered in "The Church and Homosexuals," *Christian Century,* 1 June 1977, p. 528; Jerry Falwell, in a press conference in 1979, commented: "God had created Adam and Eve, not Adam and Steve" — see *Christianity Today,* 16 November 1979, p. 48.

38. Harold Lindsell, "Homosexuals and the Church," *Christianity Today,* 28 September 1973, p. 10; see also "Can Homosexuals Inherit the Kingdom?" *Christianity Today,* 20 May 1977, pp. 26-27.

39. See "How Low Are Community Standards regarding Obscenity on Newsstands?" *Christianity Today,* 20 July 1962, p. 25; and "Obscenity and the Court," *America,* 21 July 1962, p. 521.

sin. But as time moved into the decade of the sixties, some among them tended to emphasize the structural dimension of sin as much as they did the individual dimension. Harvey Cox, for example, argued that "We must admit that we have created a set of cultural conditions in which sexual responsibility is made exceedingly difficult."[40] Through their emphasis on the social conditions of sin, liberal-leaning Christians tended to lessen the importance placed upon the sexual act itself by focusing attention on the condition that inhibited right action.

As time passed, mainline editorials tended to suggest that structural sin, as opposed to individual immorality, may be more responsible for the "twilight world" of homosexuals, where homosexuals engaged in one-night stands to satisfy their sexual longings. If cultural condemnation of homosexuals were not so prevalent, they argued, "the exploitation by desperate individuals of fellow humans would be far less prevalent."[41] These were considerably different arguments from those made by their evangelical counterparts, but both sets of arguments raised the significance of sin in their own ways.

Second Stage: Homosexuals as Diseased

Mainline Protestant leadership, in the early 1960s, started to make a distinction between homosexual practice and homosexual orientation. Along with this distinction, they began to view homosexuality as a disease. Though most continued to understand homosexual practice as sinful, they came to believe that the orientation itself could in many cases be cured, either through hormonal therapy or through counseling.[42]

The understanding of homosexuality as a disease caused some of these Christians to become more sympathetic to the plight of homosexuals, much like Christians came to a different understanding of alcoholism once it was defined as a disease. Delegates for the Lutheran Church in America, for example, called in 1970 for more understanding of homosexuals and claimed homosexuals were sinners "only as are all other persons — alienated from God and neighbor."[43] Conservatives, however, continued throughout this period

40. Cox, "Evangelical Ethics," p. 79.

41. "To Accept Homosexuals," *Christian Century,* 3 March 1971, p. 275.

42. Overholser, "Homosexuality: Sin or Disease?" *Christian Century,* 11 September 1963, pp. 1099-1101.

43. See Elliott Wright, "The Church and Gay Liberation," *Christian Century,* 3 March 1971, p. 282.

to emphasize the need for the homosexual to change or to choose celibacy.[44] For the strength to fulfill either of these goals, evangelicals stressed "an encounter with the saving power of Jesus Christ."[45] Considerable differences remained between the evangelical and mainline expressions on the relationship between orientation and practice.

Third Stage: Homosexuals as Disordered

In 1974 the American Psychiatric Association dropped homosexuality from its list of mental diseases. After this time some mainline leaders, usually relying on some argument related to the natural design of God's creation, began to describe the homosexual orientation as a "disordered" state. They increasingly argued that the causes of this "inadequate pattern" were usually very complex, some mixture of environment and genetics, and almost always beyond the control of the individual to do anything about them.[46] Those who came to argue this position emphasized that the person was not disordered, but the inclination, or orientation, to homosexual behavior was disordered.

This shift from degeneracy (sin) to disease (in need of cure) to disorder (a condition usually beyond a person's control and rarely changed) has allowed mainline Protestants to excuse the individual of any responsibility for the disorder itself (i.e., the condition itself is not a sin) and to recognize that, since homosexuality was not a disease, no one should expect a cure. Some Christian leaders have naturally argued that homosexuals ought to live out the sexuality that matched their given condition.[47] But the majority of mainline Protestants in the muddled middle today, though I have no statistical evidence to back up the generalization, have likely continued to understand as sinful any sexual activity that matches this disordered condition.

By 1970 evangelical editors at *Christianity Today* clearly had also begun to separate *orientation* from *practice.* Orientation, homosexuality as the disordered state of human sexuality, by itself became neutral. Practice of homosexual behavior remained sinful. This perspective continued to emphasize

44. See "Gay Demand," *Christianity Today,* 4 December 1970, p. 26; see Lindsell, p. 8.

45. Klaus Bockmuhl, "Homosexuality in Biblical Perspective," *Christianity Today,* 16 February 1973, pp. 12-18.

46. See Wall, "Methodists Face the Homosexual Issue," *Christian Century,* 12 March 1975, pp. 243-44.

47. For an early example, see Norman Pittenger, "E. M. Forster, Homosexuality and Christian Morality," *Christian Century,* 15 December 1971, pp. 1468-71.

human choice in the matter and kept the practice of homosexuality within the realm of individual sin. One could not help what one was, but one could certainly control what one did.[48] Most evangelicals continued to stress celibacy, but, as time has passed, many have become more patient and forgiving of those who have so-called relapses.[49]

By 1975, as they encountered more frequently the presence of homosexuality in their own midst, evangelicals became more aware of the complexities surrounding the issue. As Philip Yancey put it recently in one of his columns for *Christianity Today:* "It is safe to say that I have learned more about grace, forgiveness, diversity — and, yes, original sin — from my family than from all the theology books I have read. . . . Troublesome issues like divorce and homosexuality take on a different cast when you confront them not in a state legislature but in a family reunion."[50] Accompanying this change in perspective, evangelicals have, for the most part, recognized that a change in sexual preference is often very difficult, if not impossible. This understanding has enabled growing numbers of evangelicals to offer full acceptance to the nonpracticing homosexual, to affirm gifts homosexuals might use in service of the church, and, over the years, to develop ministries especially focused to serve gay individuals.[51] As evangelical editor Kenneth Kantzer put it in 1983, "We must learn to accept nonpracticing homosexuals as we would accept unmarried heterosexuals."[52] But congregational openness toward "practicing" homosexuals in the evangelical community remains, for the most part, fairly rare.

Recognizing the innocence of homosexuals with regard to orientation has led to increased activism within evangelicalism in this area. In 1976 Ralph Blair formed Evangelicals Concerned (EC), a group that denies any inconsistency between evangelical Christian faith and a monogamous homosexual

48. Separation between orientation and practice is evidenced in "Gay Demand," *Christianity Today,* 4 December 1970, p. 26.

49. "Homosexuality: Biblical Guidance through a Moral Morass," *Christianity Today,* 18 April 1980, pp. 12-13; Kantzer, "The Church and the Homosexual," *Christianity Today,* 22 April 1983, pp. 8-9; Randy Frame, "The Homosexual Lifestyle: Is There a Way Out?" *Christianity Today,* 9 August 1985, pp. 32-36.

50. Yancey, quoted in *Record* (winter 1997): 2.

51. A key essay demonstrating tolerance and the desire to minister to gays is John Stott, "Homosexual Marriage," *Christianity Today,* 22 November 1985 — Stott urges charity, but still cannot endorse homosexual marriage; see also Frame, "The Evangelical Closet," *Christianity Today,* 5 November 1990, pp. 56-57.

52. Kantzer, "Homosexuals in the Church," pp. 8-9. In addition to other essays in *Christianity Today,* see Margaret Clarkson, "Singleness: His Share for Me," *Christianity Today,* 16 February 1979, pp. 14-15.

relationship. By 1990 it boasted more than twenty chapters nationwide, and there are now some twenty-five chapters in the West alone, with other chapters scattered across the country. The national mailing list for the group is some two thousand strong. EC is a parachurch organization meeting in local chapters for prayer and Bible study and support. Most members maintain memberships in local congregations, either in traditional evangelical congregations or in MCC congregations or in newly developing independent evangelical congregations. The increased development of independent evangelical congregations with predominantly gay and lesbian constituencies seems already to be affecting activity within EC. As churches cater to the needs of these Christians, the strength of the parachurch movement is likely to drop off some. In the EC chapter in Laguna Beach, California, one of the larger chapters in the country, the slight majority of members attend mainstream evangelical churches chosen because there "is no gay-bashing from the pulpit." These pastors generally know these members are gay, though the majority of them do not condone the lifestyle in any way. They simply do not use the pulpit to condemn it either.[53]

A new phenomenon is developing among evangelicals in terms of congregational life. Across the country new independent evangelical congregations, composed nearly entirely of gay and lesbian memberships, are coming into being. These churches, numbering over thirty affiliated congregations (located in some nineteen different states), are growing out of evangelical discontent with the MCC, which many gay and lesbian evangelicals view to be too liberal. Five of these congregations have women pastors.[54] Generally these independent congregations are resistant to inclusive language with reference to God, though some try to be inclusive in language referring to human beings. They emphasize salvation alone in Jesus Christ. These congregations have formed, as of October 1996, a new Alliance of Christian Churches. This could very well be the nucleus of a new denominational group in American religion. If so, the rate of gay and lesbian acceptance among the mainstream evangelical community might actually slow as a result, and the isolated nature of church life among gays and lesbians might continue. The moderator of the

53. This perspective comes from Todd Souza, one of the leaders of Evangelicals Concerned in Laguna Beach, California. The phone interview took place 11 March 1997. Current information related to EC is found on its web site (http://www.ecwr.org).

54. A list of about twenty congregations, addresses, and pastors was faxed to me by Paul Barnes of White Rock Community Church on 11 March 1997. At that time, five of the twenty had women ministers. A current listing is found on the Alliance web page (http://members.aol.com/alliancecc); a visit to this site in March 1999 did not enable me to determine how many of these current churches have women ministers.

Alliance is the pastor of the largest congregation, White Rock Community Church in Dallas, Texas.

White Rock started in June 1991 in the form of a Bible study meeting in the home of Jerry Cook, a minister formerly affiliated with Southern Baptist life. Seven gay and lesbian individuals who were looking for a more evangelical alternative to the MCC started meeting regularly together. They sought a place where they could be affirmed in both their sexuality and their conservative faith. The Bible study lasted only three weeks before beginning to meet on Sunday mornings as a church. Within six months the group had purchased the old West Shore Presbyterian church building. Currently the congregation's membership, under the continuing leadership of Jerry Cook, stands at about seven hundred members, about five hundred of whom might be considered truly active.

Members come primarily from the Southern Baptist Convention (estimated to be about 40-45 percent) and the Roman Catholic Church (about 20-30 percent), with the remainder coming from Methodist, Presbyterian, Episcopalian, and Assemblies of God traditions, among others. It is a predominantly white congregation but contains a significant minority membership; about 5-10 percent are black and 10-15 percent are Hispanic. Though conservative in doctrine, the church ordains women deacons and women ministers. Most of these independent evangelical congregations (associated with one another through the Alliance) are much smaller, though their number is steadily increasing.[55] Jerry Cook's vision for the Alliance is for it to act as a denominational connection for these various congregations, enabling mission and evangelism to take place through cooperative efforts. He hopes to bring positive influences through heavy community involvement and service. His congregation is not an activist one. They do not seek activist publicity on local nightly newscasts. Instead they seek to minister in traditional evangelical ways and, in the process, perhaps help heterosexual people to reach a new understanding of God's gift of homosexuality.

Support among evangelical heterosexuals for the homosexual community has been slow in coming but not entirely nonexistent. Lewis Smedes, ethics professor at Fuller Theological Seminary, argued in his book *Sex for Christians* (Eerdmans, 1976) that the best option for any homosexual is change. If that is not possible, the next best option is celibacy. For homosexuals unable to maintain a lifestyle of celibacy, Smedes recommended a third option: "op-

55. Phone interview with Paul Barnes and Jerry Cook, 11 March 1997. In March 1997 membership stood at about twenty congregations; in March 1999 membership approached forty congregations.

timum homosexual morality," translating generally into developing a responsible and permanent relationship with one individual.[56] Smedes remains in a small but slowly growing minority among evangelicals at this point, but the trend seems to favor evangelicals eventually moving in this direction. Smedes has increasingly affirmed homosexuals in the twenty years since his book was published.[57]

This trend describing the relationship between sin and homosexuality contains connected subtrends as well. At least five such subtrends relate to this discussion, in which moderate liberals and evangelical moderates have moved toward a muddled middle during the last forty years, where they share some similarities and usually differ in some muddled areas.

Subtrend 1: Both affirm a difference between homosexual orientation and homosexual practice, though they are muddled about how to talk about this difference, the causes of it, and the Christian meaning of living in a disordered condition.

Subtrend 2: Both maintain that a homosexual orientation is not in itself sinful, though there are differing and usually muddled understandings about whether homosexual practice is always sinful.

Subtrend 3: Both affirm that a homosexual orientation is rarely ever changed into a heterosexual one, but are muddled about how to talk about the implications of this affirmation.

Subtrend 4: Both welcome "nonpracticing" homosexual individuals into church membership, but are muddled about how to handle "practicing" homosexuals who desire church membership. Aren't all Christians sinners? Should one sin bar one from church membership when other Christians are not quizzed about other sins when they become church members?

Subtrend 5: Both are creating significant ministries to address the problem of AIDS without connecting AIDS to sin or viewing AIDS as God's punishment for sin, but are very muddled about such things as their support for public safe-sex education, the public distribution of condoms, and other such activities that might or might not help to stem the rising tide of AIDS in this country.

These subtrends have grown out of the larger trend marking the theological shift that has occurred over the past forty years between the notion of sin and homosexuality. A second theological trend deserves discussion as well.

56. Barnes and Cook, phone interview.

57. In summer 1999 (22-25 July in Seattle), at an event sponsored by Evangelicals Concerned and entitled ConnECtion 1999 (the EC standing for Evangelicals Concerned), Lewis Smedes served as a featured speaker.

2. *There has been a shifting of theological ground over the last forty years among the leadership in both mainline and evangelical churches as those leaders have thought about the relationship between sin and crime.*

During the 1960s the question of the relationship of morality to law (sin to criminal activity) reached paramount importance on several fronts, including judicial definitions of obscenity, legislative efforts toward censorship, and the move to repeal legislative restrictions pertaining to birth control and sodomy. Birth control laws are an interesting example. Popular Catholic opposition to repealing these laws remained strong throughout the fifteen states where legislation remained on the books. In those states it was still illegal during the 1960s to use birth control. But it should be noted that Catholics in America rarely campaigned to put such laws on the books in the first place. They were Protestant laws. The tendency of Protestants to legislate sin as if it were crime was coming back to haunt them. But a majority of these same Protestants who now opposed birth control laws as inappropriate continued to support hundreds of other laws prohibiting such things as adultery, homosexuality, premarital sex, and abortion in all fifty states without recognizing that such laws also confused the relationship between sin and crime. Nineteenth-century Protestant culture had thoroughly codified its sexual ethic in legislation. The goal of pluralistic America during the 1960s and beyond has been to dismantle it.

Illinois became the first state to decriminalize homosexuality among consenting adults in 1963. Some Christians interpreted these arguments for homosexual civil rights as a frontal attack on Christian values. Their efforts, since the mid-1950s, have been focused on the losing battle, with few exceptions, of trying to close the widening gap in the law between Christian faith and American culture. Anita Bryant's victory in Dade County in 1977 capitalized on the fear many had that the legal guarantee of rights for homosexuals amounted to a social sanctioning of homosexual behavior. Some evangelicals still think along these lines.[58] In the public mind, at least for many Christian people, the endorsement of homosexual rights meant the breakdown of longstanding social structures, and the possibility of increased homosexual behavior among youth resulting from more public acceptance of it.[59] Many evangelicals feared that the government might require churches to hire gay

58. Kenneth Kantzer, "Should Roman Catholics and Evangelicals Join Ranks?" *Christianity Today,* 18 July 1994, p. 17. For support of Anita Bryant's work, see "Controversy Has Its Price," *Christianity Today,* 18 March 1977, p. 30.

59. See Roger Ard's argument in "Why the Conservatives Won in Miami," *Christian Century,* 3-10 August 1977, pp. 677-79.

ministers or gay secretaries if full civil rights for homosexuals were guaranteed by federal law.[60]

Recognizing homosexual orientation as a neutral and disordered state has enabled increasing numbers of evangelicals during the 1980s and 1990s to support civil rights legislation while continuing to deny theological legitimacy to homosexual activity.[61] Tony Campolo is one of the leading evangelical speakers who has advocated this position. He has faced considerable criticism in evangelical circles because of this position, still deemed too liberal by a majority of evangelicals today. His wife, Peggy Campolo, an evangelical leader in her own right, has sought a more liberal goal than the one defended by her husband — complete acceptance of the homosexual community. According to Ralph Blair, conditions are better than they were twenty years ago, but most visible leaders within evangelicalism continue to hedge (and some actively resist) when it comes to supporting civil rights for gays and lesbians.[62] Many evangelicals,

60. "Methodists: Choosing Love or License?" *Christianity Today,* 7 December 1979, p. 15. See also essays evidencing the belief that the Supreme Court is bringing radical secularism into public life through its actions: e.g., Carl Horn III, "Taking God to Court," *Christianity Today,* 2 January 1981, pp. 24-27.

61. Terry Muck appeared to argue against general civil rights for gay people in "Too Much of a Good Thing," *Christianity Today,* 13 May 1988, pp. 14-15. For evangelicals who support civil rights, see Letha Scanzoni, "Conservative Christians and Gay Civil Rights," *Christian Century,* 13 October 1976, pp. 857-62; see also "Gay Confrontation," *Christianity Today,* 12 March 1976, pp. 53-55. *Sojourners,* the progressive evangelical journal traditionally concerned with justice issues, totally ignored the homosexual issue until 1982, but when it finally weighed in, it offered unqualified support for the full civil rights of homosexuals. See "A Matter of Justice," *Sojourners,* July-August 1982, p. 6. Concerning the practice of homosexuality, the magazine appeared traditional. In 1985 the journal published an excerpt from Richard Foster's book *Money, Sex, and Power* (San Francisco: Harper & Row, 1985). Foster's essay assumed a traditional stance urging change or celibacy, but called for compassion and ministry toward those who make the "tragic moral choice" to practice homosexuality. The Sojourners community itself discovered a division in the house after the article was published, some of the staff of the magazine emphasizing that the essay was too conservative in its approach. See Richard Foster, "God's Gift of Sexuality," *Sojourners,* July 1985, pp. 14-19; "Listening Together," *Sojourners,* July 1986, p. 37. In 1991 the magazine published a forum that covered the broad range of opinion in evangelical circles, including an article from a former *Sojourners* staff member writing out of her own lesbian experience, and an article from Richard Hays offering a thoughtful and traditional treatment of the appropriate biblical passages. "The Need for a Better Dialogue," *Sojourners,* July 1991, pp. 11-35. This latter section includes essays by Melanie Morrison ("A Love That Won't Let Go") and Richard Hays ("Awaiting the Redemption of Our Bodies") and many others.

62. Phone interview with Ralph Blair, 11 March 1997. Peggy Campolo was the featured speaker at the 1999 Women's Retreat sponsored by Evangelicals Concerned in Seattle (21 July 1999).

however, have accepted the chasm between culture and faith as the new context for American Christianity. Larger numbers of evangelical leaders disdain legislative efforts that appear to violate the meaning of pluralism in America by attempting to impose a "Christian" morality on the rest of the country. Evangelical criticism of the fundamentalist right has brought new tensions to the once unified conservative stream of American Christianity.[63] Because of these changes among evangelicals, members of evangelical and mainline churches have begun to find new areas of commonality and agreement as they struggle to deal with the reality of pluralism. But many leaders among the mainstream of evangelicalism, though they would not actively campaign for new legislative restrictions against homosexuals in society, are not, at this point, overtly supportive of the move for gay civil rights.

For their part, mainline Christian leaders have tried, since the early 1960s, to put a positive spin on the reality of pluralism.[64] They affirmed much earlier than evangelicals the expectation of pluralism that they recognize the difference between personal Christian values and the public nature of laws. Mid-1960s' editorial advocacy for homosexual civil rights at a time when these editors so clearly viewed homosexual behavior as a sin marks the first time Protestants were able to separate so clearly their theological notions of sin from their cultural understandings of crime. Such distinctions are commonplace now in most denominational statements about homosexuality.[65] Many mainline

63. See the following essays critical of the religious right and its political agendas that began to appear in *Christianity Today* around 1980: "The Limits of Christian Influence," Current Religious Thought, John Warwick Montgomery, *Christianity Today,* 23 January 1981, pp. 60, 62; "The Concerns and Considerations of Carl F. H. Henry," interview, *Christianity Today,* 13 March 1981, pp. 18-23; "Candid Conversation with the Evangelist: Billy Graham," *Christianity Today,* 17 July 1981, pp. 18-24; "Lost Momentum: Carl F. H. Henry Looks at the Future of the Religious Right," *Christianity Today,* 4 September 1987, pp. 30-32.

64. See, for example, "Protestantism Enters Third Phase," *Christian Century,* 18 January 1961, pp. 72-75.

65. See Bennett, "Questions on the Jenkins Case," *Christianity and Crisis,* 16 November 1964, p. 223; "Reappraising Laws on Homosexuality," *Christian Century,* 26 May 1965, pp. 669-70; see also Roger Shinn, "Persecution of the Homosexual," *Christianity and Crisis,* 2 May 1966, pp. 84-85. See also the later discussions of homosexual civil rights in *Commonweal:* "The Homosexual and the Church," *Commonweal,* 6 April 1973, pp. 99-100, and "Homosexual Rights," *Commonweal,* 24 May 1974, pp. 275-76. See the current ELCA statement as an illustration of the commonplace nature of such distinctions today: *Human Sexuality: Working Draft* (Minneapolis: ELCA Distribution Service, October 1994), p. 27, par. 82. See also the editorial entitled "Equality for Homosexuals," *Christian Century,* 13 December 1967, pp. 1587-88, where the *Century* editor supports complete civil rights for homosexuals "without subscribing to the highly dubious notion so often advanced by defensive deviates that homosexuality is a desirable and/or necessarily irreversible state of

Christians have attempted to maintain an appreciation for the values expressed in both public and church spheres, even though the values of the civic arena (i.e., freedom of expression) might lead them to defend the "rights" of others to act in ways they could not themselves affirm. This trend is not limited to Protestantism, but is equally evident in Catholic circles as well.

For some in the mainline, this positive separation between sin and crime has translated into a separation between the civil rights one defends in politics and the civil rights one has in church. In 1972, for example, the General Conference of the Methodist Church affirmed civil rights for homosexuals at the same time it added a phrase to its *Social Principles* stating unequivocally that homosexuality is "incompatible with Christian teaching." In 1979 the United Methodists fired a woman, Joan L. Clark, for revealing herself to be a lesbian even though she had served with distinction for seven years as an employee of the national office of the Women's Division of the Board of Global Ministries. In 1995 another woman in the United Methodist Church, Jeanne Audrey Powers, publicly revealed her lesbianism. When she came out as a lesbian, she was an executive with the United Methodist Commission on Christian Unity and Interreligious Concerns, but was a year or so from retirement. A conservative group in United Methodist circles, the Good News Movement, immediately demanded her removal. The commission president and others supported her completely. This support was made easier, most likely, by the nearness of her retirement. But the unqualified support does indicate a somewhat changed climate among Methodist leadership since 1979.[66]

By the end of the 1970s, the gap between evangelical and mainline Christians on the issue of homosexuality had begun to close considerably. In the early 1960s American mainline leaders, both Protestant and Catholic, moved homosexuality from the category of sin to that of disease and began to support civil rights for homosexuals. Throughout the 1970s and 1980s, many have stressed homosexuality as disorder rather than disease, and others, moving further to the left, have argued that it should be understood as a completely normal form of human sexuality.[67] Conservatives, on the other hand,

---

being." By 1971 the support for civil rights was not tainted by such qualifications. In an editorial published in March of that year, the *Century* questioned the value system that made possible the graffiti published in a Chicago newsletter (and eventually placed on Leonard Matlovich's tombstone): "The government gave me a medal for killing two men, and a dishonorable discharge for loving one."

66. See "Group Seeks Censure of Lesbian Clergywoman," *Christian Century*, 30 August–6 September 1995, pp. 809-10.

67. By 1973 and 1977, both *Commonweal* and *Christianity and Crisis* had established policies of nondifferentiation between homosexuality and heterosexuality. These

opposed liberalized civil rights throughout the 1960s and continued to understand all homosexuals as sinful and in need of redemption. During the 1970s they began to alter their views to accommodate the separation of orientation from practice. Accompanying this separation, they began to recognize that a homosexual orientation could not be changed easily. And, as evidenced by Lewis Smedes, some evangelicals have concluded that, after all other options have been unsuccessfully explored, faithful homosexual relationships, though less than ideal, should be affirmed and accepted within the church. In a book published posthumously, Paul Jewett, professor at Fuller Theological Seminary during his lifetime, also indicated his concerns about the church's prohibition of homosexual marriages. Of course, the majority of evangelicals today remain opposed to committed homosexual relationships.[68] Currently, according to a recent poll, 13 percent of white evangelical Protestants favor marriage rights for gays and lesbians, compared to 27 percent of white nonevangelical Protestants, 31 percent of white Roman Catholics, and 25 percent of African American Christians.[69]

These common trends shared by evangelical and mainline Christians indicate the problems with an oversimplified "culture wars" approach to the debates about homosexuality. Polarization between the two groups on this issue was much more pronounced from the 1950s through the 1970s than it has been in the 1980s and 1990s. This does not mean that differences no longer remain between evangelical and mainline Christian culture on the question of homosexuality. Though this growing muddled middle shares the similarities marked out by these trends, it also is defined by significant differences between the more conservative and more liberal groups gathered there.

First, there are differences in approach to the Bible. Are biblical statements propositional, or are they disclosive of truth, with narratives pointing in the direction of truth but not acting as literal containers of truth? Each approach to Scripture has its own tensions. Those Christians who do not read

---

journals covered both the Catholic and Protestant mainline and liberal-leaning audiences. Father John McNeill's book had a significant impact upon Catholic thought. He finished the book in 1973, but it was not published until 1976, when the church finally allowed publication by granting the *imprimi potest.* See McNeill, *The Church and the Homosexual* (Kansas City: Sheed Andrews & McMeel, 1976). He argued that the homosexual orientation was a gift to be received with gratitude and lived out with responsibility.

68. See John R. W. Stott, "Homosexual Marriage: Why Same-Sex Partnerships Are Not a Christian Option," *Christianity Today,* 22 November 1985, pp. 21-28. See Paul King Jewett's book, *Who We Are: Our Dignity as Human,* published by Eerdmans. The reference to the book, with quotation, is from *Record* (winter 1997): 1.

69. These are the results of a nationwide poll conducted for the Pew Research Center for the People and the Press. These statistics were cited in *Record* (summer 1996): 3.

the Bible literally are often muddled about knowing how to express its authority; those who read it literally seem to have no trouble muddling through an avoidance of its authority when they need to. The conservative understands the Bible to condemn homosexuality, but it also condemns divorce and remarriage, says women should be silent in the church, and seems to condone slavery. In all these cases, however, many of these conservatives have had no trouble finding muddled rationalizations. Part of the muddle for the middle is the fact that there are rarely hard consistencies in either the mainline or evangelical camps.

Second, the more liberal-leaning one is in the middle, the more one emphasizes sexuality as represented in relationships rather than in actions; the more conservative one is, the more one tends to emphasize the application of rules or principles to sexual acts. Third, the more liberal middle emphasizes dehumanization as the culprit in sexual sin, while the more conservative side tends to emphasize sexual activity outside of marriage as the culprit. Fourth and finally, the more liberal middle uses arguments from nature to support fulfillment of homosexual orientation within committed relationships; the more conservative middle uses arguments from nature to oppose homosexual practice in any form.

Conclusion

These differences are serious and significant, but they do not present clear evidence of a Christian culture at war with itself on this issue. If current denominational activities surrounding homosexuality reveal anything, they reveal the desire of the muddled middle that this issue go away. Most people in the muddled middle, in other words, do not want to talk about it. Many are fearful, because of strong rhetoric from the minorities on the left and the right, that the unity of the church itself depends upon a strategy of deferral or avoidance. But this realistic problem of the church's life demands a realistic solution. And if led to examine their own theological commitments, most in the muddled middle would affirm the belief that the unity and future of the church rests ultimately in God's hands and not their own.

The denominational debates among the mainline (which today includes many evangelical voices) have dominated general conferences and assemblies during the late 1970s, the 1980s, and the 1990s. Only the United Church of Christ and the Unitarian Universalist Association have taken general church actions declaring positive views of the ordination of homosexuals. In June 1996 the Unitarians voted to endorse the legalization of same-sex marriages.[70] A number of associations in the United Church of Christ, largely congregational in its polity, still refuse to ordain "self-avowed and practicing" homosexuals. Among some other denominations, regions or areas are acting independently of the general structures and moving to ordain homosexuals. For example, this is true of a few of the regions in the Christian Church (Disciples of Christ), though those regions do not publicize it. It is also true of some Presbyterian Church (USA) congregations known as "More Light Presbyterians" whose ordinations have withstood challenges in the church's courts.[71] Some dioceses in the Episcopal Church also ordain homosexuals. Obviously Roman Catholics, with their emphasis on celibacy for clergy, have a different perspective than Protestant groups. It is significant, however, that the U.S. bishops issued a pastoral letter in 1997, "Always Our Children," that urged Catholic parents to practice love and acceptance of gay sons and lesbian daughters.[72]

As evidenced by first drafts of denominational statements on sexuality published by the Presbyterians, Lutherans, and Episcopalians, some Christians are showing signs of abandoning connections between sin and homosexual practice between committed partners, and some are advocating a new ethic of sexuality for heterosexual single people as well. This perhaps should not be surprising in light of recent public surveys indicating that the general public in America finds itself increasingly accepting of the gay lifestyle and the issues surrounding it. Increasing depiction of gay lifestyles on popular television shows indicates this trend as well.[73] Denominational rejections of these various sexuality reports also indicate, conversely, that the majority in

70. See the report in "Unitarians Endorse Same-Sex Marriages," *Christian Century,* 28 August–4 September 1996, p. 807.

71. More Light Presbyterians began on 1 January 1999, when More Light Churches Network merged with Presbyterians for Lesbian and Gay Concerns. Ultimate origin for the group is traced to 1974, when David Sindt formed a gay caucus. Sindt was an ordained Presbyterian minister who began to identify himself as gay in the early 1970s. Current information on More Light Presbyterians can be obtained on the organization's web site (http://www.mlp.org). More than ninety-five congregations have been involved in ordinations of gay and lesbian ministers as members of the More Light Churches Network.

72. See "Bishops Urge Parents of Homosexuals to Accept Their Children, Themselves, Church Teaching on Human Dignity," web site of National Conference of Bishops (http://www.nccbuscc.org/comm/archives/97-208.htm).

73. See "Gay Families Come Out," a cover story in *Newsweek,* 4 November 1996, pp. 50-57. See also Patrick McCormick, "Out of the Closet and into Your Living Room," *U.S. Catholic,* April 1998, pp. 45-48. See also Lydia Saad, "Majority of Americans Unfazed by Ellen's 'Coming Out' Episode," *Gallup Poll Monthly,* April 1997, pp. 24-26.

the Christian muddled middle remain unwilling to make these moves without more discussion and clarification.

Meanwhile, Presbyterians and Episcopalians have refused to take actions that could have reinforced conservative positions on same-sex marriages (Presbyterians) and the ordination of homosexuals (Episcopalians).[74] In fact, in their 1996 General Assembly, Presbyterians voted to "go to court in support of 'committed same-sex' partners" who seek equal civil rights. But in the same assembly they voted to add an amendment to their *Book of Order* denying ordination to "practicing" homosexuals without explicitly addressing the question. The amendment forbids ordination of ministers, elders, and deacons who fail to live "either in fidelity within the covenant of marriage between a man and a woman, or chastity in singleness." The vote was seriously split, revealing how closely divided the group is on the issue.[75] The majority of the church's 172 presbyteries approved the amendment in early 1997, but significant numbers of presbyteries voted against it. Many of the presbyteries voting for it did so by putting together only narrow margins. In the Dallas area, for example, generally considered conservative within the Presbyterian church, the Grace Presbytery passed the amendment by a vote of 238-217, a 21-vote margin.[76]

This debate will not end soon within the Presbyterian church. But there is a hopeful sign that reasoned articulation of how faith relates to these issues might bring more visible consensus within the church concerning these issues. A number of people voting one way or the other remain generally confused because of the complexity of the issues involved and their own uncertainty as to how to relate their Christian faith to the contested issues. The *Presbyterian Panel,* a polling of ministers, elders, and members of the Presbyterian Church (USA) on the controversial social and theological issues in the church, indicates that the very liberal and very conservative ends of the spectrum account for only about 10 to 15 percent of the church's membership, though they are among the loudest groups in the church's debate on the is-

74. See the discussion of the dismissal of the heresy trial against Bishop Walter Righter for ordaining a homosexual: William L. Sachs, "Procedural Abyss: After the Righter Trial," *Christian Century,* 19-26 June 1996, pp. 644-46. See the discussion of the amendment that would have prohibited ministers from conducting same-sex unions: "Presbyterians Consider Same-Sex Unions," *Christian Century,* 17 May 1995, pp. 534-35. Presbyterian presbyteries refused to pass the amendment in 1995.

75. See "Presbyterian Conflicts," *Christian Century,* 17-24 July 1996, pp. 709-10.

76. For statistics on the Grace Presbytery, see Jim Jones, "Don't Expect Sexuality Issue to Go Away," *Fort Worth Star-Telegram,* 23 March 1997; for commentary on the Presbyterian situation, see John P. Burgess, "Sexuality, Mortality and the Presbyterian Debate," *Christian Century,* 5 March 1997, pp. 246-49.

sues. In other words, "the remaining 70-80% find themselves within the bell curve" where "the vast majority remains inarticulate."[77] These are all signs of the muddle of the middle.

In 1998 the 210th General Assembly of the Presbyterian Church (USA) approved an overture that affirmed the Presbyterian commitment to inclusivity in the following way: "Standing in the tradition of breaking down the barriers erected to exclude people based on their condition such as age, race, class, gender, and sexual orientation, the PC (U.S.A.) commits itself not to exclude anyone categorically in considering those called to ordained service in the church but to consider the lives and behaviors of candidates as individuals."[78] This language represents a sort of "middle" perspective in that it allows for a differentiation between homosexual orientation and the behavior attached to that orientation. Presumably, it would allow some in the church to ordain a nonpracticing homosexual while refusing to ordain a self-avowed practicing homosexual.

A recent Presbyterian case regarding the ordination of an elder in a local congregation illustrates the point. First Presbyterian Church of Stamford, Connecticut, examined and approved Wayne Osborne for ordination in the congregation as an elder. His installation in the congregation was to take place on 14 June 1998. Two members of the church, Mairi Hair and James McCallum, filed a complaint with the Presbyterian Judicial Commission of Southern New England (PJC). A stay of enforcement was granted which temporarily prevented the installation. After investigation, the PJC found that, though Wayne Osborne had openly admitted being in a committed homosexual relationship, he had not openly admitted he was in any kind of sexual relationship. When asked "Is this a sexually active partnership?" Osborne responded, "I decline to answer this question." No factual knowledge of a sexual relationship existed; therefore, the PJC found in favor of Osborne and the congregation.[79]

In light of the 1998 General Assembly action, the Presbytery of Milwaukee has proposed, for a second year, an overture calling for an amendment to be sent to presbyteries posing the question: "Shall G-6.0106b be stricken from the Book of Order?" This is the section of the *Book of Order,* passed in 1997, that re-

77. Milton J Coalter, John M. Mulder, and Louis B. Weeks, *Vital Signs: The Promise of Mainstream Protestantism* (Grand Rapids: Eerdmans, 1996), p. 120.

78. This overture is quoted from the listing of action from the 210th General Assembly found at the Presbyterian Church (USA) web site (http://www.pcusa.org/pcusa/ga210/ovt/action.html).

79. See "Permanent Judicial Commission of the Presbytery of Southern New England," Remedial Case No. R-1998-1, on the web site with url of http://www.pforum.org/Stamford/majority.htm.

quires all those "called to office in the church" to "live either in fidelity within the covenant of marriage between a man and a woman, or chastity in singleness." Anyone "refusing to repent of any self-acknowledged practice which the confessions call sin shall not be ordained and/or installed as deacons, elders, or ministers of the Word and Sacrament."[80] In rationale supporting the overture, the Presbytery of Milwaukee emphasized that the "210th General Assembly (1998) approved an authoritative interpretation of the *Constitution,* affirming the denomination's commitment to consider the lives and behaviors of candidates for ordination as individuals and not to exclude anyone categorically." Whether or not Presbyterians are willing, in light of the 1998 action, to revisit the national debate of 1997 remains to be seen.[81]

The Evangelical Lutheran Church in America voted to have a statement on human sexuality presented during the 1997 assembly even though the Church Council had taken action recommending no statement be provided. The voting members of the assembly wanted to keep the issue in front of the church and to press for some clear word for the churches. The statement will "lift up those areas in which there is clarity and wide agreement . . . to provide a public ethical witness." The 1995 assembly voted to express "a caring welcome for gay and lesbian persons," an action that followed an earlier resolution, approved 856-129: "gay and lesbian people, as individuals created by God, are welcome to participate fully in the life of the congregations of the ELCA."[82] These actions indicate the tendency of the Lutherans to want to steer a middle course. Currently, all the mainline denominations remain active in their studies of human sexuality and the role of homosexuality within it. Most of them remain committed to the struggle to address this complex topic, but still are confused as to the best way to proceed.

The United Methodist Church (UMC) has witnessed among the most heated debates concerning this topic in the last few years. The phrase "incompatible with Christian teaching," since 1972, has blocked the possibility of ordination for homosexuals in the United Methodist Church. In 1984 the *Book of Discipline* became explicit in this regard: "Since the practice of homosexuality is incompatible with Christian teaching, self-avowed practicing homo-

80. See G-6.0106b, *The Constitution of the Presbyterian Church (U.S.A.) Part II Book of Order Annotated Edition, 1998-1999* (Louisville: Geneva Press, 1998), pp. 111-12. This paragraph was proposed for the *Book of Order* in 1996 and ratified in 1997.

81. See Overture 99-2, on Presbyterian web site http://www.pcusa.org/ga211/ovt99/ovt99-02.htm. A similar overture was rejected in 1998 (see overture 98-37) by a vote of 412-98. See "Presbyterians Decide Not to Talk about Sex," *Christian Century,* 1-8 July 1998, pp. 640-41.

82. See "Sexuality: Unfinished Business," *Lutheran,* October 1995, pp. 12-13.

sexuals are not to be accepted as candidates, ordained as ministers, or appointed to serve in the United Methodist Church."[83] Though attempts have been made at various times throughout the last fifteen years or so to strike this language, none have been successful.

More recently, Methodists have been struggling over the issue of gay and lesbian unions. The 1996 General Conference, following the trend in the church, added a new sentence to the *Social Principles* of the UMC: "Ceremonies that celebrate homosexual unions shall not be conducted by our ministers and shall not be conducted in our churches."[84] In the past, a large number of United Methodist ministers have understood the *Social Principles* to be instructive rather than binding. In August of 1998, following the trial and acquittal of Jimmy Creech, a minister from Omaha, Nebraska, brought to trial for performing a same-sex ceremony for two women, the Judicial Council of the UMC declared that the sentence in the *Social Principles* "has the effect of church law, notwithstanding its placement in §65.C and, therefore, governs the conduct of the ministerial office. Conduct in violation of this prohibition renders a pastor liable to a charge of disobedience to the Order and Discipline of the United Methodist Church under §2624 of the *Discipline*."[85]

In response to these actions, more than 1,430 clergy and over 500 laity have signed statements supporting the blessing of homosexual unions and the full rights of gays and lesbians in the United Methodist Church.[86] Perhaps the most telling response to the action of the Judicial Council organized shortly after Donald Fado, minister of Saint Mark's United Methodist Church in Sacramento, California, preached a sermon entitled "Ecclesiastical Disobedience" on World Communion Sunday (4 October 1998). Fado pointed out the irony of the UMC policy:

83. *The Book of Discipline of the United Methodist Church, 1984* (Nashville: United Methodist Publishing House, 1984), p. 189.

84. See §65C of *The United Methodist Social Principles*, found on the UMC web site (http://www.umc-gbcs.org/sp.htm).

85. See "Prohibition against Performing Homosexual Unions Ruled Enforceable," United Methodist News Service, on the Affirmation web site (http://www.umaffirm.org/cornet/jcrules.html#833). On the Jimmy Creech trial, see "Talk of Schism after Creech Trial," *Christian Century*, 22-29 April 1998, pp. 421-22; and "UMC Bishops' Stance Draws Praise, Criticism," *Christian Century*, 20-27 May 1998, pp. 521-22.

86. An organization called In All Things Charity has emerged as a movement to counter these developments in the UMC. Details concerning the statements signed are found on the organization's web site (http://www.brdwyumc.org/IATC/). Another movement publicly welcoming all persons, regardless of sexual orientation, the Reconciling Movement, claims more than 14,000 UMC members, including 148 congregations, 23 campus ministries, and 6 conferences.

> As a United Methodist Minister, I'm free to do a wedding ceremony for any heterosexuals. It doesn't matter if they've been married 755 times, and only married a day at a time. They trust me to use my good judgment. They let me have the decision of whether to utter prayers and vows for any group I want, unless it happens to be two people of the same sex who wish to have vows of fidelity. I can come to your home and offer prayers of blessings for the house. I can even bless your place of business, regardless of what it is. I can even bless your automobile. I can bless your animals. But I cannot bless you if you are two people of the same sex who want to make a vow to God of fidelity to each other. There is no other such exclusion in my ministry. It is clearly a case of homophobia and contrary to our tradition. In no way should any minister be required to offer such vows of holy union; but likewise in no way should such ministry of inclusion be forbidden by our church.

Fado then stated that he chose to act in protest to the UMC policies on this matter. He called upon other ministers to join him in performing a ceremony of union at the earliest possible opportunity as an "act of ecclesiastical disobedience." Two women, Jeanne Barnett and Ellie Charlton, later asked Reverend Fado to perform their ceremony. Accompanied by over 90 Methodist ministers and 13 ministers from other denominations, Fado performed the "holy union" at the Sacramento Convention Center on 16 January 1999. Since the ceremony, a total of 157 UMC clergy have signed on as supporters of the defiant action. The first minister to be charged for participating is David M. Holmes from Council Bluffs, Iowa. Methodists have not yet taken further action. Another minister, Greg Dell, who co-officiated at the service, stood trial 25 March 1999, but the original charges in his case stem from his blessing of a union between two males performed on 19 September 1998. The denomination's "Jurisdictional Committee on Appeals" upheld the decision of the Church Trial Court to suspend Dell from active ministry. The ruling, handed down on 17 September 1999, stated that the suspension would end 30 June 2000.[87] Other trials will no doubt follow. Methodists will be forced to deal with this issue seriously in their next General Conference, scheduled for the year 2000. The Methodist setting is the most contentious, but perhaps it is also the setting that, due to these recent dramatic actions by large numbers of influential ministers, might have to produce the most creative solutions within the next few years in order to hold things together for those furthest from the middle on these issues.[88]

87. See "Penalty Upheld for Ousted Pastor," at http://www.umaffirm.org/cornews/dell20.html.

88. The sermon by Don Fado and other materials related to this event are

Perhaps a hopeful trend in fact does exist in the history of how Christian editors have dealt with homosexuality and human sexuality over the past forty years. As leaders of very different Christian groups, these editors have ended up sharing a great deal more in common than they might have imagined decades ago. Movement has been slow, but it has been in the same direction. Even though these Christians approach the Bible differently and live out of somewhat competing moral visions, both evangelical and mainline Christians in these more middle contexts profess the transcendence, grace, and judgment of God, and define their roles as essentially inclusive of both prophetic and pastoral responsibilities. Both oppose iconic confusion between the symbols of Christianity and culture, and both profess to reject priestly attempts to legislate a particular religious vision of America, whether these attempts come from more liberal or more conservative fringes. The nurturing of such possibilities may prove much more fruitful to the formation of a common and humane public life in America than the current fixation with the language of culture wars. Perhaps our only real hope of resolving the issues surrounding the homosexual debate is to encourage the large throng of people in the muddled middle to seek theological clarity by learning first to speak more directly to one another.

The move by these journals, over these decades, in the direction of some kind of middle position on the issue of homosexuality raises a necessary question. Are their moves market driven?[89] Perhaps these independent journals have learned to model the same impulses toward self-survival that H. Richard Niebuhr accused denominations of perfecting.[90] After all, the one journal *(Christianity and Crisis)* that did not reflect much of a move toward the middle did not survive. Whatever hope this muddled middle may present in terms of fostering an ecumenical dialogue (within and between denominations) on the subject of homosexuality, it must be self-critical about its own position at the same time it seeks ways to be faithful to its pluralistic sense of the gospel. Its church leadership, journals, and churches will need to protect,

---

found on various web sites (http://www.umaffirm.org/spiritual/donfado.html; http://www.brdwyumc.org/IATC/PressRelease_10_21.html; and http://www.umaffirm.org/cornews/calstate.html).

89. See, for example, David Wells, *No Place for Truth; or, Whatever Happened to Evangelical Theology?* (Grand Rapids: Eerdmans, 1993), pp. 207-11, and Mark Noll, *The Scandal of the Evangelical Mind* (Grand Rapids: Eerdmans, 1994), pp. 15, 221-22, where both address the self-survival mechanism and cultural consumerism present in the history of *Christianity Today.*

90. See H. Richard Niebuhr, *Social Sources of Denominationalism* (New York: New American Library, 1975), p. 21.

and listen to, the fringe voices of those prophets, left and right, who by the very nature of their positions abhor the middle.

The task remains, therefore, one of muddling through, of recognizing our own complicity and sin and tendencies toward self-righteousness, of acknowledging God's judgment while trusting in God's mercy, and of assuming a willingness to risk further complicity for the sake of bringing our response to homosexuality in line with our responsibility to the gospel. There can be little doubt, however, that muddling through is more hopeful than letting the language of culture wars control all future debates. If the church continues to rethink this issue in ways comparable to the movement of the past forty years, future imaginary time travelers will find our own time as foreign to them as the 1950s now seem to us.

CHAPTER 2

Same-Sex Eros: Paul and the Greco-Roman Tradition

WILLIAM R. SCHOEDEL

The historical contextualizing of our theme inevitably suggests a relativization of the views of Paul and other early Christians about same-sex eros. This is particularly true when arguments strike us as obsolete in the light of later knowledge or experience. At the same time, some points associated with the criticism of same-sex eros still elicit serious attention, and our discussion must also try to show why this is so.

The background to Paul's comments on same-sex eros will be set by focusing on discussions in three ancient authors who share a negative view of such practices — Plato, Philo, and Clement of Alexandria. This will provide a reasonably suitable framework for the relevant philosophical, medical, and popular elements involved.

It remains unclear how much of this tradition actually lies in the background of Paul's attack on same-sex eros in Romans. I shall argue, however, that Paul's first letter to the Corinthians reveals habits of thought on related issues that help us make judgments on this matter. The conclusion will be that Paul was familiar with many of the features of the tradition and that his views reflect whatever strengths or weaknesses may be assigned to such arguments.

I. Roots

A. *Plato's* Laws

We begin with Plato's last and most conservative writing, the *Laws*, because it was looked back to by many in antiquity who opposed same-sex eros. It is alluded to by Philo and quoted at length by Clement of Alexandria. It uses the expression "contrary to nature" in the same form that it appears in Romans 1:26 to describe same-sex eros (cf. *Laws* 636c, 841d).

Near the beginning of the *Laws*, Plato's Athenian tempers his praise for the organization of the Spartan community by criticizing the separation of sexes that fosters same-sex eros, males with males (meaning the normally approved sexual relation of mature men with adolescent boys) and females with females (636bc). Two features of the argument are generally highlighted: (1) that for Plato the city requires marriages that produce children (772de, 838d-839d); (2) that only sexual pleasure for the purpose of procreation is "granted by nature" (636c). A presupposition of these arguments is the view that the obvious purpose of male and female sexual parts is procreation: in the myth that Plato tells at the end of his *Timaeus* to explain sexual differentiation, male and female sexual organs and the desire of sexual intercourse are created as appendages to humans so that the species might maintain its immortality in time (90e-91d).[1]

It is sometimes argued that Plato's judgment of same-sex eros is not as negative as it may appear today, since he tars it with the same brush that he tars heterosexual eros: both are problematic because excessive pleasure tends to characterize both (841ae). The pederast, then, "was not a monster."[2] That is true. What controls the discussion is demographic need and the desirability of order and control (legitimacy is important to Plato). At the same time, Plato deepens the charge against same-sex eros in a number of ways: (1) he insists (probably wrongly) that animals do not exhibit comparable behavior (836bc; cf. 840d); (2) he asserts that same-sex eros of the type under discussion should be stigmatized as being as unacceptable as incest, though he is fully conscious of how difficult it will be to convince people of that (838ac);

1. Francis MacDonald Cornford, *Plato's Cosmology: The "Timaeus" of Plato* (London: Routledge & Kegan Paul, 1937), pp. 291-93, 355-57.

2. Paul Veyne, "Homosexuality in Ancient Rome," in *Western Sexuality: Practice and Precept in Past and Present Times,* ed. Philippe Ariès and André Bégin, trans. Anthony Forster (Oxford: Blackwell, 1985), pp. 28-29; see also K. J. Dover, *Greek Homosexuality: Updated and with a New Postscript* (Cambridge: Harvard University Press, 1978, 1989), pp. 167-68.

(3) third, he says that, while the active partner surrenders to pleasure, the passive partner imitates the female and in fact becomes womanish (836de); or similarly, that the adolescents who are victimized by same-sex eros are those who have given themselves up to "a soft *(malthakon)* and not hard *(stereon)* life." The latter point is made not in the *Laws* but in the *Phaedrus* (239c) where Socrates attacks pederasty in a speech that is only partly withdrawn later. The passage is of some importance since an attack on softness and effeminacy has been seen as the special mark of the later Stoic and Christian attitude toward same-sex eros.[3] At the very least, Plato provides abundant resources for those who go beyond an emphasis on the procreative function of sex for the benefit of the state to an emphasis on the perversity of same-sex eros as such. The special significance of the *Laws* in the discussion is that Plato has in view the pederasty that the majority found acceptable.

Qualifications of the significance of Plato's appeal to nature lie in a somewhat different direction. Plato himself is acutely aware of the fact that nature may describe simply what is instead of what ought to be. In these same pages he quotes disapprovingly Pindar's famous dictum that by "nature's own appointment" the strong rule the weak (*Laws* 690b). Plato replaces the polarity with one of his own: it is the wise who rule the ignorant (and this time animals serve as one illustration of the discredited principle of the rule of the strong over the weak). And in fact, he argues, it is the governing role of wisdom that should be named "nature's own ordinance" (690bc). Plato, in short, appeals to nature in a higher sense. He is aware, then, that mutually incompatible claims emerge when various forms of governing and being governed are examined (690d, 714e). Plato's very definition of sexual normality in terms of the avoidance of excessive pleasure clearly depends on an analysis of the virtues that goes beyond what biological impulses by themselves might suggest.

Plato's appeal to nature, then, lacks a certain finality: nature does not necessarily coincide with virtue. Precisely such finality tends to characterize usage at the time of writers like Philo and Paul. The reason for that may be illustrated in the following way. Plato knew that "everyone is naturally his own friend." But he sees this as a violent attachment to self that leads to misdeeds of every kind (731e). Later the Stoics, whose influence on popular philosophy was strong, similarly taught that self-preservation was the basic law of human nature (Diogenes Laertius, 7.85). But since in Stoic thought nature is God, self-preservation cannot stand opposed to the universal order of things. Coherence is achieved by arguing that self-preservation means different things

3. Philippe Ariès, "St. Paul and the Flesh," in *Western Sexuality*, pp. 36-39.

at different levels of nature (7.86). Thus, for example, since rationality characterizes human beings, self-preservation is not antithetical to suicide, for suicide represents the preservation of rational self-determination (cf. Epictetus, *Discourses* 3.24.95-102). The appeal to nature is not cleared of all ambiguity in this way, but in such a context it will carry greater weight.

An underlying element in the logic of both the Platonic and Stoic appeal to nature is its teleological presuppositions: wise men aim at the highest good and do what must be done to achieve it; at the same time, they pursue their goals within a world that also displays purpose. Where nature is flatly identified with God, as in Stoic thought, the emphasis on purpose in the physical realm is correspondingly more elaborate and detailed. Thus it is characteristic of medical writers under Stoic influence that purposes for each and every part of the body are found and carefully defined.[4] Same-sex eros does not fare well in such contexts. In particular, I shall argue that those who appeal to nature against same-sex eros find it convenient to concentrate on the more or less obvious uses of the orifices of the body to suggest the proper channel for the more diffused sexual impulses of the body.

B. Plato's Symposium

Before saying a word about how such themes filter down to people like Paul and Philo, a famous but often neglected passage from Plato's *Symposium* requires brief attention: the mythological account of the emergence of sexual differentiation presented by Aristophanes. In the beginning, human beings of three types were to be found: male, female, and hermaphrodites. When they rose up against the gods, Zeus split them down the middle. Subsequently each half yearns desperately for the other. The hermaphrodites account for heterosexual love. "But the woman who is a slice of the original female is attracted by women rather than by men . . . , while men who are slices of the male are followers of the male . . ." (191e).

Aristophanes does not speak for Plato here, and it is not clear how seriously the speech is to be taken. Yet it sets in place a number of points of importance to this paper.

1. The wide variety of forms of sexuality in antiquity did not necessarily exclude the identification of distinct sexual orientations persisting at a

4. P. H. Schrijvers, *Eine medizinische Erklärung der männlichen Homosexualität aus der Antike (Caelius Aurelianus De morbis chronicis IV 9)* (Amsterdam: B. R. Grüner, 1985), pp. 17-25.

deep level (in 192e and 193d the strength of the sexual bond is explained mythologically in terms of the restoration of "the ancient nature" of the creature involved).[5] We shall find that at least some of the forms of same-sex eros were explained in the medical literature as more or less deep-seated aberrations and that it was not hard for Jews and Christians to generalize the analysis.

2. The image of the hermaphrodite was given powerful poetic form by this passage and served not only to explain mythologically heterosexual love but to support notions of sexuality as a continuum between male and female poles. Philo and Clement, as we shall see, find the latter notion unacceptable.

3. Aristophanes names women and men (in that order) in his account of homoerotic love. At the same time, he goes on (192ab) to discuss in greater detail only the men involved and unconsciously reveals the wider range of sexual options that remain open to them: he argues that the adolescents involved in pederasty become the most effective leaders "since they are by nature the most virile" (note that here "by nature" refers only to the nature of a group), but that when they become fully mature, they attend to the begetting of children not "by nature" but "by law (or custom)" (echoing views of the Sophists on nature and law).[6]

The latter point is of some immediate interest for the reader of Romans 1:26-27, where Paul also refers to same-sex eros of women and men (in that order). We should hesitate before finding that too unusual. How much else in this picture may lie in the background of the discussion known to Paul is unclear. But it is obvious that he would not have agreed with the point of Aristophanes (unless he read it as satire) that precisely such adolescents emerge as the most effective leaders "since they are by nature the most virile" (192a). We shall also see that Paul is more likely to have had in view nature in a normative sense and would have been as uncomfortable with the opposition between nature and law (or custom) as was Plato himself (though for different reasons).

5. This is a major theme also of Bernadette J. Brooten, *Love between Women: Early Christian Responses to Female Homoeroticism* (Chicago and London: University of Chicago Press, 1996). This study became available to me only after the completion of the research for this paper. Both Brooten and I find problematic the common view that sexual orientation was not recognized in the ancient world.

6. The asymmetry in the (male) treatment of male and female homoerotic love is a major theme in the study by Brooten referred to in the preceding note.

C. 4 Maccabees on Nature and Law

We choose one passage to highlight the convergence of nature and law in the world of Paul and Philo: 4 Maccabees 5:14-38. In this passage Eleazar is explaining to the Syrian king, Antiochus, why Jews abhor pork in spite of the fact that "nature has granted it us" (5:8). Eleazar tries to show that the Jewish religion is rational since "the Creator of the world in giving the law has conformed it to (our) nature" (5:25). And in a further explanation that sounds like budding dietary theory, we learn that God "commanded us to eat what was adapted to our souls and forbade us to eat flesh opposed to our souls" (5:26). Conceivably the implication of these lines is that "the dietary observances serve as discipline and symbol for general ethical conduct, as in Philo and Aristeas."[7] We shall return to this later in this paper.

4 Maccabees is shot through with themes of the popular philosophy of the day. Nevertheless, it also retains a sense of God as the one who commands and elicits obedience. Even in such an ethic of obligation, however, it is assumed (as Kant was to argue) that ought implies can. God, then, will not command what is impossible; or as Deuteronomy 30:11 puts it, "this commandment . . . is not too hard for you, nor is it too far away" (NRSV). It is in this connection that an appeal to nature may play a role in the framework of biblical ethics. That role will be a subordinate one (as it is in Rom. 1:18-32), but it is not without importance.

D. Romans 1:18-32 and Desire

One important component of the attack on same-sex eros (in Plato and later in Philo) is missing in Paul: the emphasis on procreativity as the mark of what is natural in sexual relations. It should not be overlooked, however, that in Romans 1:26-27 same-sex eros is associated with "degrading passions" and shameless "desire for one another." Criticism of pleasure for its own sake may not have been far from Paul's mind. Similarly, Paul's judgment that it is better to marry than to burn (1 Cor. 7:9), whatever its exact implications may be, scarcely adds up to a celebration of pleasure. At the same time, Paul does not mention procreation as an aim of heterosexual relations in 1 Corinthians 7:1-7 (where a mutuality of man and woman in marriage comparable to that recommended by Musonius Rufus and Plutarch is highlighted); and he does not

7. Moses Hadas, *The Third and Fourth Books of Maccabees,* Dropsie College Edition, Jewish Apocryphal Literature (New York: Harper & Brothers, 1953), p. 174.

mention children among the distracting anxieties that marriage brings in 1 Corinthians 7:32-35. But he does take children for granted as a component of marriage when he warns against moving too quickly to divorce (1 Cor. 7:12-16). Paul's lack of attention to procreation is generally (and, I suspect, rightly) explained as arising from his expectation of the coming of the end of the age (1 Cor. 7:29-31). That, however, need not indicate that he had an atypical view of marriage and its purposes other than its partial irrelevance at the end of the age. What it may well explain is why he makes nothing of what he took for granted. Later we shall also see that even when, as in Philo, the procreative function of sex is advanced, it is the abhorrence of pleasure for the sake of pleasure or the abhorrence of impurity that provides the real impetus to the rejection of same-sex eros.

II. Context

A. Philo

It is common knowledge that the link drawn by Paul between idolatry and immorality in Romans 1:18-32 echoes Hellenistic Jewish themes that appear also in the Wisdom of Solomon 13–14. But that source refers only briefly to "sexual perversion" along with "disorder in marriage, adultery, and debauchery" (14:26) in this connection. We must go to Josephus and especially Philo to gain a fuller picture of how Jews in the Hellenistic world expressed opposition to same-sex eros and how they used such opposition to mark themselves off from the nations of the earth. Here we consider briefly three passages in Philo that explore the issue: *De Abrahamo* (hereafter *Ab*) 133-41; *De vita contemplativa* (hereafter *VCon*) 48-53; and *De specialibus legibus* (hereafter *SLeg*) 3.37-50.

Philo shares with Plato's *Laws* opposition to those who in their sexual relations sow their seed "on stony and stubborn places" (*VCon* 62; cf. *Laws* 838e). Thus he opposes pleasure for its own sake and sex that does not aim at procreation or contribute to the demographic health of the world. He goes beyond Plato, however, in his discussion of the presumed damage done to both partners in same-sex eros. The crucial importance of Philo in this connection is that he is the one person who shows himself fully conversant with normal Greco-Roman views of pederasty and who at the same time knows how to turn the argument to the disadvantage of pederasty. His discussion also shows how it was found possible to move toward a blanket criticism of same-sex eros and to characterize it negatively in terms of the purity concerns of the Hebrew Bible. The blanket rejection of homoerotic love in Jewish and early Christian literature must at least sometimes presuppose such an analysis of the phenomenon.

The more obvious damage presumably done by pederasty is outlined in Philo's description of the banquets of the pagan world as contrasted with those of the Jewish Therapeutae in *De vita contemplativa* 48-63. Philo is keenly aware of the importance of social context in fostering types of behavior, and in this connection he succeeds in catching the atmosphere of elegant decadence that he thinks characterizes the pagan meals (50-51). In this connection Philo even finds elements of Plato's *Symposium* offensive. On the other hand, like the Plato of the *Laws,* he is appalled especially by the feminization of the youth that is involved, and like Plato he rejects pleasure pursued for its own sake. Here a distinction is made that is worth noting: when the two sexes madly pursue each other for pleasure, their behavior is morally wrong yet within the bounds of "the laws of nature" (59). That of course cannot be said for the love between two males. Here the tension in the concept of nature noted in our discussion of Plato's *Laws* reemerges. Nature and virtue do not always coincide.

Philo adds something new in this connection when he rejects the love of males with males even though they "only" differ in age (59). The "only" is important here. For the difference in age made all the difference in the Greco-Roman view. Philo is subtly suggesting that the normal abhorrence for the love of adult males can with equal propriety be extended to pederasty. The unequally aged lovers *are* monsters.

The damage done to the adolescent, as we have seen, is his feminization (60). But the adult male lover is also damaged. Here Philo mentions the latter's total preoccupation with love, the wasting away of his body, and the neglect of his property (61). As an attendant ill, Philo mentions the loss of population that results from preoccupation with this form of love (62; cf. *Ab* 136). Here we can sense Philo searching for a criticism of the adult male lover as decisive as his criticism of the feminized adolescent. In fact, however, he speaks here of damages that are in a sense external to the adult male lover. More decisive points of criticism emerge in the two other passages with which we are concerned.

Before moving on to these, we note one other feature of the discussion in *De vita contemplativa.* Philo rejects the mythical inventions of Aristophanes in Plato's *Symposium* (*VCon* 63). One implication of this is that Philo (like Clement of Alexandria after him) refuses to recognize any sexually ambivalent image. Surely connected with this is the unambivalent opposition to same-sex eros.

The deeper reasons for Philo's opposition to same-sex eros begin to emerge from his discussion of the sins of the Sodomites in *De Abrahamo* 133-41. Here again the excessive search for pleasure is the problem. Such excess leads to throwing off "the law of nature." This time the term "law of nature" is used in a somewhat wider sense. For a growing crescendo of moral ills is involved: drinking heavily, eating gourmet foods, engaging in forbidden forms of sexual intercourse. The latter include the mad lust for women (in particular, violating the wife of one's neighbor) and then finally the love of males for males. The love of males for males is described in terms of "the active partners not respecting the common nature with their passive partners" (135). The damage involved, then, is deeper than inattention to health and property. How much deeper remains unclear here but will become apparent in a moment.

First, however, note that Philo believes that such excess leads to damage at the biological level. When the men involved (i.e., the Sodomites) return to their wives and attempt to produce children, they "were shown to be incapable of engendering any but imperfect offspring" (135). The line may mean that they proved "incapable of any but a sterile seed" (Loeb).[8] There are medical parallels, or near parallels, for the former idea but not (as far as I have found) for the latter. Thus Soranus, in his gynecological treatise, states that drunkenness at the time of intercourse leads to no conception or to the risk that "by reason of the bad material contributed [by a drunken woman] the seed too may change for the worse" (*Gynecology* 1.10.38).[9] And Galen, in a discussion of the habits of men and women at the time of intercourse, warns that overindulgence in drink and food leads to faulty procreation.[10] Elsewhere Galen explains physiologically how too frequent coitus by a male can lead to the blockage of the emission of semen.[11] Clearly the moralists could look for support from the scientists of the period.

A final step is taken in Philo's discussion of same-sex eros in *De specialibus legibus* 3.37-50. One characteristic of this passage is that Philo

8. In *SLeg* 3.32 Philo uses the same terminology to refer (it seems) to the sterility of semen sent into a menstruating woman. That is rather different, however, from attaching sterility to the seed itself.

9. *Soranus' Gynecology,* trans. Owsei Tempkin, with N. J. Eastman, L. Edelstein, and A. F. Guttmacher (Baltimore: Johns Hopkins University Press, 1956), p. 37.

10. Galen, *De usu partium* 14.7 (ed. Helmreich, 2.308) with Galen's own cross-reference to 11.10 (ed. Helmreich, 2.143-44). For a magisterial translation of the treatise, see Margaret Tallmadge May, *Galen: On the Usefulness of the Parts of the Body,* 2 vols. (Ithaca, N.Y.: Cornell University Press, 1968).

11. Galen, *De usu partium* 14.11 (ed. Helmreich, 2.323).

seeks to spread his criticism evenly between the active and passive partner. The passive partner is guilty of fostering effeminacy in himself, whereas the active partner not only pursues an unnatural pleasure that depopulates the earth but also (and more importantly, as Philo himself says) contributes to the feminization of the youth (3.37-39). A special point is made of the social pressure occasioned by the adulation of effeminate young men in the public celebrations honoring the pagan gods (3.40-41).

The crucial point, however, is that here Philo invokes the Levitical language of impurity to flesh out his opposition to pederasty. The treatment of such evils in terms of "pollutions" and "defilements" serves at first to express admiration for the wisdom of Moses in erecting an imposing bulwark against such practices (3.42). The way in which Plato falls back on the category of incest in the *Laws* (as a more or less pedagogical move) seems comparable. There can be no doubt, however, that a sensitivity to the terrors of impurity underlies Philo's discussion of the whole issue. Especially telling here is the fact that he sets up another string of mounting excesses of pleasure that issues this time in the horror of bestiality, and that he refers to Greek mythology (Pasiphaë in particular) in this connection to drive the horror of the practice home (3.43). Philo also has a lengthy discussion of the care that Jewish animal herders exercise to prevent animals of different kinds from mating for fear of "breaking the stricture of nature whose concern it is to preserve the higher kinds from being bastardized" (3.46). Here a link between purity and clear differentiations in the natural world is recognized. Where the borders become blurred, defilement is the result.

The link in Philo between purity concerns and criticism based on traditional philosophical analysis can perhaps now be stated: pleasure madly pursued to its limits dissolves the borders that set apart the pure from the impure. Philo, we could say, experienced the vehemence of undisciplined pleasure as a kind of defilement. Pleasure and impurity, then, represent the leading themes in his criticism of same-sex eros. He does not lose sight of procreativity in this connection, but that concern recedes into the background.

Some of the details in Philo's treatment of the topic suggest that he was also following discussions in the medical literature.

B. Medical Perspectives

At least twice Philo refers to the feminization of young males as "the disease of effeminacy" (*VCon* 60; *Ab* 136). He takes the word "disease" more or less literally, as we shall see.

The main clue here is the statement that the *empyreuma* of the male sex is not allowed to develop when young men submit to same-sex eros (*SLeg* 3.37). The word *empyreuma* refers to a "live coal covered with ashes" that needs to be fanned into flame. It is used metaphorically here for the power of heat that (according to a broad stream of ancient medical theory) characterizes males, as opposed to the power of cold that characterizes females.[12] Such theories were often invoked to explain sexual differentiation, including the phenomenon of same-sex eros. A basic text here is the pseudo-Aristotelian *Problemata* 4.26 (879a36-880a5).[13]

The aim of *Problemata* is to explain why some (adult) males are willing to continue playing the passive role in same-sex eros and why some of these adopt both active and passive roles whereas others adopt only the passive role. The presumed anomaly of such behavior on the part of mature males (as opposed to adolescents) is presented in terms of a physiological abnormality: the ducts that convey sperm "are not in their natural condition," the sperm (some or all, depending on the individual) finds its way to the area of the anus, "the part in which it is collected desires friction," and such individuals seek penetration of the anus to satisfy their desire. But such desire is not easily satisfied since they are "unnaturally constituted" and diffuse their sperm abnormally. "The result is that they suffer from unsatisfied desires, like women; for the moisture is scanty and has not enough force to find its way out and quickly cools" (879b28-30). Here, as in Philo, a male who does not develop naturally sinks back into a more or less undifferentiated state comparable to that of women; and that state is one characterized by the power of cold (linked with insatiability) rather than of heat (linked with the power to satisfy desire). Philo, of course, is speaking of adolescents, and he knows nothing of abnormal ducts; but the role of male heat in both instances is comparable.

Also note that *Problemata,* like Philo, recognizes the role of socialization in producing individuals who pursue same-sex eros. Sometimes, says *Problemata,* this "disease *(pathos)*" is the result of "habit *(ethos)*" (879b). Ad-

12. Maryanne Cline Horowitz, "Aristotle and Women," *Journal of the History of Biology* 9 (1976): 183-213; David L. Balch, "The Gospel versus Greek Biological and Political Theories of Living 'According to Nature' (Rom 1:26-27; 1 Cor 6:9)," in *The Church and Human Sexuality: A Lutheran Perspective* (Chicago: Division for Church in Society, Evangelical Lutheran Church in America), pp. 24-25; Thomas Laqueur, "Orgasm, Generation, and the Politics of Reproductive Biology," *Representations* 14 (1986): 1-41.

13. For a translation see E. S. Forster, *Problemata,* vol. 7 in *The Works of Aristotle,* ed. W. D. Ross (Oxford: Clarendon, 1927). For commentary see Dover, pp. 169-70; Félix Buffière, *Eros adolescent: la pédérastie dans la Grèce antique* (Paris: Société d'edition "les belles lettres," 1980), pp. 438-49.

olescents who submit sexually to adult males often continue such behavior when they mature because of frequent repetition of the act and the pleasure associated with it. In fact, it becomes second nature to them (879b36): habit *(ethos)* functions as nature *(physis)*. The text notes finally that "all this is more likely to occur in the case of one who is both lustful and soft."

Philo goes beyond medical opinion in suggesting that the feminization of males who play the passive role as adolescents is likely to have long-range consequences for all of them. The last line quoted above, however, could be taken as a tacit admission by the author of *Problemata* that almost any such male is at risk, and Philo may be exploiting such a theme. In any event, Philo believes that feminized behavior prevents the natural development of the male heat and leads to the consequent loss of courage in the individual as he matures. The fit between Philo and *Problemata* is not perfect, but there is enough here to indicate the scientific context of Philo's remarks.

We note finally that the discussion in *Problemata* is initiated by the remark that "for every secretion there is a place into which it is naturally voided" (879a36-879b1). This emphasis on the obviousness of the function of the orifices of the body will become increasingly important for our study. An ancient Jewish or Christian critic of *Problemata* could well have asked why this principle did not rule out pederasty as well as the prostitution of an adult male to another male. What Greco-Roman society took for granted in the politics of sex — the right of the adult male to penetrate not only a wife but male and female slaves or a young male favorite — will carry no weight in the new environment.

Somewhat more light can be shed on the medical dimensions of the passage by another ancient text devoted to the problem of same-sex eros. This is a section from a lost work of Soranus (active in the days of Trajan and Hadrian) mediated to us through a translation or paraphrase made by Caelius Aurelianus in the fifth century. The translation or paraphrase is apparently basically reliable. The relevant passage is found in *De morbis chronicis* (hereafter *DMC*) 4.9.131-37 of Caelius Aurelianus. Fortunately this very difficult text has been carefully studied by P. H. Schrijvers, on whom we depend here.[14]

Soranus seems in part to have been correcting the views of *Problemata* which we have just discussed. In particular, he locates the unnatural disease of same-sex eros (by which he means, of course, only those who continue to play the passive role after maturity) not in the body (as does *Problemata*) but in the "mind *(mens)*" (4.131, 132) or "spirit *(animus)*" (4.134). A similar point

14. N. 4 above (see now also Brooten, pp. 146-73). For text and translation I have used I. E. Drabkin, *Caelius Aurelianus: On Acute Diseases and on Chronic Diseases* (Chicago: University of Chicago Press, 1950).

of view seems to be represented in Philo when he speaks of "the disease of effeminacy in their souls" (*VCon* 60) and of "degeneration in their souls" as well as emasculation of the bodies of adolescents (*Ab* 136). The shift allows for the introduction of highly negative moral judgments both in Philo and Soranus. And the language suggests that people could change perverse sexual behavior if only they would.

But what exactly is "a disease of the mind"? Elsewhere Soranus rejects the view of those who regard mania as first a disease of the soul and then of the body, "because no philosopher has set forth a cure for it" (*DMC* 1.154). Soranus's view is that mania is a loss of reason arising from a bodily cause (1.145). In his twin treatise, *De morbis acutis* (hereafter *DMA*), he explicitly raises the question whether "rabies (hydrophobia) is a disease of the soul *(animae)* or of the body" (3.109-11). Again Soranus scoffs at those who regard rabies (because of the element of fear involved) as a disease of the soul. He prefers to compare it to mania and melancholy. In short, Soranus seems to regard a disease of the soul as something rather immediately within our control, that is, as something that can be reasoned away.

It must be noted, however, that there was disagreement about the role of body and mind in various diseases even when the illness seems a deep-rooted one. Similarly there was disagreement about the causes of adult male prostitution. Thus Soranus himself, in his chapter on the pathics, goes on to discuss accounts of the condition that ascribe it either *(a)* to biological factors at the time of birth (*DMC* 4.134-35) or *(b)* to inherited biological weakness (4.135-37). With regard to the first of these possibilities, Soranus harks back to embryological theories of Parmenides. The details are difficult, and we need not pursue them here. Concerning the second possibility, Soranus makes these interesting remarks:

> Many leaders of the medical schools of thought say that the disease is inherited and therefore comes down to posterity with the seed — not indeed thereby condemning nature (who teaches the limits of her purity by means of the other animals, for they have been called her mirror by the wise), but condemning the human race because it held on so strongly to such vices once introduced that they could not be purged by any healing and left no place for renewal, and the fault of the mind became greater, because very many inherited or acquired effects weaken and wane with their bodies — such as gout, epilepsy, madness — and thus without doubt as life declines become milder. (4.135-36)

Typically when Soranus deals with the views of the leaders of different schools of thought, he is cautious or hostile (cf. *DMC* 1.116, 171; 3.11, 97,

137; 4.61, 80, 98; 5.19; *DMA* 1.22, 40, 45, 99; 2.82; 3.25, 171). Here, however, he seems more open than usual to the suggestions made by others. In any event, there clearly were others who regarded the condition of the pathics as a disease more or less deeply rooted biologically and reinforced by bad socialization. What is unclear is whether any of them would also have referred to it as a disease of the soul or mind. That is not impossible, however, if they remembered the treatment of disease near the end of Plato's *Timaeus* (86b-87b). There Plato distinguishes diseases of the mind from diseases of the body, traces the former (all forms of folly such as madness and stupidity and in particular excessive pleasures and pains) to bad upbringing or a defective inherited constitution of the body, and blames society at large rather than individuals (since "no one is willingly bad") without at the same time denying the need to attempt to set things right again.[15] Since Philo stresses the overwhelming power of pleasure in the lives of those men who (like the Sodomites) moved on from the violation of females to that of males and were found to reproduce imperfectly (*Ab* 135), a similar conception of a psychological disorder socially engendered or reinforced and genetically transmitted may be presupposed. The exact scientific implications of Philo's comments can probably not be recovered. What is clear is that he finds the disorder more widely spread than did the medical sources under discussion: both the adolescents who play the passive role and bisexual men who play the active role are included in his condemnation. The special problem of the adult male who continues to play the passive role is no longer the focus of the discussion. Here again, however, Soranus (like *Problemata*) makes a special point at the end of his discussion that could be taken to lead in a direction welcome to a person like Philo. Soranus is trying to explain why older bisexual men often unexpectedly become worse than before in their acceptance of the passive role. The solution is that they have lost the genuine male form of eros (the ability to penetrate) and are left with the passive role. Somewhat similarly, says Soranus, the genuine male form of eros has not yet fully developed in the case of adolescents so that they actually enjoy passive sex with older men. Such an analysis (if a person like Philo knew it) could easily be taken to put all male adolescents at risk.

This suggests that in the world of Philo the models for male and female same-sex eros were converging so that the blanket condemnation normally reserved for same-sex eros among females was being stretched to include all forms of same-sex eros among males. Note that Soranus was soon explicitly to compare women who practice dual sexual roles (passive with men, active

15. Cornford, pp. 343-49.

with women) with (mature) men who play dual sex roles (passive with men, active with women), though not unexpectedly he speaks in both instances only of people who adopt the presumed normal role unenthusiastically and unconsciously overlooks the more restricted range of sexual choices that remains for women (*DMC* 4.132-33). Note also that the power of undisciplined behavior such as drunkenness backed up by "shameful custom," not of physiological abnormalities, serve as the explanatory categories in the case of such women. Similarly, as we have seen, indulgence in drink and food is linked by Philo with the lust of bisexual men (*Ab* 135). It seems possible, then, that a shift of emphasis from physical abnormality to psychological disorder aided the tendency in Jewish and Christian sources of the period to go still further and to deal with all forms of homosexuality as species of the same abnormality. The usual distinctions faded when (with Plato) the avoidance of excessive pleasure became the central concern and when (at the same time) any significant distinction between the nature of adolescent males and mature males was challenged. Adolescent males may seem soft and smooth like women, but medical knowledge could be used to show that the heat associated with their essential sexual nature as males was threatened by their feminization.[16]

A few additional points from Soranus are worth noting to illustrate further the emerging picture: *(a)* animals do not exhibit homosexual behavior (*DMC* 4.136); *(b)* the parts of our body have definite and obvious purposes (4.131), though it is probably Caelius Aurelianus and not Soranus who appeals to "divine Providence" in this connection;[17] and *(c)* insatiety characterizes the disease (4.131). Soranus helps us understand the deep impact that standard themes of this kind had across a wide range of materials.

Finally, Soranus's reference to the embryology of Parmenides to explain the condition of the pathics (4.134-35) reminds us that some ancient medical theorists found a biological basis for conflicted sexuality that could hardly be welcome to Jews like Philo or the early Christians. Exactly what Parmenides had in mind must be left to the specialists.[18] Schrijvers thinks something like it reappears in the church father Lactantius (*De opificio dei* 12). The latter is

16. Philo speaks of "the disease of effeminacy in their souls" (*VCon* 60) and of the "degeneration in their souls" as well as the emasculation of the bodies of adolescent males (*Ab* 136). The presupposition is that males will sink back into the more undifferentiated nature of the female from which maturity normally releases them. As Aristotle had put it, "now a boy is like a woman in form, and the woman is as it were an impotent male . . ." (*De generatione animalium* 1.20, 728a17).

17. Schrijvers, pp. 19-23.

18. Schrijvers, pp. 42-46, 52-62.

trying to explain merely why some men have in themselves "something of the feminine beyond what suits the dignity of a man" (such as prettiness, delicacy, helplessness) and some women, "something of the masculine beyond what the character of the sex allows" (such as strength, dark complexion, hairiness, boldness). So unconscious is he of the issues possibly involved that he takes these things simply as one more proof of the wonders of human nature for which we should praise the Creator.

It is worth pausing, then, to see what others may have made of such phenomena. One classic solution to the problem of sexual differentiation is set out in the Hippocratic treatise *De victu* 1.28-29. Here it is presupposed *(a)* that both the male and the female parent contribute sperm in conception and *(b)* that both male and female sperm contain a male and female element. Further it is presupposed *(c)* that one or the other, the male or the female element, will "predominate" in the union of the two. This opens up a wide range of possibilities when it comes to determining the character of the offspring. Thus the male element in the male may go together with the male element in the female, dominate it, and produce offspring of a certain kind: purely male in this instance. And so on. There is no need to work out all the variations here.

What results is the emergence of *two intersexes* on *each side* of the divide between the *purely male* pole and the *purely female* pole.

Male intersex 1 will lack the full range of male characteristics (brilliance and strength!).

Male intersex 2 will display feminine characteristics to such a degree that we can talk about an "androgyne" (literally, male + female). Some have taken this to mean "hermaphrodite" (as in Plato's *Symposium*). But the context (as we shall see in a moment) favors a less dramatic reference to a highly "effeminate" male.[19]

Similarly, female intersex 1 lacks the full range of feminine characteristics (the purely female is "most feminine and fair"). Members of this intersex are more forward than is expected of women, but are still well behaved.

Female intersex 2 (corresponding to male intersex 2) is called "manly" (members of this intersex do not seem to be hermaphrodites in any real sense). They are "more daring" than the more conventional female intersex 1.

The biology is democratic enough, with male and female elements of apparently equal strength. But the description of the emerging types conforms to what many today would regard as nothing more than socially constructed sexual stereotypes. In any event, such theorizing supported a notion

19. As, for example, in one of our basic texts from Philo (*VCon* 60).

of sexuality as a continuum between two poles whether or not the stronger sense of the term "androgyne" is adopted.

Jews like Philo and the early Christians took for granted the "stereotypes" involved, but rejected the associated notion of sexuality as a continuum.

C. Philo and 1 Corinthians 11:2-15 on Hair

One detail of Philo's description of the unnatural adornments used by adolescents to attract men demands attention: they "plait and tightly bind the hair of their head, for they have thick long hair which is either not cut at all or has only the forelocks cut . . ." (*VCon* 51). Such a remark helps us understand what lies in the background when Paul in 1 Corinthians 11:2-15 argues that nature itself teaches us that a man should have short hair and a woman long hair (11:14-15). I am not suggesting (though some have) that Paul has partly in view the problem of same-sex eros in this text. Instead, the passage helps us understand certain habits of his thought that probably do shed light on how he would have responded to the issue of same-sex eros.

It is necessary, first of all, to correct an apparently widespread view in New Testament scholarship that the term "nature" here simply means "custom." It is true that the word "law *(nomos)*" often refers simply to what is customary. And it is true that the expression "unwritten law" sometimes refers to the law of nature and sometimes to the traditional practices of a community (a dual usage that appears also in Philo).[20] But when writers of the period appeal to nature as a guide, they are referring *(a)* to the biologically and/or culturally determined character of individuals or groups (as we have seen) or *(b)* to what ought to be in the light of the universal order of things (as we have also seen). When an appeal to nature involves moral judgments (as in 1 Cor. 11), it is clear that we are dealing with nature as a normative conception that has in view the universal order of things. It is true, of course, that here Paul's view of nature will seem to us to fall back not on nature but on custom. What this means, however, is that from our point of view Paul mistakes custom for nature, not that he uses the term "nature" in the sense of custom. What can be readily agreed to is that nature in Paul's world plays no overarching role comparable to that found in the Greco-Roman philosophical tradition. But he had apparently read enough in Hellenistic Jewish materials to recognize that the appeal to nature could at times serve to illuminate what he took to be the will of God.

20. Harry Austryn Wolfson, *Philo,* 2 vols. (Cambridge: Harvard University Press, 1947), 2:174, 181.

Why, then, did Paul think that short hair in men and long hair in women expressed the will of nature? The answer is that, in spite of more ancient practices to the contrary, this was the pattern that had imposed itself for the most part in Greco-Roman society.[21] Thus it is taken so much for granted by people like Paul and Philo that they assume it to be natural. A few Stoics like Musonius Rufus realized that if an appeal to nature includes the fact that men's hair grows long if left to itself, then men too ought to let their hair grow long.[22] But this does not occur to the majority. Why not? The answer, I believe, is that in this period (and still today?) women were associated with what is smooth and soft, whereas men were associated with what is rough and hard.[23] Long hair, then, was seen to complement the general smoothness and softness of women, and short hair was seen to complement the general roughness and hardness of men. It can be argued that what was at stake was a male mystique that felt threatened by softness and effeminacy. A selection of comments on hair from ancient sources relevant to the problem of same-sex eros will indicate how important an indicator hair could be in mapping the world of relations between the sexes.

The classic text here is a passage from Epictetus on personal adornment addressed to youths who come to the philosopher with hair and body elaborately cultivated (*Discourses* 3.1). The main problem is the hair on the body that such young men routinely plucked to achieve an attractive smoothness (see also 3.22.10). It is women, says the philosopher, who are "smooth by nature" (3.1.27) whereas men are hairy: "and if [an individual man] is not naturally so, he is a freak" (3.1.28). Epictetus regards it as dreadful that any normal man would try to turn himself into a woman in this way. In response to the retort that women like smooth men,[24] Epictetus asks whether his interlocutor would become a catamite (one of the terms used for men who continued to

21. E. Steininger, "Haartrach und Haarschmuch," in *Paulys Real-Encyclopädie der classischen Altertumswissenschaft,* ed. G. Wissowa and W. Kroll, vol. 7 (Stuttgart: J. V. Metzler, 1912), p. 2112.

22. Musonius (quoting Zeno) allows for clipping strands of hair only when they get in the way of normal activities (O. Hense, *C. Musonii Rufi reliquiae* [Leipzig: B. G. Teubner, 1905], p. 115).

23. According to Pseudo-Lucian (in the defense of heterosexual love), when a boy is about twenty years of age, his limbs become hard, his beard becomes rough instead of soft, and his thighs sprout ugly hairs; whereas a woman has hair like a luxuriant meadow, yet is hairless [*sic*] on the rest of her body (*Amores* 26). The point is that women last longer as attractive sexual objects than men.

24. One of Lucian's female prostitutes similarly favors a smooth and beardless (though nonpaying) customer over a bristly older (though paying) customer (*Dialogue of the Courtesans* 7.2). Her mother is not pleased.

play the passive role in same-sex eros after they had matured) if it turned out that women liked catamites (3.1.32). The exchange indicates that an effeminate lifestyle was not necessarily linked with abnormal same-sex eros (these young men were sexually "normal"), but at the same time that the two phenomena were closely associated in people's minds. A striking image for Epictetus's view of masculine dignity is provided by his statement (found also in Musonius Rufus)[25] that the beard sets the male apart from the female like the lion's mane and the cock's comb (3.1.45; cf. 1.16.9-14).

Epictetus would probably have followed his teacher Musonius Rufus in also forbidding the cutting of head hair beyond what was necessary. But (to complicate matters) Stoics (as opposed to the more flamboyant Cynics) were often associated with "close-cropped" hair (with the head all but shaved) as a mark of austerity.[26] I assume that such Stoics and even men who cut their hair short and shaved their beards would generally share the underlying assumptions of Epictetus about the differences between male and female. Philo, as we have seen, did not hesitate to include long (and elaborately dressed) hair in his catalogue of unnatural adornments used by adolescent boys to attract men (*VCon* 51). Many, then, simply took it for granted that cutting the hair fostered a proper male image. Indeed, in some circles the "close-cropped" (almost shaven) head was the most virile of all. Lucian describes a woman who takes off her wig to show a shaven head like the most manly of athletes as she prepares to play the man's role (with the help of a dildo?) in bed with another woman (*Dialogue of the Courtesans* 5.3). Similarly a male lover is shocked to discover that his beloved, a woman, is not only smooth and soft like a woman but also apparently has had her head shaved. It turns out that she had been ill, had lost her hair, and had covered her head during the day with a wig. She is very concerned that he should not tell anyone about her bald head (12.4)! The significance of the shaved head in a more sober context is suggested by Plutarch in his description of the way women in ancient Sparta were prepared before marriage to meet their husbands (men

25. Hense, p. 114.

26. Lucian presents his typical Stoic as having "close-cropped" hair (*Philosophers for Sale* 20). See Karl Friedrich Hermann, *Lehrbuch der griechischen Pivatalterthümer* (Heidelberg: J. C. B. Mohr, 1852), pp. 109, 112-13; E. Pottier, Maurice Albert, and E. Saglio, "Coma," in *Dictionnaire des antiquités Grecques et Romaines,* ed. Ch. Daremberg and Edm. Saglio, vol. 1, pt. 2 (Paris: Hachette, 1887), p. 1366 (on Marcus Aurelius). Note that in a lengthy discussion of hair, Galen seems unable to decide whether hair on the head belongs to the category of hair *(a)* that is naturally long because it is planted in soft and moist parts of the body or *(b)* that is short because it grows from places with a hard substructure (*De usu partium* 11.14; ed. Helmreich, 2.160-61).

who, it should be remembered, spent most of their time with other men): these women had their heads shaved and were dressed in men's clothing (*Lycurgus* 15.3)!

Paul's somewhat brutal suggestion that women who do not wear a veil, or, to follow more recent interpretations, do not wear their hair properly bound up,[27] should be shorn or shaved (1 Cor. 11:5-7) presupposes the same link between short hair and being a man. And it seems to reflect some of the anxieties that accompany the reaction to hair styles in the materials that we have reviewed. The passage may make more sense, then, if instead of thinking that women in Corinth were letting their long hair hang loose, they had taken to cutting their hair short. Paul, then, would reflect the general view that the close-cropped (almost shaven) head represented the extreme form of the normal short hair worn by men.[28] Is it not easier to take the term "uncovered" in 1 Corinthians 11:5, 13 as a reference to short hair than to unbound long hair? As many commentators have suggested, Paul was probably struggling with practices that had grown in part out of his own teaching that in Christ the polarity of male and female has been overcome (Gal. 3:28). What better way to demonstrate that than by cutting the hair short, as men usually did?[29]

The difficulty with this interpretation, of course, is that Paul clearly distinguishes an "uncovered" woman from one who is shorn or shaved (1 Cor. 11:6). How could he call for a woman with short hair to have her hair cut short (or shaved)? I remain impressed, however, by the fact that the whole discussion comes to a climax in the contrast between women as naturally long haired and men as naturally short haired (11:14-15). Does that not determine the general thrust of the passage? If I am correct in thinking so, the solution may be that these women of Corinth were cutting their hair shorter than usual, that is, short enough to shock but not so short that Paul could not call for further shearing or shaving of them. If that seems artificial (and it does not fit 11:6 as comfortably as I would like), I fear that we must fall back

27. Wolfgang Schrage, *Der erste Brief an die Korinther,* Evangelisch-Katholisches Kommentar zum Neuen Testament 7, 2 vols. (Solothurn und Düsseldorf: Benziger Verlag; Neukirchen-Vluyn: Neukirchener Verlag, 1991, 1995), 2:491-92.

28. Pottier, Albert, and Saglio, p. 1365.

29. In his criticism of unscrupulous spiritual guides, Lucian presents three Cynic philosophers with "close-cropped" hair (atypical for Cynics). With them is the errant wife of a former host of one of the men. She also wears her hair "close-cropped" in the Spartan style (cf. Plutarch, *Lycurgus* 15.3) and appears "male in looks and very masculine" (*Runaways* 27). Here, then, is at least one woman who was making a social statement by the adoption of a male hair style.

on the traditional view that Paul was speaking of women who rejected the veil (however difficult that may be for other reasons). In any event, Paul clearly falls back on conventional notions about hair styles to mark the distinction between the sexes, sharpens that distinction by ascribing it not to custom but to nature, and associates such sexual markers with the subordination of women to the authority of men.

Not all were alarmed by the feminization of men by means of their hair styles. Philostratus, for example, later spoke for many when he advised young men who had entered maturity to shave their beards (letting "art" do what "nature" once did) and let their hair grow long and curly (*Letter* 58). Those who have become rough need not hesitate to restore smoothness by artificial means. Clearly Paul would have disapproved of that attitude long before it had reached any such point. For although his criticism of men who are "soft *(malakoi)*" could cover anything from mere effeminacy to the adoption of the passive role in same-sex eros (1 Cor. 6:9), it is reasonably clear from the statement what his reaction to passivity in same-sex unions would have been even if it was merely effeminacy that was intended. Moreover, the term *malakoi* is surely colored by its association with the (unusual) term *arsenokoitai* (male + bed) that seems to have to do with same-sex eros and, as such, to serve as a general term of condemnation (colored, I think, by notions of impurity).[30] It is also worth noting that the section in *De morbis chronicis* (Soranus) discussed above is entitled *de mollibus sive subactis quos Graeci malthacos vocant,* "concerning soft [= effeminate] or passive men whom the Greeks call *malthakoi* [= effeminate/soft]." *Malthacoi* is a synonym for *malakoi.*[31] Thus the terminology may have been more precisely intended (as many now believe, following a suggestion of Robin Scroggs): Paul may have had in view the passive partner in same-sex eros

30. The verbal form of the term *arsenokoitai* occurs for the first time after Paul (and early Christian literature dependent on Paul) in the Sibylline Oracles (2:73), where it serves as an undeveloped item in a catologue of prohibitions ("do not practice homosexuality"). The passage is probably derived from a Hellenistic Jewish prototype (J. J. Collins, in James H. Charlesworth, ed., *The Old Testament Pseudepigrapha,* vol. 1, *Apocalyptic Literature and Testaments* [Garden City, N.Y.: Doubleday, 1983], p. 330). The term *arsenokoites,* then, probably represents a piece of theological vocabulary invented by Hellenistic Jews. If so, those who follow Robin Scroggs in tracing the term back to a reading of Lev. 18:22, 29, and 20:13 in Hellenistic Jewish circles are probably right. Note that Philo also alludes to these passages in his discussion of same-sex eros and impurity in *SLeg* 3.39. I conclude from this that the term was colored primarily by associations with ancient Hebrew conceptions of defilement (which tended, as we have seen, to wash out the distinctions between active and passive forms of same-sex eros).

31. Schrijvers, pp. 8-9.

when he referred to the *malakoi,* and the active partner when he referred to the *arsenokoitai.* But such a distinction, even if intended, may not have meant all that much to Paul.[32]

III. Echo

A. Clement of Alexandria

In a long section of his *Paedagogus* (hereafter *Paed*), Clement of Alexandria summarizes much of the negative criticism of same-sex eros that we have met, yet adds points that help us orient the discussion as a whole and that throw additional light on the world of Paul (2.10; subsections 83.1–115.5 in Stählin's edition).

Clement has found the relevant quotations from Plato's *Laws* and interspersed them with the relevant Old Testament passages from Leviticus (90.4–91.2). Clement also shows his opposition to pleasure for its own sake and his insistence on procreativity by echoing Philo's rejection (in *SLeg* 3.32-36) of intercourse with a menstruating woman (*Paed* 92.1-2). Other negative comments on same-sex eros discussed by Clement come from Plato's *Phaedrus* (86.2; 89.2), Paul's Romans (86.3), and the (forged) Sibylline Oracles (99.1-2). More unusual are his discussion of the details of the physiology of the womb (to show the uselessness and thus immorality of sex during pregnancy) and a reference to the womb as "thirsting for procreativity" (92.3–93.1). The latter expression echoes a widespread view that goes back to Plato's *Timaeus* (91c). In Plato it is part of the myth that the philosopher tells to account for the emergence of sexual differentiation and of sexual desire as a necessary though lower form of eros. Clement employs the theme in a medically more sober form that at the same time reflects, if not consciously encourages, the widespread view of the subordinate role of women in ancient society.[33]

32. Schrage, 1:431-32. The passages in Leviticus from which the term *arsenokoites* is presumably derived have to do with what the Greeks would call the active partner in same-sex eros. Nevertheless, I believe (as indicated in n. 30) that the term reflects a background in which the distinction between active and passive forms of same-sex eros had eroded.

33. For the theme in its medical context see Giulia Sissa, *Greek Virginity,* trans. Arthur Goldhammer (Cambridge: Harvard University Press, 1990), pp. 44-45, 198.

B. Clement and Barnabas

It is another source discussed by Clement that takes us back nearer to the world of Paul: Barnabas, *Epistle* 10.6-7. This passage is part of an interpretation of the law of Moses that attempts to make sense of it in allegorical terms from a Hellenistic-Jewish-Christian point of view. The law against eating hares (Lev. 11:6 [11:5 LXX]; Deut. 14:7) is taken as directed against the destruction (corruption?) of children (pederasty?) because the hare adds a new anal hole each year to accommodate excessive defecation. And the law against eating hyenas (not actually in the law of Moses) is taken as directed against adultery (and homosexuality) because the hyena changes its sex each year.[34] Clement more or less reverses the interpretation in Barnabas by connecting hares with sexual excess in general and hyenas with homosexuality.

Clement changes the interpretation in the first place because he cannot accept the notion implied by Barnabas that animals change their nature. He is particularly alarmed by the view that hyenas change their sex annually. He knows from Aristotle (*Historia animalium* 8.49, 632b15-25) that some birds change color and voice (*Paed* 84.1). But this, he comments, is a mere affect and does not alter the creature's nature. Clement also depends on Aristotle's proof (*Historia animalium* 6.32, 579b15-29; *De generatione animalium* 3.6, 757a3-13) that hyenas do not actually change their sex annually (*Paed* 85.2–86.1). Similarly, he insists that hyenas are not "hermaphrodites" and rejects the whole notion of "this third androgynous nature between male and female" (85.2). This is a very revealing comment. Gradations between male and female were recognized by many, and the knowledge of the existence of hermaphrodites was widespread. Clement's certainty about the will of nature in sexual matters depends in part on positing clean lines of demarcation. We might say that he echoes in more rationalized terms the rejection in the biblical food laws of anything that blurs the lines between the distinct forms of animal life. Not unexpectedly, then, he sometimes uses the language of impurity when (with reference to sexual contact and Paul's comments on it in 1 Cor. 6:15, 19) he opposes letting "that which is holy to be defiled" (100.1). But he more often speaks more clinically. Thus he names the orifices of the body and describes their proper purposes in clear and restrictive terms (87.1). And when he describes the physiology of the womb, he explicitly comments that there is no need to be embarrassed at mentioning the organs of reproduction

34. For the difficulties in interpretation see Robert A. Kraft, *The Didache and Barnabas,* vol. 3 of *The Apostolic Fathers,* ed. Robert M. Grant (New York: Thomas Nelson & Sons, 1965), pp. 111-12.

which God was not embarrassed to create (92.3).[35] The way in which Clement introduces the theological theme at this point shows, however, that his clinical language and his selection of medical perspectives serve to reinforce his sense of the body as clearly mapped territory. In this he brings to less ambiguous expression what seems to be implied in more popular comments on same-sex eros by his Jewish and Christian predecessors.

C. Barnabas, Aristeas, Paul

A discussion of a third prohibition follows in Barnabas, this time against eating weasels (10.8). The prohibition, we are told, is directed at persons (men and women) who induce sexual orgasm through the mouth since the weasel conceives through its mouth. The closest parallel to that is provided by the Hellenistic Jewish author (Pseudo-)Aristeas, in his famous *Letter* about the Septuagint and the nature of the Jewish religion. The Egyptians who interview the Jewish scholars want to know why distinctions are made in the Bible between animals, "since there is one creation only" (128). The Jews agree that indeed things are "similarly constituted" (143). Consequently, they admonish, "do not fall into the degrading view that Moses enacted this legislation for the sake of mice and weasels or such creatures" (144). Instead Moses had in view various virtues and vices that these creatures symbolize (homosexuality and other sexual sins are mentioned in 152). Weasels are particularly nasty: they conceive through the ear and produce offspring through the mouth (165).[36]

Now it is obvious that Paul knew this kind of interpretation of the law of Moses. In 1 Corinthians 9:9 he quotes Deuteronomy 25:4 ("muzzle not the ox as it threshes") and asks: "surely God is not concerned with oxen?" The striking similarity in argument here between Aristeas ("do not fall into the degrading view that . . .") and Paul ("surely God is not concerned about . . .") and the fact that Paul is making a personal ad hoc application of the method (with reference to the payment of spiritual leaders) indicate that the apostle

35. The Greeks and Romans had a wide range of euphemisms for sex and other natural functions (I. Opelt, "Euphemismus," in *Reallexikon für Antike und Christentum,* vol. 6 [Stuttgart: Anton Hiersemann, 1966], pp. 950-52). Aristotle took it for granted that if the physiology of the body was examined without considering the purposes intended by its various parts, the investigation could not be undertaken "without much disgust" (*De partibus animalium* 1.5, 645a 28).

36. This too had been corrected by Aristotle (*De generatione animalium* 756b8-12; cf. Sissa, pp. 69-70).

breathed the same intellectual atmosphere as Aristeas when thinking about the role of animals in biblical law. There is a very good chance, then, that Paul, like Barnabas, would also have heard and accepted Hellenistic Jewish applications of these laws that defined the proper uses of the orifices of the body. Paul, however, would have been among those Jews whom Philo criticizes for having gone too far, that is, for taking the allegorical interpretation of cultic laws as an excuse for ignoring the actual observance of them (*De migratione Abrahami* 89-93). Indeed, Paul would have understood and appreciated the thrust of the question asked by the Syrians in 4 Maccabees and the Egyptians in Aristeas about how a distinction between foods could be maintained in the face of the belief in God the creator of all things (cf. 1 Cor. 8:4-6: "concerning food offered to idols . . . we know . . . that there is but one God"). Paul's conception of sacrifice as "rational (spiritual) service" (Rom. 12:1) and of circumcision as a "circumcision of the heart" (Rom. 2:29) would very likely have been joined by a longer list of allegorical reinterpretations of cultic law.

IV. Paul, Romans, 1 Corinthians

We have assumed throughout this paper the traditional view that Paul attacks same-sex eros in Romans 1:18-32. Arguments to the contrary have, I believe, been sufficiently answered.[37] Note that Paul's reference here to the "use" of a man or woman employs a euphemism for sexual contact common in the period.[38] One interesting parallel even speaks of the normal "eros of women and men" as a love that "uses nature" (Plutarch, *Dialogue on Love* 5, 751c). Paul's reference to a "natural use" as opposed to a use that is "against nature" (Rom. 1:26-27) reflects some such line of thought. If we are right in thinking that Philo illuminates the associations that such language would have had for Paul, the apostle would very likely have connected unnatural sexual "use" with the biblical notion of impurity. Philo, in fact, uses the verb "to use" in the sexual sense when he describes the horrors of intercourse with animals that in his view crown the defilement of same-sex eros (*SLeg* 3.50).

The suggestion that Paul is speaking only of same-sex acts performed by those who are by nature heterosexual is a possibility that finds some support in at least one of the passages from Philo dealt with above (cf. *Ab* 135). But such a

37. Richard B. Hays, "Relations Natural and Unnatural: A Response to John Boswell's Exegesis of Romans 1," *Journal of Religious Ethics* 14 (1986): 184-215.

38. Opelt, p. 951.

phenomenon does not excuse some other form of same-sex eros in the mind of a person like Philo. Moreover, we would expect Paul to make that form of the argument more explicit if he intended it, and we would want to see how it fit into the purpose of this section of his letter. Paul's wholesale attack on Greco-Roman culture makes better sense if, like Josephus and Philo, he lumps all forms of same-sex eros together as a mark of Gentile decadence.

Philo's discussion of same-sex eros also helps us understand the significance of Paul's emphasis on same-sex eros as a result of "degrading passions" (Rom. 1:26-27). Precisely the mad quest for pleasure (according to Philo) leads to behavior that breaks all the boundaries and leads to impure forms of intercourse. There can be no sharp distinction here between *(a)* the unnatural as the excess "use" of natural impulses and *(b)* the unnatural as an affront to the apparent purposes of the parts of the created order. The distinction was recognized, as we have seen. But people like Philo and the Greco-Roman philosophers on which he depended did their best to minimize it. And the euphemistic use of the term "use" should not tempt us to think that Paul was focusing only on what is unnatural as an excess use of natural impulses.

That Paul resorts here to a theme standard in the literature of the period and that he speaks of things "according to nature" and "contrary to nature" as fully normative concepts gains some support not only from 1 Corinthians 11:14 (as we have interpreted it above) but also from Romans 2:11-16, where (as some see it) the written law of Moses is compared with "the unwritten law" in the sense of the natural law in its fully normative sense.[39] The use of the expressions "according to nature" and "contrary to nature" in Romans 11:24, where they have to do with branches naturally growing on trees (= Jews) as opposed to branches grafted into trees (= Gentile believers), does not change the picture in the earlier part of the letter. The usage in Romans 11:24 is analogous to the distinction made between what is "by nature *(physei)*" and what is "by determination *(thesei)*" when applied to the place of a person in the family or the city, that is, whether one has been born into it or has been adopted into it.[40] In such situations no moral judgment is being passed on adoption, though the priority of nature over invention is presupposed. The point, however, is that such a usage runs along lines that are independent of the appeal to nature as a normative concept. The one cannot be

39. Ulrich Wilckens, *Der Brief an die Römer,* Evangelisch-Katholischer Kommentar zum Neuen Testament 6, 3 vols. (Cologne: Benziger; Neukirchen-Vluyn: Neukirchener Verlag, 1978, 1980, 1982), 1:133-34.

40. LSJ, s.v. *thesis,* III.

used to interpret the other except at a level deeper than that which is relevant in the contexts that we have before us.

How visceral Paul's reaction to same-sex eros may have been can, I believe, be determined by how he deals with certain sexual issues in his first letter to the Corinthians. Paul's arguments in this letter revolve fundamentally around the poles of "knowledge" and "love." The claims of *gnosis* are downplayed and the claims of *agape* are highlighted. Yet the claims of knowledge are not completely disallowed, and the guidance provided by love quietly yields place at important points to the fear of impurity. The use of the language of impurity also in Romans 1:24 with reference to same-sex eros provides a link between the two discussions.[41]

Paul's complex development of these themes in 1 Corinthians is associated especially with his treatment of the problem of meat offered to idols (1 Cor. 8–10) and his discussion of sexual issues (especially 1 Cor. 6:12-20). These two bodies of material are connected by his quotation in both sections of slogans used by opponents whom he calls "the strong" and by a certain preoccupation with food in both sections.

We begin with the problem of meat offered to idols. The strong have knowledge (8:1) and argue that monotheism destroys the fear of cultic contamination from eating such meat (8:4). They are confident, then, that "all things are permitted" (10:23). Paul allows the truth of such statements up to a point. He himself had, it appears, taught them that circumcision is nothing and uncircumcision nothing (cf. 7:19), and almost surely had gone on from there to argue against the literal observance of the biblical food laws. Like the Syrians in 4 Maccabees and the Egyptians in Aristeas, Paul is able to de-mystify such matters by appealing to the lordship of God the creator of all things. The strong, I suggest, had picked up such points and sharpened them. Whether they did so under the influence of an incipient Gnosticism[42] or under the impact of popular culture[43] (particularly the popular teaching of the

41. I assume that Paul's use of the language of impurity has been to some extent rationalized and ethicized. I also assume, however, that what once made it potent still hovers in the background (cf. Paul Ricoeur, *The Symbolism of Evil* [Boston: Beacon Press, 1969], pp. 29-40, 70-99). For an exaggerated, though interesting and suggestive, account of the role of purity language in 1 Corinthians, see Dale B. Martin, *The Corinthian Body* (New Haven and London: Yale University Press, 1995). For an implausible, though also challenging, effort to rid Paul of any serious commitment to purity language, see L. William Countryman, *Dirt, Greed, and Sex: Sexual Ethics in the New Testament and Their Implications for Today* (Philadelphia: Fortress, 1988), pp. 97-123, 190-220.

42. See Schrage, 2:216-21.

43. Martin, pp. 66, 71-72.

Cynics and Stoics) is debated. The latter seems to me more likely, and that judgment admittedly favors the approach taken here. But I do not think that too much one way or the other depends on it.

Although Paul sometimes seems to admit the claims of such knowledge with considerable enthusiasm (especially in 10:23–11:1), he is basically concerned to convince the strong to give up the sense of superiority that their knowledge fosters and to let love determine a retreat from flaunting their freedom. But there is another element in the argument. At some point and for some reason that is difficult to determine, Paul flatly forbids the strong to eat meat offered to idols (10:1-22). We cannot resolve the apparent contradiction here. The point is to recognize that suddenly the fear of cultic contamination plays a decisive role (10:14-22). Paul de-mystifies only up to a point.

Similarly Paul admits that "all things are permitted" in the sexual sphere only up to a point (6:12). Indeed, he seeks to show that in this sphere some (the strong?) have totally misapplied freedom. The argument has been made that sex is like food: both represent bodily needs that require satisfaction (6:13). Such a link between food and sex plays a role particularly in the Cynic sphere.[44] The point was to satisfy such needs in order to move on to the more important task of shaping one's life as a wise man marked by virtue and intelligence. Paul does not seem to know quite what to do with the argument. But it is hard to escape the conclusion that, especially with his talk of the body as a "temple of the Holy Spirit within you" (6:19 NRSV), he is falling back on the language of impurity to oppose it. Sex, then, is *not* like food because illicit sex pollutes in a way that food does not. At the same time, Paul is stumbling toward something else as well. The language of holiness has been transformed here at least to the extent that it is no longer a matter of mysterious powers associated with bodily effluences like menstrual blood or semen. There is some justification in the claim that in this passage Paul has discovered that human beings do not *have* a body but *are* body.[45] Yet clearly the image of the temple indicates that this (new) sense of the body as a psychosomatic unity owes something to (archaic) notions of purity and impurity.

If this passage is taken to throw light on what Paul's reaction to same-sex eros would have been, we must ask to what extent ideas of purity and impurity played a role in the evaluations of same-sex eros. We have found traces

44. A somewhat extreme example is provided by a well-known story about Diogenes the Cynic: while masturbating in public he told people that "he wished it were as easy to relieve hunger by rubbing the belly" (Diogenes Laertius, 6.46). In another story about Diogenes, his eating in public and masturbating in public are dealt with as comparable issues (6.69).

45. Schrage, 2:22.

of such a connection as far back as Plato with his comparison in the *Laws* between pederasty and incest. But it is in the classic attack on same-sex eros of the fourth century B.C.E., Aeschines' *Against Timarchus,* that we find the most striking evidence. Here the male prostitute (a male who continues to play the passive role beyond adolescence) is forbidden to serve as archon or as priest. That is forbidden because the male prostitute is "not pure in body" (19; 188). Indeed, the law quoted by Aeschines states that he is "not even to walk within the parts of the market place sprinkled with lustral water" (21). Thus complaints of illegality, shamefulness, and immorality against the male prostitute are reinforced by the charge of cultic impurity. The parallel is all the more striking because the speech contains a string of passages in which the male prostitute's evil is described as a matter of "sinning against his own body" (22; 39; 94; 107; 159). Similarly the man in 1 Corinthians 6:18 who visits (female) prostitutes is said to "sin against his own body." Aeschines once uses this expression to describe the male prostitute who not only violates the wives of others but goes on to violate his own body (107). The complaint made by Philo against the bisexual man who not only violates his neighbor's wife but goes on to "mount males without respect for the common (sexual) nature which the active partner shares with the passive" (*Ab* 135) seems comparable. Against such a background, Paul's comments on heterosexual contact with prostitutes surely suggest what his reaction to same-sex eros would have been.

Conclusion

The emergence of the view of the body as clearly mapped territory reflects concerns that *(a)* impinge on it from the social and political sphere (the need for reproduction and the importance of discipline and order) and *(b)* are shaped by deeper cultural and religious impulses (the "male mystique" of antiquity and the primordial fear of impurity). In evaluating it in the light of later experience, it should be noted that the biological views that lurk in the background of the discussion are not only out of date by contemporary standards, but also that in Hellenistic Judaism and early Christianity points were selected from the scientific and medical tradition in such a way that a sense of the indeterminateness of the sexual impulses was almost totally lost. It is also important to remain aware of the teleological thinking that lurks in the background and to recognize it for what it is: a mode of thought at home in Greco-Roman science and philosophy but of secondary interest in a tradition that speaks of God addressing his creatures as an "I" addresses a "thou." In such a tradition, of course, God may be thought of simply as arbitrarily insisting on his will; but he may also be thought of as creating new covenants with his people. Paul's rejection of the purity rules as they affect food suggests that his insights in this regard could profitably be pushed further in the sphere of sexuality. It is surely not unimaginable that a God who seeks the outcast would call those to him whose sexual orientation sets them apart from the majority. Paul's discovery that a human being does not have a body but is body also points us in a useful direction: our sexuality is not some sort of addendum that can be easily set to one side.

At the same time, we need to recognize that the Jewish and early Christian rejection of same-sex eros was but one aspect of a new conception of the family. The male could not now express his authority by penetrating at will not only a wife but also his male and female slaves or a young male favorite. Sexual politics were undergoing a deep sea-change. And a good deal can still be said in favor of the new model of the family that was emerging. At the same time, we have seen that the new model tended to ignore aspects of the physiological and psychological realities of sexuality. Today, then, an accommodation is in order. Ironically, many defenders of what has now become the traditional family do not see that the call of gay couples for status as families is in fact a recognition of the basic strength of the traditional model. Surely that call should be welcomed.

CHAPTER 3

The Use, Misuse, and Abuse of Science in the Ecclesiastical Homosexuality Debates[1]

STANTON L. JONES AND MARK A. YARHOUSE

The Christian church has historically looked upon homosexual acts as intrinsically immoral.[2] The relational context, intentions behind, or consequences of these acts have not affected the fundamental moral evaluation — for instance, if those acts occurred in a loving, monogamous relationship or in an impersonal or promiscuous context. Such acts were deemed immoral by their very nature.

The American Christian church today, especially the mainline denominations, finds itself embroiled in a heated debate surrounding the morality of homosexuality and homosexual behavior. In the heat of this debate, both traditionalists and proponents for change from the historic or traditional position of the church are turning to the behavioral sciences in the hope that findings from this source will shape the discussion or inform our moral reasonings.

1. The middle section of this chapter appears, in somewhat expanded form, as S. Jones and M. Yarhouse, "Science and the Ecclesiastical Homosexuality Debates," *Christian Scholar's Review* 26 (1997): 446-77. Readers desiring full citations of all important studies should refer to that document.

2. W. S. Stafford, "Sexual Norms in the Medieval Church," and J. W. Trigg, "Human Sexuality and the Fathers of the Church," both in *A Wholesome Example: Sexual Morality and the Episcopal Church,* ed. R. W. Prichard (Alexandria, Va.: Charter Printing, 1992); General Synod of the Church of England, *Issues in Human Sexuality: A Statement by the House of Bishops of the General Synod of the Church of England* (Harrisburg, Pa.: Morehouse, 1991).

The purposes of this article are threefold: we will (1) draw upon mainline denominational documents to examine the purposes to which proponents of change from the traditional standard seem to be putting the findings and theories of the behavioral and physical sciences; (2) briefly summarize the status of the major scientific findings which are available to date; and (3) briefly examine the formal relevance of contemporary scientific research to the moral debate, especially to the traditional moral stance. We hope to demonstrate that: (1) the purposes to which the supposed "scientific findings" are pressed by proponents of change in the ethical debate are of questionable legitimacy; (2) the actual scientific findings in this area are more complex and puzzling than is usually acknowledged (and implicitly that they are often selectively reported or misinterpreted in their popular use); and (3) when properly interpreted, the scientific findings to date, and indeed the strongest possible findings that can be imagined by extrapolating from current findings, neither entail nor logically support the types of ethical conclusions which are being drawn from those findings. Parenthetically, we would suggest that though our survey in this paper is largely limited to the literature of proponents of change from the traditional view, the use of "scientific findings" by traditionalist authors is generally equally questionable; this manuscript is by no means an apologetic for the use of science by conservatives.

Purposes for Which Scientific Findings and Theories Are Used

The casual and imprecise way in which scientific findings are often brought into the debates about homosexuality, the frequent failure to cite specific studies, and the frequent failure of authors to describe explicitly the bearings of the findings upon the moral argument in question — each poses challenges to the clear explication of the use being made of such citations. Rarely are specific findings cited with a clear statement that a particular ethical position is thereby validated or obviated. Instead, vague and imprecise statements of "science has found X" are quickly followed by declarations that "and therefore it must be true that Y." The literature advocating change from the church's traditional stand, as we will attempt to show in what follows, seems to draw upon the findings of the behavioral sciences for at least two main reasons: (1) to undermine the assumptions that seem to be behind the traditional moral judgment that the church has pressed, and thus undermine the traditional view itself; and (2) to support the removal of homosexual acts as such from the category of acts that can be judged as immoral in and of themselves.

Undermining Traditional Assumptions

Behavioral science findings often are interjected into the moral debate surrounding homosexuality not to formally support any particular view, but rather in an attempt to undermine the traditionalist's view, or more specifically, to undermine the supposed assumptions behind the traditional Christian condemnation of homosexual behavior. Proponents for the moral acceptability of homosexual relations sometimes exaggerate the traditionalist's position for the purposes of presenting a caricature of the traditional Christian view of morality so that the exaggeration itself can be rejected with the apparent support of scientific data.

One such caricature of the traditional Christian condemnation of homosexual behavior is the charge that traditionalists view all experiences and expressions of homosexual orientation as deliberate and willful. For example, the leader's manual for a recent Episcopal "sexuality dialogue" process distinguished four positions on the morality of homosexuality. The first position was a caricature of the traditional view of the nature and moral status of homosexual acts: "All homosexual acts are sin, first, because they violate the strictures of Scripture and, second, because they are a willful perversion of the natural order."[3] The phrase "willful perversion" is important because it brings into the debate issues of isolated acts versus proclivities or orientations, willful choice versus involuntary conditions and acts, and normalcy versus perversity. According to this account of the traditionalist position, its focus is on specific acts, each of which is willfully chosen. An "orientation" becomes nothing more than a descriptive phrase to define persons who have certain patterns of willfully choosing perverse acts that summatively constitute their homosexuality. If this part of the caricature is accepted, if the traditionalist view of sin is conceived as a willful violation of moral law and as motivated by rebellion as opposed to other concerns, then the concept of "orientation" may be a persuasive, even devastating, rebuttal when a debate arises on whether or not homosexuals choose their sexual identity. All that proponents of gay-affirming morality have to do to demolish this caricature, and to succeed in refuting the traditionalist's view, is to

3. Committee on the Study of Human Sexuality for Province VII of the Episcopal Church, *Human Sexuality: A Christian Perspective: A Study Course and Leader's Guide Prepared for Province VII* (1992), p. 63.

produce evidence from the behavioral sciences of a more robust concept of orientation as an enduring pattern of preferred erotic objects (thus obliterating the naive focus upon acts), and of predisposing influences on behavior (thus obliterating the idea that the behavior is willful).

For example, a Lutheran working draft pointed out that "many Christians have questioned the Church's traditional teaching. They have argued that gay and lesbian persons are 'by nature' attracted to persons of the same gender." Implicitly relying upon current scientific knowledge, the authors went on to argue that "Scripture passages address only homosexual behavior and . . . not . . . the concept of 'sexual orientation.'"[4] The assumption, of course, is that if there is a large body of scientific data implicating biological or genetic factors predisposing one to homosexual proclivities, traditional condemnation of homosexual behavior will be dismissed as irrelevant or antiquated. In other words, the larger the body of scientific data on biological or genetic factors predisposing one to homosexual proclivities, the worse off will be the traditional condemnation of homosexual behavior.

If "willful" is an important word, then so too is "perversion," a word that at once brings into the debate the issue of what is "natural" or "normal." The prevalence of homosexuality or homosexual behavior is implicitly presented as relevant to determining what is natural or normal, in that "perversions" are assumed by their very nature to be statistically unusual, and one would be on risky (not to mention judgmental) ground to call what a substantial percentage of people do a "perversion." In a Presbyterian report on human sexuality, ten "myths" are listed which need to be dispelled. The first is that "Gays and lesbians constitute only a small segment of the general population and are an urban phenomenon," to which the report replies: "Research from several sectors indicates that at least 10 percent of the American population or approximately 22 million persons are predominantly gay or lesbian."[5] Even more pointedly, Episcopal bishop John Spong recently stated: "If the best scientific data seems to put the figure of gay and lesbian people in the world at about 10% of the population . . . then you and I need to realize that 10% is such a large percentage that it could hardly be accidental."[6] In other

4. Evangelical Lutheran Church in America, *Human Sexuality Working Draft: A Possible Social Statement of the Evangelical Lutheran Church in America* (Chicago: The Division for Church and Society of the Evangelical Lutheran Church in America, 1994), p. 21.

5. Presbyterian Church in the United States of America, *Keeping Body and Soul Together: Sexuality, Spirituality, and Social Justice,* Reports to the 203rd General Assembly, Part I (Louisville, Ky.: Stated Clerk of the General Assembly, 1991), p. 49.

6. J. S. Spong and J. Howe, audiotaped debate at the Virginia Protestant Episcopal Seminary (February 1992), Truro Tape Ministries, 10520 Main St., Fairfax, VA 22030.

words, data on prevalence is seen as directly relevant to the moral debate if the conservative view claims that homosexuality is extremely rare and consequently unnatural and immoral. If the traditional account can be faithfully represented as saying that homosexuality is immoral *because* it is a perversion, and if perversions by their nature are unusual or rare, then proponents of moral acceptance of homosexual relations can substantially weaken the perceived validity of the traditionalist argument by citing reports of higher statistical frequency.

Proponents also assume that the status of homosexuality as a pathology is relevant to the credibility of the traditionalist's moral argument. In 1974 the American Psychiatric Association (APA) removed homosexuality as a pathological psychiatric condition from its authoritative *Diagnostic and Statistical Manual.* Some believe that the traditional account claims that both homosexuality and homosexual behavior are immoral because they are pathological, and thus the status of homosexuality as a mental disorder becomes relevant to the moral debate. In a section of a report from the Methodist church, the issue of pathology is framed in a way which conflates moral status, etiology, and status as a pathology: "If it is possible to determine that homosexual orientation is caused exclusively by physical factors, such as the genetic makeup, then this might suggest that homosexuality is neither sin nor a sickness." Further, "If it could be shown that homosexuality is generally a symptom of unmet emotional needs or difficulties in social adjustment, then this might point to problems in relating to God and other persons. But if that cannot generally be shown, homosexuality may be compatible with life in grace."[7] The parameters for the argument are set: because traditionalists are caricatured as saying that homosexual behavior is immoral because homosexuality is a pathology, appeals to the status of homosexuality as nonpathological according to the APA's diagnostic manual will make the traditionalist's position appear invalid.

Finally, the possibility of change from homosexual to heterosexual orientation is often a part of the caricature of the traditionalist's position. The Episcopal leader's manual cited earlier portrays traditionalists as believing that "The orientation of all homosexual persons can be modified to conform to the heterosexual norm through conversion and healing."[8] To the degree this is truly a core assertion, the effectiveness of "conversion" therapies be-

7. United Methodist Church, *Report of the Committee to Study Homosexuality to the General Council on Ministries of the United Methodist Church* (Dayton, Ohio: General Council on Ministries, 1991), p. 13.

8. Province VII of the Episcopal Church, p. 63.

comes relevant to the moral debate. If the behavioral sciences can show that sexual orientation is in fact immutable, or that change is at least tremendously difficult for the majority, then the traditionalist position appears untenable.

To review, the behavioral sciences are being used in the debate on homosexual morality to refute a caricature of the traditionalist's position. The caricature includes issues such as isolated acts versus orientation, willful choice versus biological determinism, normalcy versus perversity, and the mutability versus immutability of sexual orientation. If the credibility and indeed the rationality of the traditionalist's position can be called into question by allusion to the findings of science, this would seem by implication to lend credence to the conclusion that there is no well-founded justification for regarding homosexual acts in any way other than as morally neutral in themselves. These arguments seem mistaken both in the claims that are made about "what science says" and in terms of the inaccuracy of the caricatures presented of the traditionalist view.

Homosexual Acts as Morally Indeterminate Events

The behavioral and physical sciences are also brought into the current moral debate to give implicit support to the view that homosexual acts are morally neutral, in the sense that they are not members of the class of acts that can be properly judged immoral in and of themselves. Most agree that many acts are intrinsically neutral and thus best judged as moral under certain conditions and immoral under others, and not as unequivocally immoral by their nature. For example, one might judge marital penile-vaginal intercourse to be moral in a consensual, loving, committed marital relationship but immoral in an abusive marriage where a husband physically coerces his wife into submitting to sex. The behavioral sciences are often used in an attempt to support moving homosexual acts from that class of acts that can be properly judged as immoral in and of themselves to that class of acts whose moral qualities are constituted by the personal qualities that characterize those acts and the by-products of the acts. There may be merit to such a consequentialist ethic, but importing it into the discussion via the findings of science is another matter.

Proponents for the morality of homosexual behavior sometimes attempt to tie homosexual orientation and its expression in behavior closer to the essential core of the identity of the person, and thereby make a case that homosexual behavior is itself morally neutral. A link between the etiology of homosexuality as a sexual orientation and the morality of homosexual behavior is presumed in this argument, and supposed scientific findings are a primary vehicle for making this connection of homosexual behavior to core identity.

There are two fundamental viewpoints in the contemporary debate about what "homosexuality" is: essentialist and social constructionist.[9] Essentialists argue that the term "homosexual" is a proper qualifier for a person's inner core nature or self, and that sexual orientation is intimately intertwined with one's true identity as a human being: "The category *homosexual* describes an aspect of the person that corresponds to some objective core or inner essence of the person."[10] We might say that the essentialist argues that "homosexual" is a real and critically important descriptor of a person in some manner parallel to that individual being a "female" or a "human being" (which are assumed to be real, enduring, and somewhat transcendent categorizations). This is perhaps the position taken by most proponents of gay-affirming moral systems, who would argue that expression of that identity is essential to human wholeness. The debate concerning the essentialist construct of "homosexuality" is important to defenders of gay-affirming morality because it is believed that if proponents can produce evidence that homosexual behavior is a manifestation of some inner essence, is relatively stable over time, and is characteristic of a distinct segment of the population, then the appropriateness of moral judgment is called into question. Social constructionists, on the other hand, suggest that although the existence of same-gender sexual behaviors, attractions, and so forth cannot be disputed, our intellectual construction of two categories of people on the basis of behaviors and attractions (heterosexual and homosexual) is a historical and cultural artifact which is nonenduring. The ancient tendency to categorize sexual actors more by who penetrates and who was penetrated than by gender is often used as an example of this.[11] Most social constructionists are, nevertheless, broadly sup-

9. E. O. Laumann, J. H. Gagnon, R. T. Michael, and S. Michaels, *The Social Organization of Sexuality* (Chicago: University of Chicago Press, 1994); B. Risman and P. Schwartz, "Sociological Research on Male and Female Homosexuality," *Annual Review of Sociology* 14 (1988): 125-47. For a discussion of the relationship between extrapolations from an essentialist view of sexual orientation and a materialist anthropology, see M. A. Yarhouse and S. L. Jones, "A Critique of Materialist Assumptions in Interpretations of Research on Homosexuality," *Christian Scholar's Review* 26 (1997): 478-95.

10. Laumann et al., p. 285.

11. In the constructionist view, our modern tendency to take the concept of homosexuality as an identity ("I am gay") is a peculiarity of our culture and not universally true. In support of this position, note that homosexual behavior occurs to some extent in all

portive of modification in our moral and civil responses toward homosexuality, in that our moral and civil codes are viewed as every bit a social construction as are our views of sexual orientation. Some have characterized the essentialist view as by far the more widespread one at a popular level and the one most likely to be operative as a background assumption in contemporary moral debate about "homosexuality," even though the constructionist view is the more likely background assumption of the scientist doing research on this family of phenomena.[12] Neither the essentialist nor the constructionist view is intrinsically more supportive of a traditional sexual ethic.

The committee majority in a Presbyterian report argued in a way that relied upon essentialist presuppositions when it framed the issue of sexual and spiritual wholeness. In response to moralities calling for persons to refrain from homosexual behavior, the committee said that "the church requires that gays and lesbians deny, rather than affirm, their God-given sexuality . . . they are expected not to 'practice' their sexuality, or in other words, to refrain from experiencing the deep love and intimacy made possible by God in our creation." Homosexuality, a particular manifestation of sexuality, is viewed as essential to one's core identity; in this case it is intertwined with one's need for sexual self-actualization. By intimately tying sexuality or sexual identity to one's experience of God, homosexual behavior becomes a prerequisite to self-actualization in one's encounter with God: "A genuinely incarnational, gracious theology affirms that our sexuality is integral to our relationship with God and others. Sexual wholeness is deeply connected to spiritual wholeness. When we affirm that gays and lesbians are part of God's

---

known human cultures, but the form it takes varies from culture to culture. Carrier has summarized many cross-cultural studies by saying that "homosexual behavior seems to occur for two main reasons: lack of available other-sex partners or as part of a culturally defined ritual. Neither of these causes can be invoked for understanding homosexual orientation in our society. Although homosexual behavior seems to exist in all societies, the concept of homosexual orientation as a lifelong and stable pattern does not, and is in fact rare in preindustrial societies"; J. Carrier, "Homosexual Behavior in Cross-Cultural Perspective," in *Homosexual Behavior: A Modern Reappraisal,* ed. J. Marmor (New York: Basic Books, 1980), pp. 100-122, quote p. 118. It seems clear that the view of homosexual behavior embraced by a society shapes subsequent behavior. The decisions of the church on this matter are important, as ecclesiastical decisions contribute to shaping culture. Greenberg's massive study is the landmark work of this constructionist approach; the interested reader should see Browning for a readable review of Greenberg's work with implications for the church; D. Greenberg, *The Construction of Homosexuality* (Chicago: University of Chicago Press, 1988); D. Browning, "Rethinking Homosexuality," *Christian Century,* 11 October 1989, pp. 911-16.

12. Laumann et al., *Social Organization of Sexuality.*

good creation and that they, like heterosexuals, deserve to enjoy God's good gifts of intimate sexual relationships, then we experience in new ways what it means to be faithful disciples of Jesus Christ."[13] The committee further asserts that homosexuality finds its place under the larger rubric of sexuality, which, it is argued, is fundamental to spiritual and psychological self-actualization. Sexuality is no longer primarily for uniting in marriage, but rather is a way of self-discovery or maturity. The form of sexual expression no longer matters; what is important is one's sexual self-actualization, which is an extension of the essentialist's fundamental presuppositions. Acts are neutral; it is the ends they accomplish that are to be evaluated morally.

All of these arguments have as their point of convergence the etiology of homosexuality — specifically, the question of a "willful" experience of homosexuality versus a "determined" experience of homosexuality. With the help of the behavioral sciences, this convergence points, it seems, toward the assertion that homosexual acts can no longer legitimately be deemed intrinsically immoral; rather, homosexual acts must be viewed as morally neutral in and of themselves. For example, some have argued implicitly that demonstration of nonvolitional etiology obviates moral condemnation of a behavior pattern: "Expert opinion is largely agreed . . . that a sexual orientation is not, in the vast majority of cases, voluntary in the sense of a self-conscious choice. . . . If it is granted that a homosexual orientation is involuntary . . . it is unjust to present celibacy as a calling."[14] Similarly, in an edited volume promoting ecclesiastical dialogue, another author argued that scientific findings regarding etiology validate an incipient essentialism which in turn invalidates classic injunctions to embrace celibacy: "some churches, in the face of psychological evidence that sexual orientation is not freely chosen, have begun to distinguish between homosexual orientation — which they agree, is not morally culpable — and homosexual activity, which is always morally wrong insofar as it is freely chosen. This compromise is intrinsically unstable. . . . Only a sadistic God would create hundreds of thousands of humans to be inherently homosexual and then deny them the right to sexual intimacy."[15]

Further, consider the way in which Sedgwick brings the behavioral sciences into his discussion of sexual morality: "Studies from the natural sciences suggest that homosexuality is an outcome of both biological and social

13. Presbyterian Church (cited n. 5), p. 54.

14. Protestant Episcopal Church, Standing Commission on Human Affairs, *Blue Book* of the Episcopal Church General Convention (1991), pp. 199, 202.

15. J. J. McNeill, "Homosexuality: Challenging the Church to Grow," in *Homosexuality in the Church,* ed. Jeffrey S. Siker (Louisville: Westminster/John Knox, 1994), pp. 49-60, quote p. 53.

factors. Homosexuality is not simply a matter of arrested development but a variable form of sexual identity in animals and human beings. Homosexual relations would then be moral as those relationships realize or embody the broader values of pleasure, mutuality, and generativity in their interrelationship."[16] Sedgwick suggests, on the basis of "studies" from the "sciences," that homosexual acts are generally not in a class of acts that can be properly judged immoral in and of themselves. He claims he can shift the moral focus off the acts themselves because of what the behavioral sciences have to say about causation, and about homosexuality not being the result of "arrested development" but rather as intrinsic to "sexual identity."

Traditionalists and proponents of change often make interestingly similar arguments which make use of empirical findings. For example, a Methodist committee argues that "If it could be shown that homosexual persons are not more likely than heterosexual persons to have emotional problems, to be self-centered, to be promiscuous, to be exploitative of sexual partners and others, to be less creative contributors to the good of the community, then this may help reassure us that such flaws are not caused by homosexuality. If homosexual persons are found more likely than heterosexual persons to manifest such problems, then a deeper search for the connecting links may be called for."[17] They suggest, in other words, that acts themselves cannot be evaluated morally, but rather the state of wholeness or disorder from which they proceed. After a selective review of the evidence on this question, the majority of the committee concludes that homosexual and heterosexual subpopulations do not differ in the base rate occurrence of "such problems" and asserts that the "present state of knowledge and insight in the biblical, theological, ethical, biological, psychological and sociological fields does not provide a satisfactory basis upon which the church can responsibly maintain the condemnation of all homosexual practice."[18] This approach presumes the moral neutrality of same-gender sexual behavior and searches for empirical evidences related to the ancillary qualities which would aid moral evaluation of homosexual practice generally in a manner akin to that proposed by Sedgwick. The committee states that many studies show that homosexuals experience no significant "emotional problems" and no greater rates of promiscuity (both of which are, in fact, contrary to the research data) and are no less con-

16. T. Sedgwick, "Christian Ethics and Human Sexuality: Mapping the Conversation," in *Continuing the Dialogues: Sexuality: A Divine Gift* (New York: Task Force on Human Sexuality, Education for Mission and Ministry Unit, The Episcopal Church, 1988), pp. 1-14, quote p. 11.

17. United Methodist Church (cited n. 7), p. 13.

18. United Methodist Church, p. 28.

tributors to society, and thus that moral condemnation of homosexual behavior is inexcusable. The committee relies upon criteria that the behavioral sciences might in fact purport to measure (thus utilizing the prominence of the scientific community) to reach the conclusion that homosexual behavior is morally neutral.

Conservatives have been known to argue similarly. Focus on the Family published a document on homosexuality in which the author addresses the issue of "what matters morally." The author argues that "the issue before us is whether or not people's lives are better — physically, psychologically, and socially — as a result of homosexuality. . . . If we find, through the best empirical, scientific research available, that certain kinds of sexual behavior endanger the welfare of people, then such behavior and lifestyles cannot be deemed good."[19] Again, this approach presumes the moral neutrality of homosexual behavior and searches for empirical evidences related to the ancillary qualities which would aid moral evaluation of homosexual practice generally. Focus on the Family's review of the empirical evidence yields substantially different results than that of the Committee to Study Homosexuality in the Methodist church.

As was mentioned earlier, some proponents for the morality of homosexual relations point out that the American Psychiatric Association has removed homosexuality from its official diagnostic nomenclature of mental disorders. Proponents argue from this fact to suggest (or prescribe) something about the morality of homosexual acts. For example, one document stated: "The scientific evidence is sufficient to support the contention that homosexuality is not pathological or otherwise an inversion, developmental

19. As this quote from L. Burtoft, *The Social Significance of Homosexuality: Questions and Answers* (Colorado Springs: Public Policy Division, Focus on the Family, 1994), p. 31, suggests, the caricature we mentioned earlier is at times an exaggeration of weaknesses demonstrated by some traditionalists. Apart from the fact that the caricature is an exaggeration and that few traditionalists have ever been completely guilty of such an extreme position, the critique does point to a weakness in the way some traditionalists have understood the relationship between scientific findings and morality. Like many caricatures, this one contains an element of truth. The element of truth in the critic's charge is that traditionalists have given evidence of moral argumentation in a way that confuses what can be thought of as primary factors and supporting data or secondary factors. The assumption underlying this tendency to confuse primary and secondary factors may be due to the tendency among some traditionalists to hold that the more arguments for the condemnation of homosexual behavior, the better. Traditionalists at times may confuse primary moral considerations, which are grounded in God's intention for sexual expression as seen in Scripture, with secondary moral considerations, which may include scientific findings on prevalence, etiology, status as a mental disorder, and the likelihood of change from homosexuality to heterosexuality. When this confusion occurs, traditionalists are usually guilty of giving too much weight to secondary moral considerations.

failure, or deviant form of life as such, but is rather a human variant, one that can be healthy and whole."[20] The removal of a behavioral pattern from a list of designated psychopathologies, however, bears no necessary logical relation to endorsement of that pattern as healthy, whole, or a normal variant.

Conclusion

We might summarize the foregoing section by asserting, as before, that advocates for the morality of homosexual behavior rely on scientific findings to bolster arguments that homosexual acts can no longer legitimately be deemed intrinsically immoral; rather, homosexual acts must be viewed as morally blameless in and of themselves. Formal arguments are not developed, however, to justify the quick extrapolation from scientific findings and theories to the implicit or explicit declaration of the moral neutrality of homosexual behavior.

Status of Our Scientific Knowledge

As the previous section indicates, findings and theories from the behavioral and physical sciences appear repeatedly in the denominational study documents of our mainline denominations, and are typically used to argue for change in the moral stances of our churches and of our society toward homosexual persons and behavior. Citations of the scientific findings on homosexuality in these debates continue to be poorly grounded in the primary literature. For that reason, we here offer an abbreviated review[21] of the contemporary status of this scientific research under the major headings which continue to best describe the types of evidences cited, namely, (1) prevalence, (2) etiology, (3) status as a mental disorder, and (4) efficacy of change methods.[22] In offering this review,

20. United Methodist Church, pp. 27-28.

21. See n. 1 — this section is an abbreviated presentation of Jones and Yarhouse, "Science and the Ecclesiastical Homosexuality Debates."

22. We used these headings in a previous work — S. L. Jones and D. Workman, "Homosexuality: The Behavioral Sciences and the Church," *Journal of Psychology and Theology* 17 (1989): 213-25. One other area in which scientific evidences are potentially relevant to ethical valuation will not be examined here, that being evidences related to the health risks of homosexual behavior. This controversial literature is briefly examined in T. Schmidt, *Straight and Narrow? Compassion and Clarity in the Homosexuality Debate* (Downers Grove, Ill.: InterVarsity, 1995).

we hope to increase awareness that the actual scientific findings in this area are more complex and puzzling than is usually acknowledged, and to discourage future selective or simplistic reporting of such findings.

We note at the outset that research on sexual orientation generally or homosexuality specifically is plagued by pernicious problems. One problem is the diversity of persons to whom the description "homosexual" is applied and the question of whether to categorize people by behavior (which behaviors and to what degree?), self-identification, or some other variable. Individual and subgroup differences may be sacrificed when the generic labels "homosexual" or "gay and lesbian" are used. The essentialist/social constructionist debate, as discussed earlier, further clouds these definitional issues. Essentialist assumptions — basically that sexual orientation is a stable and fundamental aspect of human character which is accurately described by the taxonomy of our contemporary understanding — are common on the part of both researchers and research participants alike and considerably complicate how we understand the data generated.[23] Constructionists such as Haldeman, in contrast, argue that our contemporary taxonomies are social constructions, and thus that the "categories of homosexual, heterosexual, and bisexual, considered by many researchers as fixed and dichotomous, are in reality very fluid for many";[24] if so, the dichotomous "gay and straight" or trichotomous "gay, straight, and bi" may not be the firm foundation for asking questions which many imagine. A second problem has been the research focus upon male homosexuals (gays), with very little in comparison being done with lesbians. A third problem is the difficulty or impossibility of obtaining a random and representative sample of homosexual individuals; many of the most famous studies were performed on convenience samples of questionable representativeness.[25] Fourth, failure to replicate findings has plagued research in this area.

23. Laumann et al., *Social Organization of Sexuality.*

24. D. C. Haldeman, "The Practice and Ethics of Sexual Orientation Conversion Therapy," *Journal of Consulting and Clinical Psychology* 62 (1994): 221-27, quote p. 222. For more formal presentations of constructivism, see P. Blumstein and P. Schwartz, "Intimate Relationships and the Creation of Sexuality," in *Homosexuality/Heterosexuality: Concepts of Sexual Orientation,* ed. D. P. McWhirter et al. (New York: Oxford University Press, 1990); Greenberg, *The Construction of Homosexuality;* and Laumann et al., *Social Organization of Sexuality.*

25. E.g., A. P. Bell and M. S. Weinberg, *Homosexualities: A Study of Diversity among Men and Women* (New York: Simon & Schuster, 1978); D. P. McWhirter and A. M. Mattison, *The Male Couple: How Relationships Develop* (Englewood Cliffs, N.J.: Prentice-Hall, 1984).

Prevalence

The apocryphal prevalence estimate that "10 percent of the adult population is homosexual" appears frequently in church documents. One denominational report listed ten "myths" it aspired to dispel, the first being that "Gays and lesbians constitute only a small segment of the general population and are an urban phenomenon," to which the authors replied, "Research from several sectors indicates that at least 10 percent of the American population or approximately 22 million persons are predominantly gay or lesbian."[26] This apocryphal 10 percent figure has been attributed to the Kinsey study of males, where he reported that 4 percent of white males were exclusively homosexual throughout life after adolescence, and that a total of 10 percent of white males were mostly or exclusively homosexual during at least a three-year period between the ages of sixteen and fifty-five.[27] Kinsey's data appear to have overrepresented male homosexuality due to sampling biases in his research, including the oversampling of prison inmates and members of gay-affirming organizations.[28]

Numerous recent and more credible studies have produced remarkably consistent and much lower prevalence estimates than has been commonly assumed. We will summarize this data in two ways: first according to self-identification as homosexual and second according to occurrence of same-gender sexual behavior. When prevalence is defined by self-identification of sexual orientation by the respondent, prevalence estimates range from 2 to 4 percent. Laumann et al., in the best survey study to date, found that 2.0 percent of men and 0.9 percent of women self-identified as homosexual, with an additional 0.8 and 0.5 percent, respectively, self-identifying as bisexual and 0.3 and 0.1 percent as "other." They also inquired of the degree to which respondents were attracted to members of the same sex, finding 6.2 percent of men and 4.4 percent of women reporting such attraction, independent of heterosexual attraction, and of the degree to which they found the idea of sex with a same-gender partner appealing, finding 4.5 percent of men and 5.6 percent of women reporting this appealing.[29] Harry similarly found that 2.4 percent of a national probability sample of men described themselves as homosexual, but added that if all respondents who described themselves to be

26. Presbyterian Church, p. 49.

27. A. Kinsey, W. Pomeroy, and C. Martin, *Sexual Behavior in the Human Male* (Philadelphia: Saunders, 1948).

28. J. Reisman and E. Eichel, *Kinsey, Sex, and Fraud: The Indoctrination of a People* (Lafayette, La.: Huntington House, 1990).

29. Laumann et al., *Social Organization of Sexuality.*

bisexual and all subjects who refused to answer that particular survey question were also classified as homosexual (both dubious assumptions), then up to 5.7 percent of the sample could be described as homosexual.[30]

Studies of the prevalence of homosexuality grounded in same-gender sexual behavior yield the lowest estimates of prevalence; the best recent studies which utilized national probability surveys are summarized in table 1 (p. 87). Most authors described their findings as "lower bound" estimates of the prevalence of homosexual behavior, given likely reluctance on the part of survey respondents to admit to stigmatized behavior patterns.

Numerous findings are striking. One is the gap between the approximately 1 percent of males who engaged exclusively in same-sex behavior in the past year and the 1.5 to 2.7 percent which experienced any same-sex behavior in the past year. This gap may be partially explained by a separate and surprising finding that 42 percent of the self-identifying gay or bisexual men in a national probability sample were married to women.[31] The low frequency of male lifetime homosexual experience in table 1 compared to Kinsey's estimate of 37 percent, and the impossibility of his 10 percent estimate of three-year exclusive male homosexual experience, are both remarkable.

The "myth" that "Gays and lesbians constitute only a small segment of the general population and are an urban phenomenon" may not be a myth after all. The population percentage of gays and lesbians is certainly smaller than previously estimated. Curiously, it is precisely because homosexuality is predominantly an urban phenomenon (whether by migration or subculture

30. J. Harry, "A Probability Sample of Gay Males," *Journal of Homosexuality* 19 (1990): 89-104. In considerable contrast to both Harry and Laumann et al., R. L. Sell, J. A. Wells, and D. Wypij, "The Prevalence of Homosexual Behavior and Attraction in the United States, the United Kingdom, and France: Results of National Population-Based Samples," *Archives of Sexual Behavior* 24 (1995): 235-48, reported the highly provocative statistics that 20.8 percent of males and 17.8 percent of females in the United States (and similar incidences for the United Kingdom and France) report either sexual attraction toward or behavior with persons of the same gender. This remarkably higher statistic appears to be an artifact of a questionable survey design which forced respondents who had never engaged in homosexual behavior to choose between the items "I have absolutely never felt any sexual attraction towards someone of my own sex" and "I have felt attracted towards someone of my own sex, but never had any sexual contact with anyone." It would appear that this question forced anyone with the vaguest attraction in adolescence to respond to the latter stem, resulting in a considerable inflation of their reported incidences of same-gender attraction. A reluctant rejection of the former stem hardly constitutes a declaration of stable same-gender attraction.

31. Harry, "Probability Sample."

Table 1: Frequency Reports of Same-Gender Sexual Behavior over Various Time Periods from Major National Probability Survey Studies

Study	Exclusive Same-Gender Sex in Last ___ Years	Occurrence of Same-Gender Sex in Last Year	Occurrence in Last ___ Years	Occurrence Since Adulthood (Age __)	Occurrence Since Puberty (or Lifetime)
Billy et al. (1993) Males Only	1.1% in last 10 years		2.3% in last 10 years		
Fay et al. (1989) Males Only		1.6–2%		6.7% since age 19; (3.3% occasionally or fairly often)	20.3%
Laumann et al. (1994) Males		2.7%	4.1% in last 5 years	4.9% since age 18	9.1%
Laumann et al. (1994) Females		1.3%	2.2% in last 5 years	4.1% since age 18	4.3%
Rogers & Turner (1991) Males Only		Study 1 — 1.9% Study 2 — 1.2% Study 3 — 2.4% Study 4 — 2.0%		All since 18 Study 1 — 4.8% Study 2 — 4.9% Study 3 — N/A Study 4 — 6.7%	
Sell et al. (1995) Males	last 5 years: US — 0.82% UK — 1.15% Fr. — 0.72%		last 5 years: US — 5.42% UK — 3.51% Fr. — 9.94%		
Sell et al. (1995) Females	last 5 years: US — 0.27% UK — 0.54% Fr. — 0.14%		last 5 years: US — 2.96% UK — 1.54% Fr. — 3.02%		
Spira et al. (1993) Males Only (France)		1.1%			4.1%
Stall et al. (1990) Males Only	0.8% in last 5 years	1.4% in last 5 years			
Wellings et al. (1994) Males (Britain)		1.1%			6.1%
Wellings et al. (1994) Females (Britain)		0.4%			3.4%

disinhibition)[32] that it may seem to some that 10 percent of the population is gay. A probability sample[33] of males in major urban centers (which was not representative of the country at large) was recently compared to a national probability sample, and found that the percentages of men who had had sex only with other males in the last five years rose from 1.4 percent (national) to 3.7 percent (urban), with an additional 2.0 percent in the urban sample having had sexual relations with both men and women in the last five years. Similarly, Laumann et al. selectively examined respondents who lived in the twelve major urban centers of the United States, and found that self-identification as either homosexual or bisexual increased to 9.2 percent of men and 2.6 percent of women, with reports of any same-sex behavior since puberty increasing to 15.8 percent of men and 4.6 percent of women. There is some validity to the perception that homosexuality is more common in urban settings.

Conclusion

The rate of homosexuality as a stable life orientation in our culture is certainly not 10 percent. There is good evidence to suggest that less than 3 percent, and perhaps less than 2 percent, of males are homosexually active in a given year. The rate of males who engage in sustained homosexual practice over a significant period of adult life is probably less than 5 percent of the male population, and the rate of men who manifest a sustained and exclusive commitment to homosexual practice is certainly less than 3 percent. Female homosexuality continues to be estimated at approximately half or less of the male rates; it appears to characterize less than 2 percent of the female population. So when the genders are combined, homosexuality almost certainly characterizes less than 3 percent of the population, and the correct percentage combining men and women might be lower even than 2 percent.

What Causes Homosexual Orientation?

The etiology of homosexual behavior and orientation figures prominently in ecclesiastical debates, as we demonstrated earlier. Much of this casual discus-

32. Laumann et al., pp. 306-9.

33. R. Stall, J. Gagnon, T. Coates, J. Catania, and J. Wiley, "Prevalence of Men Who Have Sex with Men in the United States," in J. Catania (chairperson), *Results from the First National AIDS Behavioral Survey* (symposium presented at the convention of the American Psychological Association, San Francisco, August 1990).

sion springs from the caricature of the traditionalist position as asserting that homosexuality is always a "willful perversion"; hence, if homosexuality can be shown to be neither "willful" (by showing that development of the orientation is nonvoluntary) nor a "perversion" (by showing that the orientation is somehow "natural" to the person), the traditionalist case loses credibility.

The past decade has witnessed a dramatic swing toward biological theories for the etiology of homosexuality. The major proposed causes for a homosexual orientation have included genetic, prenatal hormonal, adult (postnatal) hormonal, and psychological factors. The following is a brief summary of the current state of the evidence for each.[34]

Genetic Factors

Judgments about the viability of a hypothesized genetic "cause" of homosexuality have been on a roller coaster in the last four decades, and are currently in favor. Genetic studies look for concordance for homosexuality between siblings (or other family members); concordance is the rate at which two siblings both show the characteristic being studied, and greater concordance between more closely genetically related siblings presumably indicates greater genetic causation. Recently, research into the actual chromosomal foundations for such correlations has begun. It appears that there is strong evidence of some genetic influence on the development of homosexual proclivity for some subpopulation of persons. The size and nature of this influence are unclear.

Bailey and Pillard published studies of male and female homosexuals which have forcefully advanced the genetic causation hypothesis. In terms of sample size and methodological sophistication, these are surely the most significant studies yet published in this area. Their study of male homosexuals reported a 52 percent concordance rate for homosexual preference among

34. For the best recent comprehensive summaries of the research on biological causation (with very different emphases and conclusions), see W. Byne and B. Parsons, "Human Sexual Orientation: The Biologic Theories Reappraised," *Archives of General Psychiatry* 50 (1993): 228-39; W. Byne, "The Biological Evidence Challenged," *Scientific American* 270 (1994): 50-55; R. Green, "The Immutability of (Homo)Sexual Orientation: Behavioral Science Implications for a Constitutional (Legal) Analysis," *Journal of Psychiatry and Law* 16 (1988): 537-75; and S. LeVay and D. Hamer, "Evidence for a Biological Influence in Male Homosexuality," *Scientific American* 270 (1994): 44-49. For more detailed Christian reactions to this literature, see, for example, S. O. Cole, "The Biological Basis of Homosexuality: A Christian Assessment," *Journal of Psychology and Theology* 23 (1995): 89-100.

monozygotic twins, a 22 percent concordance for dizygotic twins, a 9.2 percent rate for nontwin brothers, and an 11 percent rate between adoptive brothers.[35] Their study of female homosexuals reported a 48 percent concordance rate for homosexual preference among monozygotic twins, a 16 percent concordance for dizygotic twins, a 14 percent rate for nontwin sisters, and a 6 percent rate between adoptive sisters.[36] Their statistical conclusion for both studies was that genetic factors, heritability, explain the majority of the variance in sexual orientation. One other study to date has produced comparable results.[37]

We would raise several concerns about these studies, with our core concerns engendered by the large size of the genetic influence findings claimed in these studies, not by the claim of genetic influence per se. First is the issue of replication. Other recent studies of the genetic hypothesis have not produced comparable results. A study with a smaller sample size and simpler methodology than Bailey and Pillard's studies reported concordance rates for male and female homosexual identical twins mixed together of only 10 percent (if bisexuals are not counted as homosexual) or 25 percent (if bisexuals are counted as concordant with the homosexual twin);[38] the higher estimate is still half or less of the rates reported by Bailey and Pillard.[39] Research from the Minnesota Twin Project (which examines identical twins reared apart since birth) has also challenged Bailey and Pillard's findings by suggesting lower heritability rates;[40] the researchers reported that all four female monozygotic twin pairs raised apart in which there was one homosexual twin were discordant for lesbianism, one male twin pair was concordant,[41] and

35. J. M. Bailey and R. C. Pillard, "A Genetic Study of Male Sexual Orientation," *Archives of General Psychiatry* 48 (1991): 1089-96.

36. J. M. Bailey, R. C. Pillard, M. C. Neale, and Y. Agyei, "Heritable Factors Influence Sexual Orientation in Women," *Archives of General Psychiatry* 50 (1993): 217-23.

37. F. L. Whitam, M. Diamond, and J. Martin, "Homosexual Orientation in Twins: A Report on Sixty-one Pairs and Three Triplet Sets," *Archives of Sexual Behavior* 22 (1993): 187-206.

38. M. King and E. McDonald, "Homosexuals Who Are Twins: A Study of Forty-six Probands," *British Journal of Psychiatry* 160 (1992): 407-9.

39. Parenthetically, King and McDonald, "Homosexuals Who Are Twins," also reported a high likelihood of sexual relations occurring between identical twins, which the authors suggest as a possible nongenetic variable which could elevate concordance rates between monozygotic twins.

40. E. Eckert, T. Bouchard, J. Bohlen, and L. Heston, "Homosexuality in Monozygotic Twins Reared Apart," *British Journal of Psychiatry* 148 (1986): 421-25.

41. In fact, they became homosexual partners to each other immediately upon rediscovering each other.

one male twin pair was discordant.[42] The lesbian discordance in this study is quite striking in comparison to Bailey and Pillard's remarkably high concordance rates for lesbians.

Second, and of greater concern, are the sampling methods of the Bailey and Pillard studies. With the biases of Kinsey's samples in mind, we may note that subjects for the studies were recruited through openly homophilic magazines and tabloids and through general advertisements in the gay community. The ads stated that the researchers were looking for gay men and lesbians with twin or same-sex adopted siblings. Given the political sophistication of the gay community, it is conceivable that some degree of volunteer bias could have affected the results of the study. If monozygotic twins who had homosexual twin brothers and sisters were more likely to volunteer than discordant twin pairs because they believed the study would produce benefits for the gay community, substantial bias could have swayed the findings.[43]

There were numerous other problems with the Bailey and Pillard studies. There should have been only insignificant differences in the concordance rates between dizygotic twins and nontwins (these two sibling relationships share identical genetic overlap), but instead they found the dizygotic twin brothers to have twice the rate of concordance for homosexuality as nontwin brothers. Their study of lesbians produced similar (and extraordinarily high) concordance rates for dizygotic twins and nontwin sisters.

Further, the estimates of heritability generated in the study were speculative, as they had to incorporate estimates of the amount of error in the population and estimates of the base rate of homosexuality in the general population into their statistical model. How could their mathematical model produce estimates of heritability approaching 75 percent when fully half of the twin sets were discordant in sexual orientation, and when the base rates for homosexuality from these families far exceed the base rates reported in the best recent estimates of prevalence which we reviewed earlier? If the true population base rate of male homosexuality is 2 percent, then some process in these families increased the risk for male children becoming homosexual (even for nonrelated adopted brothers, who share no genes with their siblings) fivefold over the base rate (from 2 to 10 percent). If the 50 percent estimate of monozygotic twin concordance holds, which seems unlikely, then genes increased the risk for these men by an additional fivefold; this suggests

42. One twin homosexually identified, and the other was exclusively and happily heterosexual in marriage, though he had a homosexual affair from age fifteen to eighteen.

43. Interestingly, though, the King and McDonald study, "Homosexuals Who Are Twins," used an identical recruitment method and came up with markedly lower concordance rates in their sample.

equivalent effects for nature/heredity and nurture/environment. Similarly for women, if the base rate of lesbianism is 1 percent, then nonrelated adopted women were six times more likely to become lesbians by growing up in these families than in the general population, and fraternal siblings more than fourteen times more likely than the general population.

Finally, if a genetic explanation is to be accepted as the most important causal influence in homosexuality, the 50 percent nonconcordance rate between monozygotic twins begs explanation. If two individuals share 100 percent of their genetic makeup (nature) and almost 100 percent of their formative developmental experiences (nurture), how can the high rate of discordance be explained?

Only recently has the technology been developed to directly examine specific genetic sequences that may influence the development of homosexuality. In 1993 the media reported the discovery of a "sexual orientation gene" by Dean Hamer and his research team, though the authors of the research were much more circumspect in their report.[44] There were two aspects to their project. First, a pedigree analysis of seventy-six men recruited out of an AIDS treatment program who met a criterion of having a gay brother (a very select subsample of gay men) was performed, from which the researchers reported a strong pattern of homosexual orientation represented in maternal relatives but not in paternal relatives. This led to the second part of the study, which focused on subjects only from families where there was preexisting evidence of maternal transmission of homosexual orientation from the pedigree analysis. A "DNA linkage analysis" of forty pairs of homosexual brothers from this subsample was conducted, which produced a finding that thirty-three of the forty pairs shared a statistically significant concordance of the "Xq28 subtelomeric region of the long arm of the sex (X) chromosome."

A replication and extension study by the same research team reported three significant findings.[45] First, this study of a new sample of homosexual males which again met the criterion of having a gay brother and being from a family which evidenced maternal genetic transmission produced nearly identical results to the previous study, with twenty-two out of thirty-two brothers sharing identical Xq28 markers, a statistically significant concordance. Second, the original Hamer study only examined genetic material shared by gay male

44. D. H. Hamer, S. Hu, V. L. Magnuson, N. Hu, and A. M. Pattatucci, "A Linkage between DNA Markers on the X Chromosome and Male Sexual Orientation," *Science* 261 (1993): 321-27.

45. S. Hu, A. M. Pattatucci, C. Patterson, L. Li, D. W. Fulker, S. S. Cherny, L. Kruglyak, and D. H. Hamer, "Linkage between Sexual Orientation and Chromosome Xq28 in Males but Not in Females," *Nature Genetics* 11 (1995): 248-56.

siblings and did not check to see if discordant (nongay) siblings shared the exact same material; if they had, this would have suggested that the chromosomal overlap was related to a shared family trait that had little to do with sexual orientation. The second study found that heterosexual brothers were strikingly unlikely to share the same Xq28 markers, thus increasing the likelihood that the marker is indeed related to homosexual orientation. Third, a sample of lesbian sisters was also examined (though there is no evidence of maternal transmission of female homosexuality), with the result that no statistically significant effects were found; the authors conclude from this last finding that the Xq28 region is uninvolved with the occurrence of female homosexuality. The technical methodology of these studies appears to have been exceptional.

There are, naturally, problems and limitations with these studies as well. First, these findings have yet to be replicated by other research teams, and similar findings in the last decade reporting "genes for" manic depression, violence, alcoholism, and schizophrenia have often not been replicated or have been formally retracted.[46] A newspaper has reported, in fact, that Hamer et al.'s studies have actually failed attempted direct replication in a Canadian laboratory,[47] though the Hamer team has warned that their findings depend critically on exact usage of their sample inclusion criteria, which may or may not explain any specific failure to replicate. Second, and very seriously, allegations of selective reporting of data by Hamer and his collaborators to enhance statistical power have been made by a researcher on Hamer's team and are apparently in the process of being adjudicated.[48]

The major limitation (as opposed to flaw) of these studies is that they did not, contrary to the media reports about the first study, find a sexual orientation gene. They rather appear to have found a cluster of shared genetic segments which seem to relate to sexual orientation in this unusual and selective sample of male homosexuals. There are huge gaps between genotype and phenotype; i.e., there are many possible ways in which some shared genetic material (the genotype) might contribute to the highly complex and variable human

46. Byne and Parsons, "Human Sexual Orientation." Turner presented evidence in favor of Hamer et al.'s hypothesis of causation by a gene in the Xq28 region of the X chromosome by offering analyses of familial "pedigree charts" which purported to show transmission of homosexuality in a convenience sample only through the maternal side of each family, and also to show concordance of homosexuality with various chromosomally based disease processes; W. J. Turner, "Homosexuality, Type 1: An Xq28 Phenomenon," *Archives of Sexual Behavior* 24 (1995): 109-34.

47. J. Crewdson, "Study on 'Gay Gene' Challenged," *Chicago Tribune,* 25 June 1995, pp. 1, 10, 11.

48. Crewdson, "'Gay Gene' Challenged."

outcome which we call sexual orientation. It is quite clear that these studies did not find a chromosome which causes homosexual orientation: "the Xq28 region was neither necessary nor sufficient for a homosexual orientation."[49] The findings may be of a chromosome set that has a somewhat direct effect on orientation, or may be a marker for or cause of temperamental or other variables that exert their influence indirectly and thus make homosexuality more likely to occur.[50] Hu et al. acknowledge this explicitly by not calling the Xq28 region a sexual orientation locus, but a "sexual orientation related locus."[51] The region appears to relate to the development of sexual orientation for a subpopulation of men, but how it does so is as of now a mystery.

Brain Differences

We will discuss possible brain differences between homosexuals and heterosexuals as a separate category of etiological possibilities, even though the putative brain differences could be conceptualized as a by-product of developmental biological mechanisms such as genetic factors or prenatal hormone influences, or of *post hoc* biological factors such as disease processes, or of nonbiological (or, more precisely, secondarily and derivatively biological) influences such as adult behavior patterns, or of any combination of these in interaction.

Some studies infer indirectly that the brains and/or neurohormonal systems of homosexuals are different from their heterosexual peers based on neuropsychological performance studies. For instance, research suggests that male and female homosexuals are less right-handed than heterosexuals.[52] This apparent shift is statistically significant but surprisingly modest on an absolute basis, and the correlation with sexual orientation may be spurious. There is also some evidence of differing mental abilities compared to heterosexuals which may be based on different brain structures (specifically, in some studies and on some tasks male homosexuals on average perform in a manner unlike male heterosexuals and in a manner not statistically different from females or intermediate between heterosexual males and females).[53]

49. Hu et al., p. 253.

50. See Byne and Parsons, "Human Sexual Orientation," for a fine discussion of such an "interactionist" theory.

51. Hu et al., p. 250.

52. E.g., J. Lindesay, "Laterality Shift in Homosexual Men," *Neuropsychologia* 25 (1987): 965-69.

53. See Green, "Immutability of (Homo)Sexual Orientation," pp. 553-54, for a review of the pre-1987 data which dealt exclusively with males, and more recently C. M.

Finally, there have been suggestions of cerebral lateralization differences.[54] These findings can only be termed suggestive at this time, and are only indirect indicators of brain differences.

Researchers recently have been exploring the possibility that the physical structures of the brains and/or neurohormonal systems of male homosexuals are different from their heterosexual peers, being significantly "feminized," or more accurately, "not defeminized."[55] The first direct evidence of such possible differences emerged from studies which examined hormonal responses to injection with estrogen; these results are in dispute because of the questionable relevance of the response to the development of sexual orientation for humans and because there have been several major failures to replicate the original findings with humans.[56]

Most recently, attention has moved to direct dissection studies of brain differences between women and heterosexual and homosexual men. Researchers have examined seven areas of the brain for gender differences (gender dimorphism) and/or sexual orientation differences (orientation dimorphism). Findings in this area often conflict or await replication, as summarized in table 2 (p. 97).[57]

Findings on the midsagittal plane of the anterior commissure are con-

---

McCormick and S. F. Witelson, "Functional Cerebral Asymmetry and Sexual Orientation in Men and Women," *Behavioral Neuroscience* 108 (1994): 525-31.

54. L. Allen and R. A. Gorski, "Sexual Orientation and the Size of the Anterior Commissure in the Human Brain," *Proceedings of the National Academy of Science USA* 89 (1992): 7199-7202; C. M. McCormick and S. F. Witelson, "A Cognitive Profile of Homosexual Men Compared to Heterosexual Men and Women," *Psychoneuroendocrinology* 16 (1991): 459-73; McCormick and Witelson, "Functional Cerebral Asymmetry."

55. Byne and Parsons, p. 230.

56. See reviews by Green, "Immutability of (Homo)Sexual Orientation," pp. 549-52; and B. A. Gladue, "Hormones in Relationship to Homosexual/Bisexual/Heterosexual Gender Orientation," and L. J. G. Gooren, "An Appraisal of Endocrine Theories of Homosexuality and Gender Dysphoria," both in *Handbook of Sexology,* vol. 6, *The Pharmacology and Endocrinology of Sexual Function,* ed. J. M. A. Sitsen (New York: Elsevier, 1988), pp. 388-409 and 410-24, respectively. See also the replication failure of S. Hendricks, B. Graber, and J. Rodriguez-Sierra, "Neuroendocrine Responses to Exogenous Estrogen: No Difference between Heterosexual and Homosexual Men," *Psychoneuroendocrinology* 14 (1989): 177-85; see Byne and Parsons, "Human Sexual Orientation," for a general discussion of the significance of these findings.

57. For the best reviews of this area, see D. F. Swaab, L. J. G. Gooren, and M. A. Hofman, "The Human Hypothalamus in Relation to Gender and Sexual Orientation," in *Progress in Brain Research,* vol. 93, *The Human Hypothalamus in Health and Disease,* ed. D. F. Swaab, M. A. Hofman, M. Mirmiram, R. Ravid, and F. W. van Leeuwen (New York: Elsevier, 1992); or Byne and Parsons, "Human Sexual Orientation."

Table 2: Brain Differences between Heterosexual and Homosexual Men and Heterosexual Women

Study	Brain Region						
	INAH 1	INAH 2	INAH 3	INAH 4	SCN	SDNH	MPAC
Swaab & Fliers (1985)	HetM > HetF						
Allen et al. (1989)	HetM = HetF	HetM > HetF	HetM > HetF	HetM = HetF			
LeVay (1991)	HetM = HetF	HetM = HetF	HetM > (HetF & HomM)	HetM = HetF			
Swaab & Hofman (1988)						HetM = HomM; (HetM & HomM) > HetF	
Swaab & Hofman (1990)					HomM > HetM; HetM = HetF; shape spherical in HetM; elongated in HomM and HetF		
Allen & Gorski (1991)							HetF > HetM
Allen & Gorski (1992)							(HetF = HomM) > HetM
Demeter et al. (1988)							HetF < HetM

flicting. Two findings of orientation dimorphism await replication and have not as yet been contradicted by other findings. Swaab and Hofman found that the suprachiasmic nucleus (SCN) of homosexual men was larger in volume and number of neurons than that of heterosexual men, though this is an area of the brain which does not differ by gender in volume or cell count[58] and

58. As shown by D. Swaab and M. Hofman, "An Enlarged Suprachiasmatic Nucleus in Homosexual Men," *Brain Research* 537 (1990): 141-48; see also Byne, "Biological Evidence Challenged."

which appears to have no direct bearing on sexual behavior at all.[59] This obscures the meaning of the finding. The shape of this anatomical feature, as noted in the chart, did suggest parallels between females and homosexual males. The second and most widely publicized finding, that of LeVay, that the third interstitial nuclei of the anterior hypothalamus (INAH 3) of homosexual males is on average structurally more like that of heterosexual females than heterosexual males, is problematic for a number of reasons. "First, his [LeVay's] work has not been replicated, and human neuroanatomical studies of this kind have a very poor track record for reproducibility."[60] Second, the samples used by LeVay were of uncertain definition. Individuals were presumed heterosexual on the basis of no mention of sexual orientation in their medical charts; the death of a significant number of the heterosexual subjects from HIV infection so early in the AIDS crisis makes their identification as heterosexuals suspect. Third, all of his homosexual population died of AIDS, and the disease processes may have produced the noted anatomical anomalies; there is research suggesting that end-stage AIDS suppresses testosterone levels which may influence the structure of INAH 3.[61]

Even if the replication of either of these findings (or even of future unanticipated findings) is assumed, the direction of causation may be difficult to establish, as behavior both affects and is affected by brain structure and function. For example, the gay men in LeVay's study may have had smaller INAH 3 areas because of years of action peculiar to a male homosexual lifestyle rather than the structure of the INAH 3 causing them to be homosexual. Contrary to popularly shared myths, the brain is structurally plastic throughout life, and the size and nature of different brain structures are influenced by behavior.[62] The conclusion of an eminent research scientist, John Bancroft, regarding the current state of brain research on sexual orientation, seems reasonable: "The reader is entitled to be sceptical if not confused by these findings. There is either a lack of consistency or replication. There are methodological problems. . . . It certainly seems unlikely that there is any direct relationship between structure of a specific area of the brain and sexual orientation per se."[63]

59. S. LeVay, "A Difference in the Hypothalamic Structure between Heterosexual and Homosexual Men," *Science* 253 (1991): 1034-37.

60. Byne, p. 53.

61. Byne and Parsons, "Human Sexual Orientation."

62. See S. M. Breedlove, "Sexual Dimorphism in the Vertebrate Nervous System," *Journal of Neuroscience* 12 (1992): 4133-42.

63. J. Bancroft, "Homosexual Orientation: The Search for a Biological Basis," *British Journal of Psychiatry* 164 (1994): 437-40, quote p. 438.

Prenatal Hormonal Factors

Some researchers propose that human sexual orientation is largely determined between the second and fifth month of pregnancy by fetal exposure to the sex hormones. Again, hypothesized genetic and prenatal hormonal causal processes may be independent and mutually exclusive or interdependent and complementary. Several studies have administered abnormal sex hormone levels to animal fetuses in their mothers' wombs to study the effects this has on sexual differentiation and the development of sexual behavior patterns in the adult animals. It has been shown that the abnormal doses of sex hormones administered to an animal fetus at a critical developmental juncture can result in that adult animal showing inverted sexual behavior in conjunction with mating. These effects are complex and multifaceted, and have been taken by some as evidence suggesting that similar hormone variations must be causal factors in human homosexuality,[64] while others have argued that there are monumental problems in establishing the relevance of this animal research for human beings, including the highly abnormal hormone levels used to create these inversions and the vast differences between animal and human sexual behavior.[65] For example, what is called "homosexual behavior" in rats — such as lordosis in males (elevation of the rump to facilitate being mounted from behind as characterizes normal females) or mounting by females (which is characteristic behavior of the male) — occurs as a reflex which the experimental rats emit upon sexual stimulation without reference to the gender origin of the sexual stimulus.[66] A behavioral reflex which can be "mechanically" elicited is a poor analogue for human sexual orientation. Such rats do not have a "homosexual orientation" as understood for humans.

Four major types of evidence grounded in research for the prenatal hormone hypothesis in humans are cited. Some theorists argue on the basis of these evidences that homosexuality is biologically determined, while oth-

64. E.g., L. Ellis and A. Ames, "Neurohormonal Functioning and Sexual Orientation: A Theory of Homosexuality-Heterosexuality," *Psychological Bulletin* 101 (1987): 233-58.

65. E. Adkins-Regan, "Sex Hormones and Sexual Orientation in Animals," *Psychobiology* 16 (1988): 335-47; Byne and Parsons, "Human Sexual Orientation"; H. Feder, "Hormones and Sexual Behavior," *Annual Review of Psychology* 35 (1984): 165-200; W. Ricketts, "Biological Research on Homosexuality: Ansell's Cow or Occam's Razor?" *Journal of Homosexuality* 9 (1984): 65-93.

66. For example, the male rat exposed to prenatal feminizing hormones will exhibit lordosis in response to the experimenter's hand as easily as to another (normal) male rat.

ers disagree.[67] First, both the direct and indirect evidences of male homosexual brains being less defeminized than their heterosexual peers (as discussed in the previous section) are cited as evidence in favor of the prenatal hormonal hypothesis, as early hormonal exposure may be the prime mechanism producing gender-based and/or orientation-based brain differences. The lack of well-established findings in this area, as well as the speculative nature of connections to prenatal hormonal causation, is problematic.

A second type of evidence comes from "quasi experiments" on prenatal hormonal levels. Although experiments directly manipulating hormones in the womb cannot be ethically performed with human fetuses, a number of naturally and accidentally occurring medical conditions have served as quasi experiments of sorts. Studies of these unfortunate occurrences have shown that some human fetuses exposed to abnormal hormone levels during development can show altered physical development, brain functioning, gender orientation, and sexual behavior when mature.[68] For example, one recent study reported that the female children of mothers who unwittingly exposed their fetuses to elevated intrauterine levels of estrogen by taking a synthetic estrogen drug during pregnancy were disproportionately (though modestly) more likely to become bisexuals (or much less likely, lesbians) as adults.[69] Application of these studies in understanding homosexuality is questionable. First, the homosexual population shows no elevated rates of the expected physical abnormalities which often occur with prenatal hormonal aberrations. Second, the fact that certain outcomes can be created by one set of abnormal conditions (such as synthetic hormone administration) by no means leads to the conclusion that "naturally occurring" instances of the same outcome occurred because of the same abnormal conditions; the fact that delirium can be induced by striking another's head hard with a Bible hardly implicates such as a standard cause of delirium. Finally, few of the unfortunate

67. Ellis and Ames, "Neurohormonal Functioning," and Green, "Immutability of (Homo)Sexual Orientation," argue this most forcefully, while strong critics of this position include J. DeCecco, "Homosexuality's Brief Recovery: From Sickness to Health and Back Again," *Journal of Sex Research* 23 (1987): 106-29; T. Hoult, "Human Sexuality in Biological Perspective: Theoretical and Methodological Considerations," *Journal of Homosexuality* 9 (1984): 137-56; and Ricketts, "Biological Research on Homosexuality."

68. See reviews by Byne and Parsons, "Human Sexual Orientation"; Green, "Immutability of (Homo)Sexual Orientation"; Gladue, "Hormones in Relationship"; and J. Money, "Genetic and Chromosomal Aspects of Homosexual Etiology," in *Homosexual Behavior*, pp. 59-74.

69. H. F. L. Meyer-Bahlburg, A. A. Ehrhardt, L. R. Rosen, R. S. Gruuen, N. P. Veridiano, F. H. Vann, and N. F. Neuwalder, "Prenatal Estrogens and the Development of Homosexual Orientation," *Developmental Psychology* 31 (1995): 12-21.

subjects in these "quasi experiments" manifest "pure" homosexual identity in isolation from other broad disruptions of gender identity and behavior.

A third type of human evidence for prenatal causation suggests that the most powerful predictor of adult male homosexuality is striking gender nonconformity or gender inappropriateness early in childhood. Boys who are strikingly effeminate as young children appear to be much more likely to become homosexual men than their more typically masculine peers, though some effeminate children do not grow up homosexual and many homosexuals do not report gender-inappropriate behavior as children.[70] This research has been criticized on the basis, first, that it "repathologizes" homosexuality by returning it to the status of a "deviation" from the normal path of development (as evidenced by some of the researchers in this area using such terms as "atypicality," "disorder," and "abnormality" in discussing homosexuality); second, that it restigmatizes male homosexuals as effeminate, not true men, or "sissies," an image gays have been trying to shed for years;[71] and finally, that this research may be founded upon outmoded and caricatured understandings of gender behavior.[72] There is no conclusive understanding of why early gender behavior distortion occurs. Although some regard it as evidence for the prenatal hormone hypothesis, there is some evidence that the causes could be psychological. One study reported that "significantly fewer male role models were found in the family backgrounds of the severely gender-disturbed boys," and that there were more emotional problems in the families of the most disturbed boys.[73]

Finally, some researchers argue that maternal stress during pregnancy may predispose the child to homosexuality. The most frequently cited studies are those of Dorner showing that an unusual number of homosexuals were born to German women who were pregnant during World War II.[74] Similarly, a recent study of birth order found that homosexual men are likely to have an overabundance of brothers compared to sisters (by a ratio of approximately

70. J. M. Bailey and K. J. Zucker, "Childhood Sex-Typed Behavior and Sexual Orientation: A Conceptual Analysis and Quantitative Review," *Developmental Psychology* 31 (1995): 43-55; R. Green, *The "Sissy Boy" Syndrome and the Development of Homosexuality* (New Haven: Yale University Press, 1987); J. Harry, *Gay Children Grown Up: Gender Culture and Gender Deviance* (New York: Praeger, 1982); J. Harry, "Sexual Orientation as Destiny," *Journal of Homosexuality* 10 (1985): 111-24.

71. DeCecco, p. 109.

72. Risman and Schwartz, "Sociological Research."

73. G. Rekers, S. Mead, A. Rosen, and S. Brigham, "Family Correlates of Male Childhood Gender Disturbance," *Journal of Genetic Psychology* 142 (1983): 31-42, quote p. 31.

74. Discussed in Ellis and Ames, "Neurohormonal Functioning," and Green, "Immutability of (Homo)Sexual Orientation."

1.5 to 1.0) and to have been later in the birth order of their mothers;[75] the authors suggest that the mothers of homosexuals are more likely to have been stressed, which tends to result in a higher incidence of male births and which is hypothesized to create androgen insufficiency which would produce incomplete masculinization of the male fetus, resulting in adulthood in homosexuality. Such indirect evidence, while compatible with the prenatal hormone hypothesis, could also be seen as compatible with other psychological theories of causation, as noted by the authors.

Adult (Postnatal) Hormonal Factors

There is a long research tradition of investigating the possibility that male and female homosexuals have abnormal levels of certain sex hormones compared to normals. The consensus from research on males is that there are no substantial hormonal differences between homosexuals and their comparable heterosexual peers. Research which was once thought to show such differences in males has been shown to be plagued by inaccurate methods of measuring hormones and inaccurate ways of categorizing the sexual preferences of subjects in the studies.[76] The results of some studies of lesbians suggest that while most lesbians fall within the normal ranges of serum testosterone and estrogen, a subpopulation may be characterized by elevated testosterone levels. These findings could, however, be an artifact of sample selection, stress, occupational affiliation, or physical exercise patterns.[77] In any case, the general consensus is that "it is unlikely that sex hormone levels have any direct bearing on sexual orientation in adults."[78]

Psychological Causation

Though much of the research on psychological causation is based upon the clinical impressions of practicing psychoanalysts (and hence dismissed by some as contaminated by the "heterosexist biases" of the therapists), there has been a considerable amount of prospective or retrospective research on families that produce homosexual sons, though that research has fallen into disfa-

75. R. Blanchard, K. J. Zucker, S. J. Bradley, and C. S. Hume, "Birth Order and Sibling Sex Ratio in Homosexual Male Adolescents and Probably Prehomosexual Feminine Boys," *Developmental Psychology* 31 (1995): 22-30.

76. Gooren, "Appraisal of Endocrine Theories"; Byne and Parsons, p. 230; Green, "Immutability of (Homo)Sexual Orientation," pp. 543-45; Ricketts, pp. 71-76.

77. Gladue, "Hormones in Relationship."

78. Gladue, p. 393.

vor and has largely disappeared from formal academic publication.[79] The bulk of the empirical research on the families of homosexuals documents patterns that would be predicted by psychoanalytic theory, such as patterns of distant relationships with the same-gender parent or elevated incidences of same-sex play or abuse in childhood and adolescence. For example, one study reported a much higher loss of fathers and/or mothers to death or divorce in its homosexual sample than in the heterosexual sample.[80] Another reported that among those who had been sexually molested as children, 7.4 percent were gay men and 3.1 percent were lesbian women as adults, compared to those who had not been sexually molested as children, among whom 2.0 percent were gay men and 0.8 percent were lesbian women as adults; abuse appears to encourage homosexual adaptation.[81]

Many of the findings in this literature cannot be argued to support only a psychological theory. For example, proponents of the prenatal hormone hypothesis[82] would argue that all of the research documenting problematic relations between prehomosexual boys and their fathers, rather than proving that rejecting fathers cause homosexuality, instead reflects the tendency for fathers to reject their gender-inappropriate sons, with said gender inappropriateness being the cause rather than effect of father bonding difficulties. But the reverse may be true as well; some of the indirect evidence for more biological causation could be taken as supportive of psychological hypotheses as well.

It seems that there is not enough evidence to prove the psychological causation hypothesis, but there is too much evidence to dismiss it at this time. Several survey studies have produced evidence which has been taken as falsifying the notion of psychological causation, but this is problematic, as all survey or interview research is subject to the phenomenon of adult reinterpretation of the past, and also because the psychoanalytic paradigm itself, with its emphasis upon repression and the other defense mechanisms, would not deem retrospective surveys about child-rearing practices in the family of origin as a particularly useful method by which to test its hypotheses. At least some of the incentive to dismiss psychological causation at this time is based on renewed

79. See M. Siegelman, "Kinsey and Others: Empirical Input" (in *Male and Female Homosexuality: Psychological Approaches,* ed. L. Diamant [Washington: Hemisphere, 1987], pp. 33-80), for a comprehensive review of the substantial amount of research in this area.

80. M. T. Saghir and E. Robins, *Male and Female Homosexuality: A Comprehensive Investigation* (Baltimore: Williams & Wilkins, 1973), p. 139.

81. Laumann et al., p. 345; see also L. S. Doll et al., "Self-Reported Childhood and Adolescent Sexual Abuse among Adult Homosexual and Bisexual Men," *Child Abuse and Neglect* 16 (1992): 855-64.

82. E.g., Bailey and Zucker, "Childhood Sex-Typed Behavior."

enthusiasm for biological explanations. Also, much of this literature is dismissed on the presumption that all of the "old" research was done on biased samples, such as those drawn from homosexuals under psychiatric treatment. The irony in this complaint, as we have already noted, is that there has never been a study of a representative sample of homosexual persons, and much of the best contemporary biological research is performed on nonrepresentative samples. Though the substantive body of psychological causation research is aging and not being regularly renewed, it has never been refuted and still holds promise for understanding part of the causal puzzle of homosexuality.

Conclusions regarding Causation

The genetic, brain structure, and prenatal hormonal causation hypotheses are "hot" right now. Although an impressive amount of research is cited in favor of the former three hypotheses, the direct research in support of each of them is not conclusive. On the other hand, a substantive legacy of research on psychological/familial factors is being generally ignored today despite the statistically significant findings represented in that literature. It is worth noting that the recent movement toward biologic theories may be as much a product of the contemporary Zeitgeist and of political forces as any real dissatisfaction with the psychosocial theories. In reality, the biologic theories at this point "seem to have no greater explanatory value"[83] than the psychosocial models they seek to displace.

It seems most reasonable to conclude that genetic, brain structure, prenatal hormonal, and psychological/familial factors may each be a facilitating or contributing cause of homosexual orientation in some individuals. We would argue with Bancroft that if homosexual orientation "was determined solely by biological factors, it would be inconceivable that no counterpart could be found in other species" and thus that homosexual orientation must be "a consequence of a multifactorial developmental process in which biological factors play a part, but in which psychosocial factors remain crucially important."[84] Similarly, some of the most respected proponents of biological causation argue that sexual orientation appears to be a "complex characteristic" of "multifactorial or heterogeneous" origin which probably involves "a complex interaction between genetic, biological, experiential and sociocultural factors."[85] None of these influences can be presumed to be necessar-

83. Byne and Parsons, p. 236.
84. Bancroft, p. 439.
85. Hu et al., pp. 252, 252, 248.

ily operative in all homosexuals, and there is no evidence that any one factor can by itself "cause" homosexuality. The complex of factors which results in the orientation toward homosexuality probably differs from person to person. Thoughtful persons reflecting on the causation literature must strive to rid themselves of the simplistic thinking that demands a single cause for this complex phenomenon. Some of these influencing factors may be genetic in origin, but genetic influence may not mean a "sexual orientation gene"; rather, other higher-order traits may dispose some children to atypical social relationships, patterns of psychological identification, and so forth. Like Byne and Parsons (1993), we favor an interactional hypothesis for the formation of sexual orientation, one which suggests shifting ratios of influence from different sources for different persons, and with nature and nurture in constant interaction.

Does the presence of possibly powerful causative influences, be they biological or psychological/familial, render human choice utterly irrelevant to the development of sexual orientation? There appear to be a variety of factors which can provide a push in the direction of homosexuality for some persons, but there is no evidence that this "push" renders human choice utterly irrelevant. We again concur with Byne and Parsons, who argue that human choice can be construed to be one of the factors influencing the development of sexual orientation, but that this "is not meant to imply that one consciously decides one's sexual orientation. Instead, sexual orientation is assumed to be shaped and reshaped by a cascade of choices made in the context of changing circumstances in one's life and enormous social and cultural pressures,"[86] and, we would add, in the context of considerable predispositions toward certain types of preferences. And perhaps, as Baumrind and others have argued, for some people erotic proclivities really are their chosen sexual preference, as adult converts to lesbianism seem to exemplify.[87]

Many are most troubled by the concept of "choice" when it is linked to "genetic causation." We are used to thinking of genes as causing us to have things like brown eyes or wavy hair, and choice has little to do with such phenomena. But behavior genetics has produced abundant evidence of genetic influences that clearly do not render human choice irrelevant. One study of the correlations between the television viewing of adopted children and their adoptive and biological parents produced evidence of "significant genetic in-

86. Byne and Parsons, p. 237.

87. D. Baumrind, "Commentary on Sexual Orientation: Research and Social Policy Implications," *Developmental Psychology* 31 (1995): 130-36.

fluence on individual differences in children's television viewing."[88] The findings had nearly the statistical power of the heritability studies of Bailey and his colleagues reviewed earlier. This finding helps to put the genetic evidence into perspective; all of us would reject the notion that our genes make us sit for a certain number of hours in front of a television screen, but we may have a predisposition of some sort (sedentary tendencies?) which would make the choice to view television appealing to varying degrees.

Finally, we would note that a recent, highly publicized study illustrates the complex interrelationship between biological and environmental (nature and nurture) factors. Zhang and Odenwald published a study which created genetic alterations in fruit flies which produced "homosexual behavior" in the altered fruit flies.[89] Many tabloid headlines heralded the creation of a "homosexual gene." But curiously, when genetically normal or "straight" fruit flies were introduced into the habitat of the "gay" flies, they began engaging in the same type of "homosexual" behavior as the genetically altered flies. Thus, in a most biological experiment, evidence of environmental ("psychological") influence emerged once again. Clearly, Baumrind is correct in arguing that "it is impossible to disentangle the biological and the psychological contributions to the behavioral differences that constitute sexual orientation."[90]

Is Homosexuality a Psychopathology?

The view that homosexuality is not psychopathological, and in fact is judged to be a healthy lifestyle variant, is frequently cited in the mainline denominational literature, with implications drawn for the ethical argument. For example, one study stated, "If it could be shown that homosexuality is generally a symptom of unmet emotional needs or difficulties in social adjustment, then this might point to problems in relating to God and other persons. But if that cannot generally be shown, homosexuality may be compatible with life in grace." The report went on to conclude that "The scientific evidence is sufficient to support the contention that homosexuality is not pathological or

88. R. Plomin, R. Corley, J. C. DeFries, and D. W. Fulker, "Individual Differences in Television Viewing in Early Childhood: Nature as well as Nurture," *Psychological Science* 1 (1990): 371-77, quote p. 371.

89. Shang-Ding Zhang and W. F. Odenwald, "Misexpression of the White *(W)* Gene Triggers Male-Male Courtship in Drosophila," *Proceedings of the National Academy of Sciences USA* 92 (1995): 5525-29.

90. Baumrind, p. 132.

otherwise an inversion, developmental failure, or deviant form of life as such, but is rather a human variant, one that can be healthy and whole."[91] What does the evidence actually show?

There is much less new research in this category than for the previous two sections. In our earlier analysis,[92] we argued that the decision by the American Psychiatric Association to remove homosexuality as a pathological psychiatric condition per se from its *Diagnostic and Statistical Manual (DSM)* in 1974 was as much a sociopolitical action as a scientific one. We suggested that the removal of homosexual orientation from the *DSM* does not answer definitively the thorny question of the psychopathological status of homosexual behavior, nor does it constitute an endorsement of homosexual orientation or lifestyle as necessarily healthy or wholesome. We summarized some of the available evidence relating to the four standard empirical criteria used to define behavior patterns as abnormal: statistical infrequency, personal distress, maladaptiveness, and deviation from social norms. Regarding the first and last of these four criteria, since our earlier review, estimates of prevalence have more clearly suggested that homosexuality is less statistically frequent than would have been estimated in the 1980s,[93] and surveys of public opinion have continued to show for over two decades that almost 80 percent of the general public has continued to view all instances of homosexual behavior as immoral, even while support for equal civil rights for homosexuals has grown.[94] But we would like to more fully supplement our earlier analysis of the second and third factors, personal distress and maladaptiveness.

Personal Distress

Personal distress is a common but not strictly necessary aspect of psychopathology. Most people with a diagnosable condition are subjectively dis-

91. United Methodist Church, pp. 13, 27-28.

92. Jones and Workman, "Homosexuality."

93. Further, the lifetime incidence estimates of the major psychopathological disorders range from 14.3 percent for phobias and 13.8 percent for alcohol abuse and dependence, to 1.6 percent for panic and 1.5 percent for schizophrenia, to 0.1 percent for somatization disorder; see L. N. Robins, B. Z. Locke, and D. A. Regier, "An Overview of Psychiatric Disorders in America," in *Psychiatric Disorders in America: The Epidemiological Catchment Area Study,* ed. L. N. Robins and D. A. Regier (New York: Free Press, 1991), pp. 328-66, here p. 343. Thus, homosexuality is not so common as to be eliminated as a possible pathology on frequency bases alone.

94. A. Greeley, R. Michael, and T. Smith, "Americans and Their Sexual Partners," *Society* 27 (1990): 36-42; Laumann et al., *Social Organization of Sexuality.*

tressed by their problems, but the notable examples of antisocial personality disorder and alcoholism/drug addiction, with their attendant patterns of denial and minimization of distress, serve as reminders that personal distress is not always present. Reflection on this topic is also complicated by the legitimate concern that distress in a homosexual population may be exogenous (the result of persecution, rejection, lack of acceptance, and so forth) rather than endogenous.

It is often asserted in the sexuality literature that "there is no evidence of higher rates of emotional instability or psychiatric illness among homosexuals than among heterosexuals."[95] While this has been repeated so often as to assume the status of a truth that "everybody knows," the factual basis for this assertion is questionable. The two most frequently cited studies in support of this platitude merit closer examination. The first major study to challenge the prevailing view of homosexuality as intrinsically pathological was the study by Hooker,[96] who conducted psychological tests on a group of "healthy" homosexuals and a comparison group of heterosexuals, and then (to the surprise of the mental health establishment) demonstrated that skilled psychological diagnosticians could not distinguish the heterosexuals from the homosexuals on the basis of their test results. By their test findings, the homosexual sample was judged to have no different and no worse problems than heterosexuals. Given that the prevailing wisdom was that to be homosexual was necessarily to be manifestly, obviously, and deeply disturbed, Hooker's study was an apt refutation of that prevailing wisdom; she decisively refuted the absolute judgment that all homosexuals are manifestly disturbed. The study was the logical equivalent of refuting the judgment that "all women are intellectually inferior to men" by demonstrating that a select sample of intellectually gifted women outperformed a sample of men on an intelligence test.

But Hooker's study is often interpreted as having accomplished much more, not merely demonstrating that "it is not the case that all homosexuals are manifestly disturbed," but rather proving that "homosexuals are as emotionally healthy as heterosexuals" or that "homosexuality per se is not psychopathological." Logically and methodologically, her study accom-

95. W. Masters, V. Johnson, and R. Kolodny, *Human Sexuality,* 4th ed. (Glenview, Ill.: Scott Foresman and Co., 1992), p. 394; see also M. Ross, J. Paulsen, and O. Stalstrom, "Homosexuality and Mental Health," *Journal of Homosexuality* 15 (1988): 131-52.

96. E. Hooker, "The Adjustment of the Male Overt Homosexual," *Journal of Projective Techniques* 21 (1957): 18-31; also reported in E. Hooker, "The Adjustment of the Male Overt Homosexual," in *The Problem of Homosexuality in Modern Society,* ed. H. M. Ruitenbeek (New York: Dutton, 1963), pp. 141-61.

plished neither of these ends. As a necessary but not sufficient condition for assessing either of these latter claims, Hooker would have had to study a representative sample of homosexual persons; but in Hooker's own words, "It should also be stated at the outset that no assumptions are made about the random selection of either group [homosexual or heterosexual]. No one knows what a random sample of the homosexual population would be like; and even if one knew, it would be extremely difficult, if not impossible, to obtain one."[97] Hooker worked explicitly with homophilic organizations such as the Mattachine Society in the mid-1950s to recruit a sample of well-adjusted homosexual persons. Further, she explicitly required that participants not be under psychiatric or psychological treatment (it is not clear from her report if her recruits were required to not be in therapy at the time of recruitment for the study or to never have been in therapy); this insistence on a nontherapy sample may have made Hooker's sample extraordinarily nonrepresentative of homosexuals.[98] It must be emphasized that a nonrepresentative sample is only a challenge if certain types of claims are being investigated; Hooker did empirically refute the claim that all homosexuals are manifestly disturbed in a similar way that one "conversion" of a homosexual to heterosexuality refutes the absolute claim that homosexuality is "immutable." We may conclude that the Hooker study proved that a select sample of homosexuals were no more distressed than and could not be psychometrically distinguished from a heterosexual sample, but because of the nonrepresentativeness of her sample, she did not in fact prove the conclusion which some infer from her work.[99]

Contemporary research continues to suggest higher levels of distress in the homosexual population even if that conclusion is usually not stated. For example, a recent study reported on the National Lesbian Health Care Survey.[100] The authors minimized differences between homosexual and heterosexual women, arguing that the two groups were comparable except for ele-

97. Hooker, "Adjustment" (1963), p. 142.

98. We have no idea of the rate of therapy utilization in the late 1950s, but a recent study found that 77.5 percent of lesbians (vs. 28.9 percent of heterosexual women) had been in therapy; J. Bradford, C. Ryan, and E. D. Rothblum, "National Lesbian Health Care Survey: Implications for Mental Health Care," *Journal of Consulting and Clinical Psychology* 62 (1994): 228-42.

99. Similarly, the sample in the famous Saghir and Robins study was selected to minimize or exclude psychopathology; 14 percent of the male homosexual sample and 7 percent of the female homosexual sample had to be excluded because of prior psychiatric hospitalization, while no subjects recruited in the heterosexual control sample had to be excluded on that basis; Saghir and Robins, *Male and Female Homosexuality.*

100. Bradford, Ryan, and Rothblum, "Lesbian Health Care Survey."

vated use of alcohol and drugs[101] and of counseling in the lesbian sample. But their empirical results suggest differently. Bradford et al. reported that 37 percent of the lesbians surveyed had experienced serious depression in their lifetime, 11 percent were experiencing depression at the time of the survey, and 11 percent were currently in treatment for that depression; in contrast, the best estimates for the general female population are 10.2 percent lifetime incidence of major depression, 3.1 percent current major depression, and probably less than 1.0 percent obtaining treatment for that depression in the year before the survey.[102] Bradford et al. further reported that 57 percent of the lesbians surveyed had experienced thoughts about suicide in their lifetime, and that 18 percent had attempted suicide at least once; the best estimates for the general population are that 33 percent of women report lifetime "death thoughts" (a category much milder than thoughts about suicide, as it included answering yes to having "thought a lot about death" at any point in life), while the frequency of suicide attempts was so infrequent that it was not reported.[103]

Maladaptiveness

In our prior analysis, we argued that maladaptiveness can only be judged against some implicit or explicit standard, some tacit model of wholeness and health, a vision of what constitutes a "good life." Any standard of "adaptiveness" can be challenged; neither vocational success nor income nor relational stability nor even the absence of self-injurious behavior is really an utterly reliable or indubitable standard of adaptiveness. Elevated rates of depression, substance abuse, and suicide challenge the adaptiveness of homosexuality. Alternatively, the educational and vocational success, not to mention the recent

101. The elevations were quite serious; Bradford, Ryan, and Rothblum, "Lesbian Health Care Survey," reported that 30 percent of the lesbians surveyed currently abused alcohol more than once a month, 8 percent abused marijuana more than once a month, and 2 percent each abused cocaine, tranquilizers, or stimulants more than once a month. In contrast, Robins and Regier (tables 5-1 and 6-4) estimated for the general population that 4.6 percent of women had abused alcohol in their lifetime and 1.0 percent in the last month, while 4.4 percent reported lifetime abuse of marijuana and less than 1.0 percent reported current abuse, and abuse of other substances was very infrequent. Robins and Regier, eds., *Psychiatric Disorders in America.*

102. Robins and Regier, tables 4-3 and 13-5.

103. Robins and Regier, table 4-7. On suicidality among homosexual persons, see also K. Erwin, "Interpreting the Evidence: Competing Paradigms and the Emergence of Lesbian and Gay Suicide as a 'Social Fact,'" *International Journal of Health Services* 23 (1993): 437-53.

political ascendancy of gay and lesbian concerns, might be seen as supporting the adaptiveness of this orientation.

Many Christian ethicists, including some who are gay affirming, express a concern for monogamy (traditionalists for heterosexual monogamy, others for monogamy regardless of the genders of partners). This ethical concern would lead us to examine adaptiveness in terms of relational stability, though this concern might be seen as peculiarly or parochially Christian. In our earlier report we cited evidence of relational instability and sexual promiscuity among homosexuals. As mentioned in the previous section, this reality may (or may not) be a by-product of societal rejection and failure to provide social structures of support (such as marriage) to gay people. Nevertheless, research continues to suggest contrasts between homosexuals and heterosexuals, though those contrasts are not as stark as a decade ago. We will just mention a sampling of studies which we either did not cite in our prior report or which have appeared since that time. In contrast to the huge lifetime sexual partner estimates of the famous Bell and Weinberg study, Laumann et al. found that on average gay men reported 42.8 lifetime sexual partners compared to 16.5 for heterosexual men; lesbians reported almost exactly twice as many partners as the average heterosexual woman (9.4 and 4.6, respectively).[104] Several studies have examined the issue of sexual exclusivity in homosexual partnerships. A study of 156 stable, committed male homosexual couples found that none of the over 100 couples which had been together for more than five years had been sexually monogamous or exclusive. The authors argued that, for male couples, sexual monogamy is a passing stage of internalized homophobia and that what matters for male couples is emotional, not physical, faithfulness.[105] The second study, also of 156 gay couples, reported that the majority of the partners in the couples (62 percent) had had sexual encounters outside of the relationship in the year before the survey, and that the average number of extrarelational sexual partners for each member of the gay couples in the year before the survey was 7.1.[106] The largest study, of 1,000 gay and 800 lesbian couples, found a sexual "non-monogamy" occurrence rate across the life of the couple relationship of 79 percent and 19 percent respectively, and reported that only 36 percent of gay men and 71 percent of lesbians value sexual monogamy.[107] If one presupposes that the capacity to form and maintain exclusive monogamous erotic relationships is an essential adaptive capacity, then real difficulties for male homosexuals are

104. Laumann et al., p. 315.

105. McWhirter and Mattison, *The Male Couple.*

106. A. A. Deenen, L. Gijs, and A. X. van Naerssen, "Intimacy and Sexuality in Gay Male Couples," *Archives of Sexual Behavior* 23 (1994): 421-31.

107. Blumstein and Schwartz, findings cited on p. 317 and p. 319 (n. 9).

suggested by this research. If the psychological community de-emphasizes relational stability among its criteria of adaptiveness or healthy emotional adjustment (or if Christians do, as some would urge),[108] then promiscuity in the male homosexual community does not constitute maladjustment.

Conclusion

The evidence cited above falls far short of a convincing case that homosexuality in itself constitutes a psychopathological condition. The evidence also suggests that one would be on shaky grounds in proclaiming that there is no evidence that homosexuality is anything other than a healthy, normal lifestyle variant.

Is Change to Heterosexuality Impossible for the Homosexual?

The issue of change surfaces often in denominational documents. One discussion guide, playing off the idea of homosexuality as a willful perversion, portrayed traditionalists as believing that "The orientation of all homosexual persons can be modified to conform to the heterosexual norm through conversion and healing."[109] It is supposed that if conversion to heterosexuality can be shown to be impossible for some, the traditionalist case is considerably weakened.

However the orientation toward homosexual preference develops, there is substantial agreement that it is not a preference that can be easily changed by a simple act of the will. "Difficult to change" and "unlikely to change" are not the same, however, as "impossible to change." A number of authors argue that homosexual orientation is "immutable" or unchangeable[110] despite the fact that every study ever conducted on change from homosexual to heterosexual orientation has claimed some successes, though the reported success rates have never been very high.[111] Interpretations of these findings vary widely.

108. R. Williams, *Just as I Am: A Practical Guide to Being Out, Proud, and Christian* (New York: HarperPerennial, 1992).

109. Province VII of the Episcopal Church, p. 63.

110. E.g., Green, "Immutability of (Homo)Sexual Orientation"; also C. Burr, "Homosexuality and Biology," *Atlantic Monthly,* March 1993, pp. 47-65; Haldeman, "Practice and Ethics"; Harry, "Sexual Orientation as Destiny."

111. For a reasonably complete review of existing "conversion therapy" studies, see J. Nicolosi, *Reparative Therapy of Male Homosexuality* (New York: Jason Aronson, 1991). Critics are right to note that many of these studies lack methodological rigor and are basically compilations of independent clinical interventions. Reported success rates have hovered in the 33 to 50 percent range.

No new original research of real merit has emerged on the issue of change from homosexual orientation, with opinions varying as to whether this is because of the impossibility of obtaining positive results honestly or the impossibility of funding, conducting, and publishing a credible study in the current political environment. Haldeman has furnished the most wide-ranging and negative critique of the "conversion" literature to date, and so we will evaluate his critique. First, Haldeman demeans the conversion literature in an ad hominem fashion in numerous places, describing various studies as "founded on heterosexist bias."[112] Such a criticism is vacuous and historically myopic. Reviewers should assess methods, findings, and arguments, not the character or motivations of researchers; knowledge is not advanced when parties point and yell either "homophobe!" or "homophile!"

Second, he implies that the reported "conversions" are fraudulent, that those who are reported to have changed merely told the researcher therapists what they wanted to hear but never really changed at all. The clearest example of this is his dismissal of claims of religious healing of sexual orientation on the basis of anecdotes. There may indeed be substantial incentives for homosexual clients who are failing to experience change to dissimulate, feigning progress in order to disengage from therapy without disappointing or confronting the therapist. Haldeman's charge of fraud is possible. On the other hand, there is no evidence to support Haldeman's charge, and it verges on solipsism. Further, anecdotes lack any normative weight for the evaluation of therapeutic outcomes, negative or positive; if Haldeman finds it important to dismiss anecdotes of change, why should anecdotes of fraud or failure to change be given credence?

Third, he criticizes the conversion literature as naively founded upon essentialist assumptions about sexual orientation, with authors assuming naive and dichotomous views of "gays and straights." As quoted earlier, he states that "The categories of homosexual, heterosexual, and bisexual, considered by many researchers as fixed and dichotomous, are in reality very fluid for many." This is a very strong and valid argument which deserves careful attention. Nevertheless, in rebuttal of conversion findings he quickly drops back into essentialist assumptions himself, describing homosexuals and bisexuals as "apples and oranges"; clearly, he contradicts himself. He also describes heterosexuals as coming out as "lesbian or gay later in life" but fails to describe similar shifts in the other direction (because of a commitment to immutability?), admitting instead only that homosexual persons might later "engage in heterosexual behavior and relationships for a variety of personal and social

112. Haldeman, p. 223.

reasons."[113] The implication seems to be that "coming out" after a period of heterosexuality is a revelation of one's true sexual identity, while embracing heterosexual behavior after living in the gay lifestyle is a mere change of behavior.

Fourth, Haldeman attributes the putative successes of conversion efforts to the researchers having actually worked with a mixed sample of bisexuals and homosexuals, with resultant alterations in the behavior and perhaps inclinations of the bisexuals but not the homosexuals. He appears to have a partially valid point here. Much of the conversion literature does indeed presume to diagnose an individual as homosexual on the basis of any homosexual desires or action, so that a bisexual married man with diminished heterosexual satisfaction who engaged in impulsive impersonal homosexual acts might well have been labeled a homosexual in these studies, and then declared a "success" in conversion therapy when extramarital behavior stopped and heterosexual satisfaction improved.[114] We would agree with Haldeman that most of the prior research in this area lacks diagnostic rigor and sophistication. But this criticism must be contextualized by recognizing that broadly accepted, rigorous, and sophisticated definitions of what either homosexuality or bisexuality is simply do not exist. Most attempts at such definitions quickly fall into the essentialist trap which Haldeman claims to deplore. Further, Haldeman's criticism presumes that individuals who engage in sexual action with both genders are not "true homosexuals," but this conflicts with Harry's surprising finding that 42 percent of the gay or bisexual men in his national probability sample were married to women (and it was not just the bisexuals who were married).[115] Finally, it appears dangerously *post hoc* to examine past research and conclude, based on the a priori that homosexuality is immutable, that therefore any evidence of change must necessarily have occurred in a nonhomosexual (i.e., bisexual) subsample. At issue here is the question of whether the weight of evidence would lead us to believe that change is possible for some, or that change is actually impossible. The absolute claim that homosexuality is immutable needs only one contrary case (i.e., one case of change) to lead us to conclude that homosexuality is not always immutable, and hence not immutable.

Fifth, Haldeman criticizes as trivial what might be described as the

113. Haldeman, p. 222.

114. Blumstein and Schwartz, p. 309, make the same point about "diagnosis as homosexual" on the basis of isolated attractions or behaviors, but with an emphasis on such categorizations in the gay community, where homosexual attraction or action must mark one's "true" orientation.

115. Harry, "Probability Sample."

grafting of heterosexual action over a homosexual orientation without more basic change.[116] He critically quotes another author who described the change process as an "adaptation" which allows the client to function in heterosexual marriage while homosexual fantasies and attractions, and possibly behavior, never go away completely. He calls such change processes a "laboratory for heterosexual behavior, rather than a change of sexual orientation," and criticizes those who are "eager to equate heterosexual competence with orientation change."[117] In this view, any residual of homosexual attraction or action is taken as indication of treatment failure. Again, this criticism must be partially valid, in that mere behavior change (the lesbian wife who endures sexual intercourse with her husband by engaging in homosexual fantasy) falls short of a profound and pervasive change of orientation. But on the other hand, given how deeply rooted and pervasive we must understand sexual orientation to be, surely it is an overly stringent standard of success to demand that psychotherapeutic treatment of any sort must eradicate all vestiges of homosexual attraction and firmly establish heterosexual eroticism to be deemed successful. Such a stringent standard would never pass the test of generalization to other human conditions; we would not declare alcoholism treatment to be a failure on the basis of recurring attraction to or even occasional relapses into alcohol consumption, nor would we declare depression treatment unsuccessful on the basis of treated individuals needing to combat tendencies to reexperience depression. Haldeman's easy dismissal of change reports on the basis of some continuing homosexual attraction, fantasy, or even action seems impossibly harsh.

What can be concluded from the change literature? We would not share the optimistic and seemingly universal generalization of some conservative authors that "healing is possible for homosexuals who are motivated to change,"[118] if change is taken to mean complete alteration of sexual orientation to replace homosexual with heterosexual erotic orientation. Even the most optimistic empirically grounded spokespersons for change by psychological means say change is most likely when motivation is strong, when there is a history of successful heterosexual functioning, when gender identity issues are not present, and when involvement in actual homosexual practice has been minimal. Change of homosexual orientation may well be impossible for some by any natural means. Yet the obverse position that homosexuality is

116. See Green, "Immutability of (Homo)Sexual Orientation," p. 569, for similar criticisms.

117. Haldeman, p. 223.

118. B. Davies and L. Rentzel, *Coming Out of Homosexuality: New Freedom for Men and Women* (Downers Grove, Ill.: InterVarsity, 1994), p. 25.

immutable seems questionable in light of reports of successful change. In informal ecclesiastical dialogue, reports of change by psychological or supernatural means are frequently dismissed by anecdotes such as "I tried that ministry (therapy), and it was a complete failure; I know lots of people who claimed to change by that means, but they are now out in the gay lifestyle!" Yet it is standard in professional circles to recognize that such anecdotes have no power to either establish or discredit the efficacy of a change method. In that light, it is troubling that the many Christian ministries which attempt to provide opportunities for growth and healing for the homosexual person rarely if ever study and report their success rates.[119]

Conclusion

Citations of the scientific findings appear frequently, casually, and with great imprecision in ecclesiastical debates about the morality of homosexual behavior. We would argue, based upon our review, that the "findings of science" are not as clear as is commonly assumed, and that the logical implications of the findings of science are far less clear than is casually assumed in ecclesiastical study documents. We have just gone to great lengths to establish the former point; let us now expand on the latter.

To repeat the essence of an argument we have made before,[120] even if the scientific findings in the four areas we have examined were clear and unequivocal, their relevance to the moral debate would still be less than decisive. The prevalence of a particular behavior pattern has no clear relevance to the moral evaluation of that pattern; patterns which are common or uncommon may be immoral or moral. Even if the types of results which might be presumed to be more favorable to the moral acceptance of homosexual behavior were attained, namely, a high prevalence level of 10 percent or more, this would seem to only move homosexual behavior, in the evaluation of the traditionalist, from a less common to a more common sinful pattern; the high prevalence of pride, greed, and fornication seems to have little bearing on their morality.

119. For further discussion of the ethical concerns raised in the treatment of homosexual clients, see M. A. Yarhouse and S. L. Jones, "The Homosexual Client," in *Christian Counseling Ethics,* ed. R. K. Sanders (Downers Grove, Ill.: InterVarsity, 1997).

120. Jones and Yarhouse, "Recent Scientific Research"; Jones and Workman, "Homosexuality"; S. Jones, "1993 Addendum," in *Homosexuality in the Church: Both Sides of the Debate,* ed. J. S. Siker (Louisville: Westminster/John Knox, 1994), pp. 107-15.

There is a need for greater sophistication in our thinking about how etiology should influence our moral reasoning. The ecclesiastical literature often inappropriately collapses the notion of causation of probabilistic proclivities together with the causation of specific behaviors, and seems to presume that documentation of any causal influence whatsoever somehow utterly obviates moral responsibility. Both moves are unwarranted. Further, it is common to assume that "sin," as a class, can only include those behavioral choices which the person embraces in an utterly voluntary and uncoerced manner (including having no predisposition toward any particular class of acts) while knowing that the action is a violation of the law of God. This is problematic; such logic would force the church to throw out the possibility of moral evaluation of many conditions other than homosexuality which have also been shown to have contributing causes, such as antisocial personality disorder[121] and alcoholism.[122] The church's moral concern is not fundamentally with homosexual orientation (nor with a proclivity to drunkenness or violence and victimization), but with what one does with it. Only in the case of extreme biological determination at the level of individual acts would moral culpability be seen properly as eliminated. But homosexual persons are not subhuman robots whose acts are predetermined — they are moral agents who inherit tendencies from biology and environment, and who share in shaping their character by the responses they make to their tendencies and life situations. Like all persons, they must ask, "This is what I want to do, but is it what I should do?" The existence of proclivities or predispositions does not obviate the need for moral evaluation of those proclivities themselves nor the behavior they incline one toward. The shift in preferred etiological variables from psychological to biological is immaterial to the ethical debates; there is no reason to think that establishment of either type of causation (nor their conjunction in interactionist accounts) fundamentally alters human accountability for what one does with the proclivities one receives, nor that proclivities established by psychological rather than biological influences are any easier to alter or resist. The confluence of our existing evidences suggests that biological variables are involved in shaping sexual orientation for many, and even powerfully for some. These findings neither obviate moral responsibility for what is done with those proclivities nor obliterate our responsibility for

121. P. B. Sutker, F. Bugg, and J. A. West, "Antisocial Personality Disorder," in *Comprehensive Handbook of Psychopathology,* ed. H. Adams and P. Sutker, 2nd ed. (New York: Plenum, 1993), pp. 337-69.

122. K. Kendler, A. Heath, M. Neale, R. Kessler, and L. Evans, "A Population-Based Twin Study of Alcoholism in Women," *Journal of the American Medical Association* 268 (1992): 1877-82.

cultivating dispositions more in accord with God's revealed will for our lives. Research on etiology may enrich pastoral guidance by deepening our understanding of the forces which influence our behavior, but there is no compelling reason for expecting it to fundamentally transform our ethical evaluation.

Ethical pathology and psychological pathology (or abnormality) are not coterminous; there is no necessary overlap between sinfulness and status as a psychopathology. Many conditions which are "sins" are not pathologies (idolatry, pride, lust, fornication), and many conditions which are pathologies are not in themselves sins (anxiety, depression, psychosis). Thus, the status of contemporary debate on the "healthy lifestyle variant" or pathology status of homosexuality is largely irrelevant to the church's moral evaluation of homosexual behavior.

Finally, there is no direct and formal relevance of the efficacy of change methods to the moral or ecclesiastical argument. The fundamental teaching of the Christian tradition with regard to sexual ethics is that God wills chastity in marriage and celibacy outside of marriage. This standard does not require (or promise) change in orientation. It may be that the church can no more guarantee healing to egodystontic homosexuals than it can guarantee healing to married but sexually dysfunctional heterosexuals or marriage to disconsolate single heterosexuals.

Does the scientific research speak in any definitive way to the ethical and ecclesiastical debates of the Christian church? No. Kendler's comments about psychology specifically would seem applicable to all scientific research: "Psychology, conceived as either the human science of consciousness or the natural science of behavior, cannot validate moral imperatives and therefore cannot support social policies because of their presumed ethical underpinnings." Further, the church, like empirical or what Kendler calls "natural science psychology," must "abandon two seductive myths: (a) Psychology is able to identify ethical principles that should guide humankind, and (b) the logical gap between is and ought can be bridged by empirical evidence."[123] We would reject, however, the utter independence of science and ethical analysis. Good science should inform ethical analysis. Ethical and theological analysis should proceed in the context of the best understandings of the subject matter under consideration, and science can provide us with valuable insights and understandings. While science can and should inform our ethical analysis, it will not determine the outcome of that analysis.

123. H. H. Kendler, "Psychology and the Ethics of Social Policy," *American Psychologist* 48 (1993): 1046-53, quotes pp. 1050 and 1052.

We close by returning full circle. The two main reasons for the casual citation of scientific findings in this ethical debate by proponents of change in the church's traditional stance have been to undermine the assumptions that seem to be behind the traditional moral judgment and to support the removal of homosexual acts as such from the category of acts that can be judged as immoral in and of themselves. Regarding the former, when the traditionalist stance is painted as assuming that homosexuality is statistically rare, manifestly perverse and necessarily intertwined with deep pathology, and freely chosen on the basis of religious rebellion and perversity and thus easily amenable to change by the penitent, these assumptions can be seemingly demolished by recourse to scientific findings. We have shown that science does not speak as unequivocally nor univocally to these issues as is often imagined. Further, despite the discordant voices in the traditionalist camp, the distilled essence of the traditionalist argument has little to do with the caricature presented. The traditionalist argument is essentially that God has revealed that heterosexual union in marriage or chastity are the two desired outcomes with regard to genital sexual experience for which God created humans, and that God commands us to refrain from all noncommended sexual behaviors, including homosexual ones, regardless of the sources of our urges to do otherwise.

Regarding the latter reason for invoking science, that science supports the removal of homosexual acts as such from the category of acts that can be judged as immoral in and of themselves, the flow of the argument seems to be as follows: Scientific research shows essentialism to be true in a variety of ways. If homosexual identity is a "real thing," then it must be a core characteristic of the person which is in itself neutral and only suitable for moral evaluation as it is manifested in behavior. That behavior must be evaluated morally by standards generally applicable to all behavior and in the light that it is expressive of the "natural" essence of the person. There are problems with this line of reasoning at every point. Science does not prove essentialism to be true; it rather usually presumes it in the same way that political surveys assume that Republicans and Democrats are real categorizations. Further, science cannot validate or invalidate the ethical conclusions which seem so frequently drawn from essentialism. It cannot establish the ethical neutrality of homosexual orientation, cannot establish what ethical standards should be used to evaluate it, and cannot establish an ethical vision of moral normalcy.

Science will not solve the ethical debate about homosexual behavior for the church; "the moral and political issues must be resolved on other grounds,"[124] even if science can contribute positively to the church's ethical

124. Bancroft, p. 439.

deliberations. Science is often invoked in the church's debates for rhetorical rather than substantive purposes. Even if what some proponents of change regard as the most "optimistic" scientific scenario were realized — that homosexuality were found to be common, utterly unassociated with psychological distress, clearly and determinatively caused by genetic factors, and the orientation itself utterly immutable — the traditionalist vision of sexual morality would still have to be engaged on ethical and theological grounds, not on the grounds of science.

CHAPTER 4

The Bible and Science on Sexuality

CHRISTINE E. GUDORF

The Bible and Science as Interpreted Sources

This paper examines the ethical status of biblical evaluations of homosexuality in the light of scientific research, both biological and social scientific. I would reiterate some of Dr. Jones's and Dr. Yarhouse's basic points on scientific research: (1) studies of homosexuality have defined terms such as "homosexuality," "heterosexuality," and "bisexuality" very differently; (2) representative samples of homosexual persons are difficult to obtain; (3) many studies have not been confirmed or replicated; and (4) science cannot decide the morality of homosexuality for the Christian churches because the moral status of homosexuality is not a scientific question. While largely concurring with Dr. Jones's and Dr. Yarhouse's treatment of scientific research, I will dispute their position regarding fundamental Christian teaching: God's standard for homosexual persons would continue to be the same as for all persons — chastity in marriage or celibacy outside of marriage.

My understanding of the status of the Bible as a resource for Christian ethics, stated baldly, has three aspects. First, the Bible is *a* (not *the*) primary resource for Christian ethics; to approach the Bible as the sole and absolute source of revelation is idolatry, the worship of a text rather than the one true living God who was definitively revealed in Jesus Christ and continues to be revealed in history. Second, the Bible always requires interpretation. The New Testament makes clear that Jesus himself was involved in debating the interpretation of the Old Testament. All texts are context-bound, because language itself is context-bound. Third, the interpretation of biblical texts must be consistent; there can be no biblical grounds for reinterpreting biblical attitudes or teachings on other sexual or ethical issues, such as divorce, slavery, marriage, or the role of women, but insisting that biblical teaching on homosexuality is timeless, universal, uninterpreted, and exceptionless.

Neither is science, whether biological or social, without need of interpretation. Scientific research can and does suffer from design flaws and/or researcher bias, in addition to various problems in interpreting results. Results of individual studies need to be placed within the overall framework of previous research in the area; periodically, new research results which do not fit within the existing paradigm are either discredited or augmented until they suggest a new paradigm which gradually replaces the old. A period of paradigm shift regarding homosexuality has been under way for four decades, beginning in the social sciences and more recently extending to the biological sciences. To say this is not to posit the evolving paradigm for understanding homosexuality as the final scientific word; the late twentieth-century paradigm for understanding homosexuality may be no more adequate than the one it replaced. But at the moment it is this most recent paradigm which best explains the data concerning homosexuality, though, as Jones and Yarhouse point out, not without some overstatements, inconsistencies, and even internal contradictions from some proponents.

Science on Sexuality

The most fundamental insight of recent social science regarding homosexuality concerns the discovery of sexual orientation, that is, the discovery that sexual attraction in humans is neither uniformly heterosexual nor continuously plastic and fully open to manipulation by the will. Sexual orientation, understood in terms of the object of one's sexual attraction, exists on a spectrum between exclusively heterosexual and exclusively homosexual, and for most persons in this culture is fixed relatively early in life. Kinsey's research in the late forties and early fifties laid out a spectrum of sexual orientation repeatedly confirmed in studies ever since, with only minor modifications as to percentages of the populations in different areas of the spectrum.[1]

1. A. Kinsey, W. Pomeroy, and C. Martin, *Sexual Behavior in the Human Male* (Philadelphia: Saunders, 1948), pp. 636-59; and A. Kinsey, W. Pomeroy, C. Martin, and P. Gebhard, *Sexual Behavior in the Human Female* (Philadelphia: Saunders, 1953), pp. 468-69.

Though many persons with homosexual orientations have insisted that their discovery of this orientation began in early childhood, this insight arises in hindsight and is difficult to verify. Today there is general consensus that discovery of a predominantly homosexual orientation occurs during adolescence for most males and some females, and after adolescence for most females. For some males adolescent homosexual experimentation merely confirms and does not initiate the sense of being homosexual.[2] Despite the report of psychoanalyst Irving Bieber in 1962 that he had been successful in changing the sexual orientation of 27 percent of his sample of gay men,[3] later studies had far less success. Much of the success they did have seems to have been in convincing homosexual and bisexual persons not to act on their homosexual desires, a decision which often did not endure long-term.[4] While there is a great deal of controversy as to whether or not it is ever possible to reverse a sexual orientation once fixed, there is general agreement that, at the very least, sexual orientation seems extremely resistant to change, even in persons motivated strongly enough to seek out expensive and physically and/or emotionally painful change therapies.[5]

Such psychological research on sexual orientation led some denominations, for example, Roman Catholicism in 1975, to declare that homosexual orientation was not in itself sinful because it did not always seem to be personally chosen.[6] However, Rome continued to forbid acting upon this orientation, and later clarified that homosexual orientation, though not sinful, was not to be considered natural or normal, but rather disordered, in that it could easily lead to sin since it, unlike heterosexual orientation, has no legitimate outlet for sexual desire.[7] This is a relatively common position in Christianity.

2. William H. Masters, Virginia H. Johnson, and Robert C. Kolodny, *Human Sexualities* (San Francisco: Harper Collins, 1992), pp. 399-400, referring to studies by Dank, 1971; Weinberg, 1978; Cass, 1979; Stanley and Wolf, 1980; Troiden and Goode, 1980.

3. Irving Bieber, *Homosexuality: A Psychoanalytic Study* (New York: Basic Books, 1962), p. 276.

4. Janell L. Carroll and Paul Root Wolpe, *Sexuality and Gender in Society* (San Francisco: Harper Collins, 1996), p. 244.

5. R. Green, "The Immutability of (Homo)Sexual Orientation: Behavioral Science Implications for a Constitutional (Legal) Analysis," *Journal of Psychiatry and the Law* 16 (1988): 537-75.

6. See the Congregation for the Doctrine of the Faith, "Declaration on Certain Issues concerning Sexual Ethics," 29 December 1975, #8, in A. Kosnik et al., *Human Sexuality: New Directions in American Catholic Thought* (New York: Paulist, 1977), pp. 299-313.

7. Congregation for the Doctrine of the Faith, Letter to the U.S. Bishops, "On the Pastoral Care of Homosexual Persons," 31 October 1986.

The discovery of sexual orientation has greatly complicated discussion of homosexuality and, of course, heterosexuality. Scientists agree, for example, that both a celibate person whose sexual fantasy is almost exclusively with same-sex partners and a person whose sexual partners are predominantly of the same sex have a homosexual orientation. But persons with predominantly heterosexual partners and homosexual sexual fantasies are described as heterosexual, homosexual, or bisexual by different researchers.

Thus homosexuality, like all sexuality, is complex; this complexity challenges traditional Christian pastoral practice as well as ethics. The pastoral advice traditionally given to homosexual men in the church has been to marry, because the church shared with Saint Paul the assumption of original human heterosexual orientation. Such pastoral advice has created situations of great suffering for many husbands, wives, and children because sexual orientation is not a matter of a choice by the will.

Neither is it determined solely by the sex of one's partners; some persons with homosexual orientation and identity are celibate, just as some persons with heterosexual orientation are celibate. Bell and Weinberg's research revealed that 16 percent of men and 11 percent of women with homosexual orientation fit a category called "asexuals." They are loners with characteristically little or no sexual interest or activity.[8] For most contemporary Christian teaching which recognizes the existence of homosexual orientation, this asexual category represents the path of virtue for those with homosexual orientation. Yet Bell and Weinberg found asexuals had the highest incidence of suicidal thoughts, high rates of therapeutic counseling, considerable difficulty in simply coping with life, and were relatively isolated from others.[9]

Essentialism and Constructionism

Dr. Jones and Dr. Yarhouse referred to the current debate as to whether homosexuality — and heterosexuality as well — should be understood in terms of essentialism or social construction. Essentialism posits that one's sexual orientation manifests something innate, or biological/genetic, in oneself, while constructionism points to ways in which different sexual orientations are constructed through the interaction of social forces on human persons.

8. Alan P. Bell and Martin S. Weinberg, *Homosexualities* (New York: Simon & Schuster, 1978), pp. 134, 137.

9. Bell and Weinberg, pp. 173, 181-82, 184, 199-201, esp. p. 207.

There is evidence to support both sides, which usually indicates flawed construction of the categories.

The strong assumption in traditional Christianity that heterosexuality was basic to human nature and homosexuality a deliberately chosen perversity gradually gave way in the late nineteenth and early twentieth century to an understanding of homosexuality as a kind of disease with environmental causes. Thus early explanations were constructionist in their understanding of homosexuality and essentialist in their understandings of heterosexuality; in the later twentieth century constructionism has prevailed. Although Freud considered male homosexuality neither a vice nor an illness, and opposed identifying it as degenerate,[10] he also explained its source as an unresolved Oedipus complex. He proposed that an intense relationship with his mother, coupled with a distant father figure, could trigger in the young boy an association of penis-less women with fear of castration, resulting in homosexual orientation. Other psychologists as well pointed to intense relationships between boys and their affectionate (and sometimes, as for Bieber, overly intimate and seductive) mothers, often compounded by distant or absent fathers, as producing homosexual orientation in sons.[11] The basic problem with this theory of causation was that, although this pattern was more frequent among homosexual than heterosexual groups of men, the lives of many homosexual men did *not* manifest such a pattern; conversely, such a pattern was present in the lives of significant numbers of men with *heterosexual* orientation. Contemporary explanations of homosexual orientation include gender-role nonconformity, peer group interaction, and behaviorism. Gender-role nonconformity studies have shown some correlation between boys who exhibit "girlish" behavior traits and later adult homosexual orientation. Green, for example, compared fifty-six "masculine" boys with sixty-six boys who cross-dressed; played with dolls; avoided rough play; wished to be girls; were rejected, harassed, and ignored by peers; and were considerably more sickly than their peers. Three-fourths of these later exhibited homosexual or bisexual orientation, while only one of the fifty-six "masculine" boys grew up to be bisexual.[12] However, one cannot know

10. Sigmund Freud, *Three Essays on the Theory of Sexuality*, trans. James Strachey (New York: Avon Books, 1962), pp. 25-26.

11. Sandor Rado followed Freud in understanding homosexuality in terms of the Oedipus complex gone wrong, but disagreed with Freud about the naturalness of bisexuality in early childhood. See Sandor Rado, "An Adaptional View of Sexual Behavior," in *Psychoanalysis of Behavior: Collected Papers* (New York: Grune & Stratton, 1949; rev. ed, 1955), pp. 196-98, and Bieber, p. 47.

12. R. Green, *The "Sissy Boy Syndrome" and the Development of Homosexuality* (New Haven: Yale University Press, 1987), p. 99.

if the "girlish" behavior indicated some physiological/developmental difference from other boys (essentialism), or if society's reaction to these boys' unconventional behavior encouraged them to develop a homosexual orientation (constructionism).

Peer group interaction theories, such as that of Storms, observe that children whose adolescent sexual development begins early experience sexual arousal before they have much contact with the other sex; their erotic feelings, therefore, are more likely to focus on the same sex. Persons of homosexual orientation do report earlier sexual contacts than do those of heterosexual orientation. Since boys' sex drive as measured by masturbation rates seems to emerge at earlier ages than girls', this theory could also perhaps explain why there are more male homosexuals than lesbians.[13] On the other hand, the sex of partners available at the time of the onset of adolescent sex drive cannot by itself explain sexual orientation in other cultural situations. For example, according to Gilbert Herdt, Sambian boys in New Guinea are taken from their mothers at age seven and live in a communal boys' house until marriage at about age nineteen, in order to be weaned from mother's milk to men's milk (semen) so that they can develop into men. Young Sambian boys are required to fellate the older boys regularly; after puberty they are fellated by the younger boys until marriage, at which point their sexual behavior becomes exclusively heterosexual, although some adult men report homosexual fantasizing.[14]

Behaviorist theories of sexual orientation point to positive sexual experiences with one sex and uncomfortable or frightening sexual experiences with the other sex as determining the direction of sexual orientation. Fantasizing on positive sexual experiences during masturbation may further reinforce their strength. Supporting evidence comes from the research of Van Wyck, who found that those who learned to masturbate by being manually stimulated by persons of the same sex and whose first orgasm took place in a same-sex context are more likely to have a homosexual orientation as adults.[15] Again, however, it is impossible to know whether the sexual experience led to the orientation or some innate predisposition to the orientation led to the experience.

13. M. D. Storms, "Theories of Sexual Orientation," *Journal of Personality and Social Psychology* 38 (1980): 783-92; Storms, "A Theory of Erotic Orientation Development," *Psychological Review* 88 (1981): 783-92.

14. Gilbert Herdt, *Guardians of the Flutes: Idioms of Masculinity* (New York: McGraw-Hill, 1981), pp. 232-39.

15. P. Van Wyck, "Psychosocial Development of Heterosexual, Bisexual and Homosexual Behavior," *Archives of Sexual Behavior* 13 (1984): 505-45.

Recent genetic and psychological studies have been touted as supporting essentialism. Though Kallman reported in his 1952 twin study that among homosexual males who had male twins, 100 percent of the identical twins were homosexual and 12 percent of fraternal twins were homosexual, his study was largely dismissed as unreliable; 100 percent outcomes are highly suspect.[16] More recently, Bailey and his colleagues did a number of studies of twins and discovered that, beginning with a population of sexually active men with homosexual orientation, 52 percent of their identical twins, 22 percent of their fraternal twins, and 11 percent of their adoptive brothers were also homosexuals. Among females, 48 percent of the identical twins, 16 percent of the fraternal twins, and 6 percent of the adoptive sisters of lesbians were likely to share their lesbian orientation. Bailey and colleagues also found that homosexual males were more likely to have lesbian sisters and that lesbians were more likely to have homosexual brothers.[17] These studies indicate some genetic basis for sexual orientation, but also some environmental influence at work. With a solely genetic basis, 100 percent of identical twins would share homosexual orientation, and the rate of homosexuality in adoptive siblings would not exceed the incidence of homosexuality in the general population (closer to 2-4 percent than the 6-11 percent of the study).

Further genetic evidence comes from the research of Dean Hamer of the National Cancer Institute, who found that men with homosexual orientations tend to have more relatives with homosexual orientation on their mother's side than do other men. Focusing on homosexual men from such families, Hamer discovered the existence of a gene pattern, passed through the mother, which he located in thirty-three of forty gay brothers.[18] Two studies, in 1990 and 1991, by Swaab and LeVay found physiological differences in the brains of homosexual and heterosexual men, specifically in the hypothalamus.[19] However, these autopsy studies cannot disclose whether dif-

16. F. J. Kallman, "Comparative Twin Study on the Genetic Aspects of Male Homosexuality," *Journal of Nervous and Mental Disease* 115 (1952): 283-98.

17. J. M. Bailey and A. P. Bell, "Familiarity of Female and Male Homosexuality," *Behavior Genetics* 23 (1993): 313-22; J. M. Bailey and D. S. Benishay, "Familial Aggregation of Female Sexual Orientation," *American Journal of Psychiatry* 150 (1993): 272-77; J. M. Bailey and R. C. Pillard, "A Genetic Study of Male Sexual Orientation," *Archives of General Psychiatry* 48, no. 12 (1991): 1089-96, and T. Lidz, "A Reply," with response from Bailley and Pillard, 50, no. 3 (1993): 240-41.

18. D. H. Hamer et al., "A Linkage between DNA Markers on the X Chromosome and Male Sexual Orientation," *Science* 261 (1993): 321-27.

19. D. F. Swaab and M. A. Hofman, "An Enlarged Suprachiasmatic Nucleus in Homosexual Men," *Brain Research* 537 (1990): 141-48; S. LeVay, "A Difference in Hypothalamic Structure between Heterosexual and Homosexual Men," *Science* 253 (1991): 1034-37.

ferences were present from birth or developed later in life, or whether differences were due to sexual orientation rather than some intervening pathology, such as AIDS.

While these studies point to some biological foundation for sexual orientation, most point to nongenetic influences at work as well; none of them define how or to what extent sexual orientation is determined in individuals. Because these studies argue forcefully against a purely environmental or constructionist origin of homosexual orientation, they also undermine the plausibility of the heterosexist assumptions in Romans 1, in which Paul implies that homosexuality is a deviation from divine creation, as are the sins he lists in verses 29-31. Through the mid–twentieth century social science research on homosexuals similarly linked homosexuality to both criminality and various psychological pathologies, due to the way the research populations were chosen. Many studies of homosexuality done in the fifties and earlier chose research populations of homosexuals which consisted exclusively of prison inmates and patients in mental hospitals or psychiatric treatment programs. It was not surprising that results pointed to homosexuality as itself pathological and immoral.

This attitude began to radically change with Evelyn Hooker's groundbreaking 1957 work.[20] Hooker collected the life histories and conducted extensive psychological testing of thirty gay and thirty straight noninstitutionalized men matched for age, education, and IQ, and submitted the results to expert psychologists without identifying the orientation of the subjects. The raters could not distinguish between the two groups. These results were confirmed by the series of studies done by Saghir and Robins in 1973: selected nonpatient homosexuals and heterosexuals show no significant differences in terms of psychological health, criminality, dependability, or social responsibility.[21] While it is true that the homosexual individuals examined were not necessarily representative of that population, and thus one cannot conclude that the heterosexual and homosexual populations are equal in character or adjustment, these studies do suggest that sexual orientation per se is not a pathology. As Bell and Weinberg point out, there are a variety of homosexualities, just as there are a variety of heterosexualities. In their own research, coupled homosexuals were virtually indistinguishable from heterosexual marrieds in terms of sexual behavior, personal adjustment, and rela-

20. Evelyn Hooker, "The Adjustment of the Male Overt Homosexual," *Journal of Projective Techniques* 21 (1957): 18-31.

21. Marcel T. Saghir and Eli Robins, *Male and Female Homosexuality: A Comprehensive Investigation* (Baltimore: Williams & Wilkins, 1973).

tionship patterns, just as asexual homosexuals and asexual heterosexuals shared the same personal traits and social difficulties.[22]

Some types of wickedness most stereotypically attributed to those with homosexual orientation are not, in fact, characteristic of them and may even be more characteristic of those with heterosexual orientation. For example, homosexuals are often accused of seducing or molesting the young into homosexuality, but Bell and Weinberg conclude:

> the seduction of innocents far more likely involves an older male, often a relative, and a pre- or postpubescent female. Moreover, rape and sexual violence occur more frequently in a heterosexual than a homosexual context. Rape (outside of prisons) generally involves sexual attacks made by men upon women, while the relatively rare violence occurring in a homosexual context is usually the result of male youths "hunting queers" or a man's guilt and disgust over a sexual episode just concluded.[23]

Peplau studied the similarities and differences in homosexual and heterosexual relationships and found that the differences have more to do with sex (whether the partners are men or women) than with sexual orientation.[24] In the same vein, younger homosexual people are more sexually active than older homosexual people, just as are younger heterosexual people compared to older heterosexual people.[25]

However, some types of vice *are* more prevalent among homosexual

22. Bell and Weinberg, pp. 198-223, 230-31.

23. Bell and Weinberg, p. 230. While it is clear that the great majority of sex with children/youth is heterosexual (as are the majority of adult potential abusers) and that first affairs of homosexuals are with partners closer in age than in first affairs of heterosexuals, I am not aware of any study focused on comparing proportionate rates of child/youth sexual abuse by homosexuals and heterosexuals.

24. This is especially true of what many have termed "homosexual promiscuity," meaning casual sex with large numbers of partners. In fact, lesbians have the smallest number of sexual partners over a lifetime, followed by heterosexual women, followed by heterosexual men, followed by homosexual men. Studies show that while each group contains both persons with few partners and persons with many partners, because women are more likely to see sex as appropriate within committed relationships and men are more likely to separate sex from intimacy, heterosexual sex seems to be a compromise between the male and female sexual patterns (L. A. Peplau, "What Homosexuals Want in Relationships," *Psychology Today* 15 [1981]: 28-38; B. Leigh, "Reasons for Having and Avoiding Sex: Gender, Sexual Orientation and Relationship to Sexual Behavior," *Journal of Sex Research* 26 [1989]: 199-208; L. Markowitz, "Homosexuality: Are We Still in the Dark?" *Networker*, January/February 1991, pp. 27-35).

25. Bell and Weinberg, pp. 69-72.

populations. Homosexual men and women are substantially more likely to use alcohol, marijuana, and cocaine, and to have higher rates of alcoholism.[26] Persons with homosexual orientation are also more likely to have been in therapy, though, contrary to long-standing assumptions, studies of aging gay men and lesbians show no higher rates of psychopathology.[27] Higher rates of therapy are typical of more urban populations, and homosexuality is disproportionately urban in the United States. While it is possible to interpret higher rates of alcoholism and psychological therapy for homosexual persons as evidence of the sinfulness of homosexual behavior, such an argument is inherently dangerous: statistics for other minority populations, including racial minorities, migrant workers, and the most severely impoverished in general, demonstrate similar patterns, yet few would want to morally stigmatize poor, dark-skinned, or migrant populations. A link more likely than depravity between these populations and the homosexual population is discrimination and low social status. Strong cultural homophobia, which makes the lives of homosexual persons much more difficult, is generally understood as one important factor in elevated use of alcohol, drugs, and therapy among homosexual persons.

Homosexual persons are generally understood as more promiscuous than other persons. Yet histories which include many sexual partners are not universal among gay men, and 57 percent of lesbians have fewer than ten sexual partners in a lifetime (compared to 42 percent of married persons). At the same time, 41 percent of homosexual men in Bell and Weinberg's 1978 study reported over five hundred lifetime partners, while the 1993 Janus Report lists only 5 percent of married persons and 15 percent of divorced persons as having more than one hundred lifetime partners.[28] In addition, homosexual men who are coupled have casual sex outside their primary relationships at

26. D. J. McKirnan and P. L. Peterson, "Alcohol and Drug Use among Homosexual Men and Women," *Addictive Behaviors* 14 (1989): 545-53; D. P. McWhirter and A. M. Mattison, *The Male Couple: How Relationships Develop* (Englewood Cliffs, N.J.: Prentice-Hall, 1984); J. A. Lee, "Invisible Men: Canada's Aging Homosexuals: Can They Be Assimilated into Canada's 'Liberated' Gay Communities?" *Canadian Journal on Aging* 8 (1989): 79-97; A. Lipman, "Homosexual Relationships," *Generations* 10, no. 4 (1986): 51-54; S. Deevy, "Older Lesbian Women: An Invisible Minority," *Journal of Gerontological Nursing* 16 (1990): 35-39.

27. R. C. Pillard, "Sexual Orientation and Mental Disorder," *Psychiatric Annals* 18 (1988): 52-56.

28. S. S. S. Janus and C. L. Janus, *The Janus Report on Sexual Behavior* (New York: Wiley, 1993), p. 163; Bell and Weinberg, p. 308. (Bell and Weinberg's research was done between 1970 and 1978, before the AIDS crisis, which has considerably lowered incidence of casual sex in the gay population and increased the likelihood of coupled gays.)

much higher rates than any other coupled group.[29] Nevertheless, it is difficult to interpret promiscuity as evidence of the sinfulness of homosexuality in general given that the lesbian pattern is so similar to and in some measures less promiscuous than that of heterosexual women. Furthermore, the ability to maintain permanent, satisfying sexual partnerships is affected by such factors as the legal status of the partnership, attitudes of employers and society toward the partnership, and family support for the partnership. In all these factors homosexual unions are distinctly disadvantaged.[30]

Biblical Theology on Homosexuality

I leave the task of exegesis to the biblical scholars and restrict myself to biblical theological themes in Christian ethics on homosexuality.

Covenant

Covenant offers no basis for a blanket prohibition on homosexual activity. The Old Testament covenant is not the New Testament covenant; Christianity explicitly abandoned the purity laws under which homosexuality had been banned in the Old Testament. Furthermore, to the extent that an image of the Mosaic covenant did carry over into Christianity through the marital metaphor (first used for Yahweh/Israel) applied to the relationship of Christ and the church, it cannot serve to make sex/gender complementarity normative. Metaphors are one-directional; they point out similarity in one aspect of two entities. The point of the marital metaphor was to recognize in the relationship of Yahweh and Israel some key qualities which had not been conveyed in the impersonal political associations of "covenant" as treaty. Some qualities involved in both relationships have been identified as trust, intimacy, permanence, and

29. This was especially true because the open-coupled portion of the homosexual sample was proportionately larger than in the heterosexual sample; there was little difference between the close-coupled homosexual and close-coupled heterosexual groups. R. A. Isay, *Being Homosexual: Gay Men and Their Development* (New York: Farrar, Straus & Giroux, 1989); B. Leigh, "Reasons for Having and Avoiding Sex: Gender, Sexual Orientation and Relationship to Sexual Behavior," *Journal of Sex Research* 26 (1989): 199-209; Bell and Weinberg, pp. 85-94, 231.

30. Patricia Beattie Jung and Ralph F. Smith, *Heterosexism: An Ethical Challenge* (New York: SUNY Press, 1993), pp. 184-85.

complementarity, among others. It would be nonsensical to use this heterosexual metaphor to condemn intimacy between same-sex persons, since the metaphor's original use was to assert the intimacy between a masculine God and a collection of Israelite males. The fact that the official sign of the Mosaic covenant was penile circumcision makes this clear. In Christianity, although women were a part both of the group following Jesus and of the early first-century church leadership, recent biblical scholarship has illuminated how by the second century women were being pushed out of leadership positions and made to conform to prevailing patriarchal sex roles.[31] By the fourth century Augustine said with impunity in the Christian community that men are made in the image of God in themselves, but women are made in the image of God only when joined to their husbands.[32] Thus Christianity very early exhibited the same general pattern as in the Old Testament: men are the mediators between God and women, and the covenant is essentially between masculine beings. To give normative status to *heterosexuality* on the basis of a heterosexual metaphor applied to what has been almost exclusively understood as a same-sex relationship is absurd. It would make more sense to argue for acceptance of same-sex marriage, given that the biblical marital metaphor was applied to what was concretely a same-sex relationship in which the male collectivities were historically feminized under the guise of "Israel" and "church." If the marital metaphor for the covenant makes heterosexuality normative, then, since Jesus Christ was/is a male, shouldn't both Jewish and Christian covenants join the divine masculine to human females?[33] The price of attempting to literalize biblical metaphors regarding sex is absurdity.

The distinction commonly made between contract and covenant in Christian theology, based on the assumed intentions of Paul and the Israelite authors who used the marital metaphor, with contract interpreted juridically and covenant as more interpersonal, suggests that covenantal approaches define marriage as a relationship of sexual partners who pledge love and commitment to each other. Legalistic requirements of opposite sex and intention to procreate are not necessarily central.[34]

31. Elisabeth Schüssler Fiorenza, *In Memory of Her: A Feminist Theological Reconstruction of Christian Origins* (New York: Continuum, 1988), pp. 205-342.

32. Augustine, *On Christian Grace and Original Sin,* 2.40, in *The Nicene and Post-Nicene Fathers,* ed. P. Schaff (Edinburgh: T. & T. Clark; Grand Rapids: Eerdmans, 1987), pp. 251-52.

33. This is one of the questions that Howard Eilberg Schwartz explores in his provocative book, *God's Phallus and Other Problems for Men and Monotheism* (Boston: Beacon Press, 1994).

34. Jung and Smith, pp. 158-59.

One problem in advocating homosexual unions in terms of Christian marriage is that Paul does not use gender-neutral language in his discussion of marriage, but rather speaks of husbands and wives, men and women. But if gendered biblical language is always to be literally interpreted, women can only live on the margins of the church, if at all. A great gulf looms between those who find homosexual unions unacceptable because Paul's language on permissible sex is heterosexual and those who find Paul's arguments on the permissibility of marriage and sex capable of logical extension from heterosexuals to homosexuals. John Shelby Spong has observed that making all humans, regardless of sexual orientation, bound by the same rules of sexual behavior is not nearly so bold a step for the church as it took when it abandoned the teaching and example of the historical Jesus to admit Gentiles.[35]

Righteousness

Genesis and Judges

In the stories of Lot and the Levite there are no homosexual acts, only frustrated intentions and demands for same-sex sex. It is unwarranted to read God's punishment of Sodom and Gomorrah and the other tribes' punishment of Benjamin as God's response to their frustrated homosexual desires, rather than as God's response to their use of unprovoked violence — even mortal sexual violence — against guests. If the suffering that befell the citizens of Sodom, Gomorrah, and Benjamin should be interpreted as God's judgment against their intention/action of homosexual gang rape, and homosexuality is therefore banned, then consistency demands that God's justification of Lot, the Levite, and the old man of Gibeah who offered their daughters/concubine to be gang-raped and killed should be interpreted as divine approval for men's ensuring their own well-being by delivering women to abuse and death. But discerning divine intention is not simple. Myth, even historical myth, is not easily translated into rules of conduct because it is multilayered; different meanings emerge in the different contexts in which the story is read. Certainly many women reading these stories today read them with Phyllis Trible as "texts of terror,"[36] as revelations of the terrible historical blindness of past tradition to women's dignity and equality.

35. John Shelby Spong, *Living in Sin? A Bishop Rethinks Human Sexuality* (San Francisco: Harper & Row, 1988), p. 207.

36. Phyllis Trible, *Texts of Terror* (Philadelphia: Fortress, 1984).

Romans 1

Paul explains homosexual behavior both as contrary to original human nature, which he assumes was heterosexual, and as visited by God upon societies which have engaged in idolatry. He does not say that individuals become homosexual as a result of their own idolatry; such a claim would be seriously undermined both by contemporary evidence that homosexual orientation emerges in puberty or even earlier, before children are capable of the sin of idolatry, and by the fact that some homosexual individuals have demonstrated great Christian faith and love, even to following Jesus to the cross. Rather Paul claims homosexuality is a social, not an individual, consequence of a society's idolatry.

We cannot read into Paul the long tradition of Christian interpretation of "acts against nature" as referring to nonprocreative sex. Not only is there nothing in the text referring to procreation, but it is well recognized that Paul put no stress on procreation in what he regarded as the last days. Moreover, with global warming, ozone holes, and predictions of massive world hunger within the next half-century as world population increases from five to ten billion,[37] we can no longer snicker and smirk at the idea that nonprocreativity should perhaps be regarded as an important social benefit of homosexuality. Given humanity's role as God's steward of the earth, in this day and age it is no longer human nonprocreativity which must be morally defended, but procreativity itself. This is, of course, something that Paul could not have foreseen.

The concept of nature in Paul is not very clear. Paul not only describes "natural intercourse" as heterosexual and marital in Romans 1:26-27, but in Romans 2:14-15 he argues that Gentiles, despite being deprived of the revelation of the Law, have the law of God "written on their hearts, to which their own consciences also bear witness." There is in Paul, then, at least a basic natural law theology: an understanding that the will of God can be discerned within creation, independent of historical revelation.

This concept of natural law is important within Christian discussions of science and ethics, for natural law constitutes the fundamental bridge between the Bible and science as sources for ethics. One of the profound historical ironies in modern Christianity is that Catholicism, which had so many clashes with modern science within its resistance to the Enlightenment, nevertheless carried over from its medieval theology a concept of natural law

37. As an example from a voluminous literature published since the Rio Earth Summit, see Paul Harrison, "Sex and the Single Planet," *Amicus Journal*, winter 1994, pp. 17-19, 21-23, 26.

which has allowed it in the contemporary period to integrate the findings of science into theology as further revelation of the Creator embedded in the creation. Thus contemporary Catholicism teaches that in addition to Scripture and postscriptural revelation embedded in the tradition of the church, Christians can discern the will of God in the structures and working of nature, both human and nonhuman. Thus discoveries of science, once verified, contribute to understandings of God's original intention and ongoing will. There is, of course, still room for disagreements over methods of interpretation and integration of science into theology, as is clear, for example, in the dispute over official Catholic teaching on contraception, where a central issue is what weight to give to which scientific evidence.

Protestants, who carried the banner of the Enlightenment, rejected both nature as so corrupted by sin as to disfigure any original revelation, and natural law as therefore blurring necessary distinctions between Creator and created, redeemed and unredeemed, and nature and history. For traditional Protestantism, nature was the realm of paganism and pluralism, and natural law was based on a disregard for the reality of sin in the world and in the human person.

A general Protestant tendency toward the Lutheran *sola Scriptura* as a Protestant principle emerged as a response to moral corruption in late medieval Catholicism. But the rejection of natural law left Protestant theology with difficulty in dealing with historical transformations in consciousness and culture. In the United States and much of western Europe, the political legacy of the Enlightenment, democracy, has an implicit natural law basis which, together with the tremendous emphasis on science in modern Western culture, has pressured dominant Protestantism to refer to science in its ethical deliberations. Thus over the last decades Protestantism has been divided. Conservative Protestants tend to reject science as shedding any independent light on ethics or theology especially when science conflicts with scriptural interpretation. Liberal Protestants have integrated scientific findings into specific ethical and theological deliberations, but often without specifying the theological foundation for so doing. Episcopalians, heirs of the English Reformation, which retained some use of natural law despite ongoing internal opposition from "puritan" influences, and Methodists, who also originated in the Anglo-Catholic tradition and eventually adopted a quadrilateral approach to sources of revelation (Scripture, tradition, reason, and experience) which can legitimate science as human experience, bridge the Catholic/Protestant gap on natural law.

The Roman Catholic Church is engaged in internal theological debate on the legitimate appropriation of science in theology and moral theology which parallels much debate in Protestantism on the use of the Bible in theology and ethics. Arbitrary and partial selections from science and the Bible and applications of these to specific debates in support of positions already chosen are criticized, and demands for more holistic approaches to science and the Bible are common. In Protestantism a prior issue is deciding the standing of science within the theological and ethical debate. The doctrine of creation needs to be taken more seriously by treating science as a method for uncovering divine intention within creation, instead of understanding science as merely describing the temporal situation in which divine intention gets played out. In the traditionally anti-intellectual ethos of conservative American Protestantism, such a shift will not be easy.

Such a move will also depend upon some developments within the sciences themselves, including a greater openness to religion and theology, and even more fundamentally, a shifting of some emphasis from scientific method and practical applications of science in technology to the philosophy of science and the meanings of scientific discoveries.

1 Corinthians

The difficulty of translating *malakoi* and *arsenokoitai* in 1 Corinthians 6:9 has led, in turn, to the first RSV translation of both words as "homosexuals," to the revised RSV translation of both words as "sexual perverts," and to the NRSV translation as "male prostitutes, sodomites," as well as to other varying and imprecise translations. It is difficult to place any great weight on this passage. It is not even clear that *malakoi* is a sexual reference, since its basic meaning is "soft," with both cowardly and effeminate as derived meanings. The meaning of *arsenokoitai* is even more obscure.[38]

What seems to me the most fruitful method for approaching the question of the status of homosexual acts is not to argue over how to translate certain imprecise words in the Greek New Testament, but to investigate how the condemnation of homosexuality accords with the scriptural witness in general. Many find it difficult to justify the exclusion of those with homosexual orientation from the church or from ministry in the face of Jesus' inclusion of various marginalized groups of the unclean, sick, sinners, women, and children. For such Christians homosexuals seem to be the lepers of today. Yet for other Christians any association of the lepers of the gospel with homosexuals is scandalous — an obstacle to faith. What is at stake is not only different approaches to the Bible but, just as fundamentally, different images of who we

38. L. William Countryman, *Dirt, Greed, and Sex: Sexual Ethics in the New Testament and Their Implications for Today* (Philadelphia: Fortress, 1988), pp. 117-20.

mean by the term "homosexuals." Do we refer to the middle-aged gay couple who are the long-term foster parents for four orphaned Haitian sisters born HIV positive in my city, or to the stereotypic gay who prowls the bar and bathhouse scene, racking up hundreds of sexual partners? Homosexuals, like heterosexuals and other groups, exhibit variety.

Though compassion is the central virtue the Gospels attribute to Jesus,[39] Christian compassion is misplaced when it prevents recognition of, and opposition to, sin. When Jesus included in his fellowship those understood as sinners in his society, he was not setting an example of overlooking sin. He was rather both insisting on God's willingness to forgive the contrite and rejecting prevalent understandings of temporal retribution under which the poor, the sick, and other low-status unfortunates were thought to have committed sin which had brought upon them God's wrath.[40] It is not true compassion to accept sinners who have not repented their sin, for premature forgiveness encourages sin.

The primary question before us is whether homosexual acts in themselves really *are* sinful. If homosexual acts in themselves are sinful, then they are sinful for those with either homosexual or heterosexual orientation, and those with homosexual orientation must accept lifelong celibacy as a condition of church membership. If homosexual acts really are sinful, then it does not matter how many people commit them, or how difficult it is to avoid committing them; the church must witness to their sinfulness. My own Roman Catholic Church takes this position on homosexuality, as on other issues such as artificial contraception. Christian morality is not defined by majoritarian votes. But as in the contraception issue, when the personal costs of both abiding by the teaching and of failing, despite one's best efforts, to abide by the teaching are so very high, the churches have a tremendous responsibility to define sin only where there is certainty.

We have a number of ways of identifying sinful acts within the Christian tradition. One of the most common ways is to observe the consequences of various acts, to assess the act's impact on the actor, the society, the church, and the larger world. A second way is to look to God's revelation in the record of Scripture and church tradition: Is there a clear and consistent teaching from Scripture through to the present day? A third way, which often draws upon the first two, is to look for God's revelation in the voice of conscience.

Today, the social and personal consequences of homosexuality are hotly debated in church and society. The historical record shows long periods of

39. Albert Nolan, *Jesus before Christianity* (Maryknoll, N.Y.: Orbis, 1976), pp. 27-29.
40. Hugo Echegaray, *The Practice of Jesus* (Maryknoll, N.Y.: Orbis, 1984), pp. 41-43.

Christian tolerance, even acceptance of some forms of homosexuality,[41] and the biblical record displays a generally negative attitude toward homosexuality, supported largely by arguments and circumstances no longer relevant. And Christian consciences are divided.

Research on celibate clergy in the last decades has suggested that celibacy is more demanding, even more destructive, in the postmodern world than in previous ages. Not only is the proportion of vowed celibates in the Catholic clergy of North America who violate their vows of celibacy rising, but the personal toll of attempting celibacy is greater in terms of clerical alcoholism, depression, and even suicide. Some commentators include increased rates of sexual abuse of children and young adults among a minority of the clergy as another consequence of celibacy.[42] Postmodern culture is structured in ways that more or less limit intimacy to sexual relationships, especially for males. Persons who forgo sexual relationships are more often emotionally isolated, with unmet interpersonal needs for disclosure, acceptance, nurturance, and intimacy. In other cultures and in past periods, men and women have met their intimacy needs through lifelong social relationships with extended family and neighbors, primarily through same-sex friendships. The different occupations, interests, and roles of men and women in the past usually prevented marital relationships from becoming the primary, much less the sole, source of intimacy. Women's low status often impeded male-female intimacy and companionship,

41. See John Boswell, *Christianity, Social Tolerance, and Homosexuality: Gay People in Western Europe from the Beginning of the Christian Era to the Fourteenth Century* (Chicago: University of Chicago Press, 1980), and Boswell, *Same Sex Unions in Pre-Modern Europe* (New York: Vintage, 1994).

42. A very small minority — estimated to be between 0.2 and 2.0 percent (Philip Jenkins, *Pedophiles and Priests: Anatomy of a Contemporary Crisis* [New York: Oxford University Press, 1996], pp. 80-82). Recent books on clerical child abuse tend to connect celibacy and abuse in different ways. Jason Berry's *Lead Us Not into Temptation: Catholic Priests and Sexual Abuse of Children* (New York: Doubleday, 1992) understands clerical child abuse as tied to homosexuality, and celibacy as foundational for homosexuality in the Catholic priesthood (chap. 11 and p. 191). But Eleanor Burkett and Frank Bruni, in *A Gospel of Shame: Children, Sex Abuse, and the Catholic Church* (New York: Viking Press, 1993), dispute Berry, insisting that: (1) no research demonstrates a necessary connection between child sex abuse and homosexuality; (2) celibacy today seems to attract both populations (homosexuals and child sex abusers) to the priesthood; (3) some sexual abusers of same-sex children have adult other-sex partners; and (4) male child abusers are more likely to abuse young girls than boys (pp. 220-28). Some commentators point out that Protestant denominations have had recent problems with sex abuse by married clergy in similar numbers; yet among Protestants much of the abuse was with harassment of or adultery with adult women, and was less abuse of minors (Jenkins, pp. 50-52; Harold I. Lief, "Sexual Transgressions of Clergy," in *Religion and Sexual Health*, ed. Ronald M. Green [Amsterdam: Kluwer, 1992], pp. 167-82).

as evidenced in Augustine's comment that the writer of Genesis who described Eve as a helpmate of Adam must have had in mind procreation, for "If woman is not given to man for help in bearing children, for what help could she be? To till the earth together? If help were needed for that, man would have been a better help for man. The same goes for comfort in solitude. How much more pleasure is it for life and conversation when two friends live together than when a man and a woman cohabitate!"[43] But the anonymous urban, highly mobile society of postmodernity has left persons primarily reliant on sexual partners for the satisfaction of virtually all interpersonal needs.[44] Celibates are, therefore, seriously disadvantaged. This disadvantage is even greater for males than for females, since males are even more likely than females to depend solely on sexual partners for intimacy.[45] Thus the cost of discovering one's homosexual orientation, like the cost of clerical celibacy, has gone up tremendously in the Christian churches in the last century.

Sin is generally not difficult to recognize, at least by hindsight. Murder and adultery happen all around us, but few need to ask why they are sinful; their usual consequences explain their moral status. But the more likely we are to know homosexual persons, and the more we know about homosexuality, the more likely we are to question the universal sinfulness of every homosexual act.[46]

Conclusion

Though it is certainly true that the Bible has a generally negative attitude toward homosexuality, the traditional biblical texts quoted against homosexuality are not sufficiently persuasive to justify excluding all homosexual persons from either church membership or clerical roles. Leviticus's purity codes

43. From Augustine, *De genesi ad litteram* 9.5-9, in Augustine, *On Genesis: Two Books on Genesis — "Against the Manichaeans" and "On the Literal Interpretation of Genesis"* (Washington, D.C.: Catholic University Press, 1993); translation here from Uta Ranke Heinemann, *Eunuchs for the Kingdom of Heaven: Women, Sexuality, and the Catholic Church,* trans. Peter Heinegg (New York: Doubleday, 1990 [Hamburg, 1988]), p. 88.

44. Christine E. Gudorf, *Body, Sex, and Pleasure: Reconstructing Christian Sexual Ethics* (Cleveland: Pilgrim, 1994), pp. 131-32.

45. See James B. Nelson, *The Intimate Connection: Male Sexuality, Masculine Spirituality* (Philadelphia: Westminster, 1988), pp. 45-66, esp. pp. 48-49.

46. Robert Crooks and Karla Baur, *Our Sexuality,* 6th ed. (Indianapolis: Benjamin Cummings, 1993), pp. 255-57; M. Stevenson, "Tolerance for Homosexuality and Interest in Sexuality Education," *Journal of Sex Education and Therapy* 16 (1990): 194-97.

are not relevant to Christianity; the stories from Sodom and Gibeah deal with homosexuality very indirectly, if at all; and interpretations of the 1 Corinthians text involve a great deal of guesswork. Two of the most compelling arguments for church acceptance of homosexual persons can be derived from Romans 1 and 1 Corinthians.

Paul in 1 Corinthians writes that "it is better to marry than to be aflame with passion" (7:9), and "because of the temptation to immorality, each man should have his own wife and each woman her own husband" (7:2). This argument that marriage is the cure for sin has a long history in Christianity, though it is, I think, one of the poorer and most negative purposes of marriage. In the first century, when preparing for an imminent second coming took precedence over more ordinary concerns such as marriage and procreation, "better to marry than to burn" became the primary reason to marry. Later on, as expectation of an imminent second coming receded, procreation became the primary purpose of marriage but prevention of sin remained of secondary importance. In our day, when all life on our planet is at risk from massive overpopulation, the church has an obligation to de-emphasize procreation. Also, postmodern culture has developed in ways that largely deprive celibates not only of sexual gratification but also of interpersonal intimacy, making success at lifelong celibacy much more difficult. Because of the temptation to immorality, homosexual marriages should be recognized by the church.

In Romans 1, after arguing that the uncleanness of homosexual acts is one consequence of idolatry, Paul goes on to argue that another consequence of failing to acknowledge God is improper conduct, which he describes in a list of sins. Paul assumes that we can recognize sin and sinners, that a turning away from God manifests itself in a general turn toward evil conduct. If homosexual acts are evil, then we should be able to discern homosexuals by their generally evil conduct. But this is not so. The vast majority of homosexual persons in our society are still unrecognizable — closeted — even to those close to them, precisely because the quality of their actions and their lives does not distinguish them from others. Since the AIDS crisis began, many commentators have come to agree with Freud[47] and other researchers that, in the words of Rev. John McNeill:

47. Building, for example, on the opinion of Sigmund Freud, who saw homosexuals as "of high intellectual and ethical development" and "as characterized by special development of their social instinctual impulses and by their devotion to the interests of the community" (Sigmund Freud, "The Sexual Life of Human Beings," Lecture XX, *Introductory Lectures on Psychoanalysis,* in vol. 16 of *The Complete Psychological Works of Sigmund Freud,* trans. James Strachey in collaboration with Anna Freud [London: Hogarth Press, 1963], p. 304; and "Some Neurotic Mechanisms in Jealousy, Paranoia and Homosexuality" [1922], in vol. 18 of *The Complete Psychological Works,* p. 122).

> Compassion, like hospitality, is a virtue extraordinarily alive in the gay community. Gay people are involved in compassionate works of human service out of all proportion to their numbers in the community. The world has noted the recent astounding outpouring of compassion by lesbians and gay men to all persons with AIDS. . . . With the AIDS crisis, gay love and gay compassion have come out of the closet, and the world is saying: See how they love one another![48]

There are sinners in the homosexual community, just as there are sinners in the heterosexual community. But if membership in the fellowship of Christ is a major channel for the grace that brings salvation, then any exclusion is a terribly serious matter and cannot be based either in prejudice or uncertainty.

48. John J. McNeill, *Taking a Chance on God: Liberating Theology for Gays, Lesbians, and Their Lovers, Families, and Friends* (Boston: Beacon Press, 1988), p. 106.

CHAPTER 5

The Bible in Christian Ethical Deliberation concerning Homosexuality: Old Testament Contributions

PHYLLIS A. BIRD

The current debate in the church concerning the status of homosexual[1] persons, acts, and relationships requires us, as in every theological and ethical debate, to seek the counsel of Scripture, but it also requires us to clarify our understanding of the nature of Scripture and the way it informs and norms Christian ethical judgments. The debate is occasioned because changed practice and perceptions have created tensions between traditional norms and current understandings and raised questions for which existing rules and

1. For convenience I have used the terms "homosexual" and "homosexuality" to refer to the whole complex of biological and social factors relating to homoerotic attraction and relationships, recognizing that a single term does not do full justice to the range of phenomena encompassed thereby or the lack of consensus concerning etiology and expression. The term is a modern one, without correspondence in the biblical writings or in the cultures from which they stem. The hermeneutical significance of this observation is treated below. See Martti Nissinen, *Homoeroticism in the Biblical World: A Historical Perspective,* trans. Kirsi Stjerna (Minneapolis: Fortress, 1998; orig. pub. *Homoerotiikka Raamatun maailmassa* [Helsinki, 1994]), pp. v-vi, 5-17, 123-40, 142-44. This important Finnish study of homoeroticism in the biblical world became available to me in a preliminary English translation after I had completed this article. I have expanded my treatment to include discussion of Mesopotamian sources, drawn largely from Nissinen, and have included some references to his general discussion of gender roles, but I have not attempted to "update" my treatment of the OT texts by systematic inclusion of references to his interpretation — which is very close to my own.

guidelines do not provide clear answers. In a situation of uncertainty and conflict, the church seeks to discern the will of God by searching the Scriptures, probing the tradition, and seeking the counsel of science, reason, and experience. But the Bible, to which the church turns for guidance, is already present in this debate, appearing to many as the source of the conflict. On the question of homosexual practice, the Bible's word is both known and clear, or so it seems — and it is a word of unambiguous and unconditioned condemnation. Upheld through the ages by both secular and ecclesiastical authority and justified by traditional theological and scientific reason, this condemnation seems to pit the full weight of Scripture, tradition, and reason against the weak authority of divided and ambivalent experience. It has not succeeded, however, in silencing the voice of experience. Homosexuality is a subject of debate in the church today because faithful Christians who understand themselves as homosexual and seek fulfillment of their sexual needs in same-sex relationships have insisted that their identity and practice as gay men and lesbians is consonant with, and even expressive of, their identity as Christians. It is also a subject of Christian debate because other homosexual Christians, faced with a perceived conflict between biblical norms and their own sexual needs, have been driven to the tragic options of divided lives, divided consciences, denial of sexual expression, contorted rationalizations, rejection of biblical authority and the Bible itself, self-hate, and even self-destruction.

For most Christians struggling with the conflicting testimony of Scripture and homosexual experience, the conflict is understood as a conflict of revelation with experience. This perception rests, I believe, on a faulty understanding of Scripture and its relationship to experience. It treats the Bible as divine oracle or law, abstracting its words from their literary and social contexts and absolutizing them as statements of timeless rules or principles that stand over against changing social practices and values. The Bible does indeed contain attempts to formulate governing principles for a variety of ethical situations, exemplified in the Decalogue and the "love command." But these are set within contexts of deliberation concerning specific and changing demands for personal and communal righteousness and an overarching narrative of God's continuing action in creation. When the dynamics of interchange with specific historical situations are lost or when particular judgments are cast as absolutes, the Bible's ethical witness is distorted.

The Bible does not present us with a distinct mode of revelation, but a privileged locus — in which the divine self-disclosure is mediated by the same processes of tradition interacting with experience and reason that we recognize as sources of continuing revelation today. As a foundational document and as a medium of continuing communication with God, the Bible has an essential and primary place in Christian theological and ethical deliberation. But it is the starting point of the church's conversation, not the end, a conversation partner, not an oracle.

My approach to the Bible as a source of ethical guidance in the current debate is in fundamental agreement with Christopher Seitz's insistence on the two-part canon of Old and New Testament Scriptures viewed together as the relevant corpus for Christian theology and ethics. My focus on the Old Testament is dictated only by the space allotted to me and my conviction that this portion of the Christian Scriptures has been both neglected and misused. Where I differ from Seitz is in my insistence on the historical character of the biblical witness and hence my employment of historical-critical tools (including social analysis) to inquire into the ancient literary and sociohistorical contexts of the writings. I reject the view that traditional interpretation must determine Christian understanding of these texts and insist that they be allowed to speak on their own terms — however discordant this may appear either to traditional interpretations or to contemporary demands.[2]

Limits of space require me to eliminate the fuller exegetical arguments that underlie my interpretations and abbreviate treatment of texts I have dealt with in previous publications. The fundamental issues in the current debate are hermeneutical, however, rather than exegetical, so I begin with a brief statement of my understanding of the nature and authority of Scripture.

The Christian Scriptures comprise a collection of diverse documents bound together in a two-part canon, whose center is the witness to Christ as the new revelation of the God made known to Israel. As a collection of writings, the Bible is pluriform and multivocal — as are many of its constituent parts. Thus the Bible is characterized by an irreducible pluralism that requires constructive effort to grasp the unity within the diversity and discern the pattern(s) that gives coherence to the whole. While the church has an interpretive tradition that shapes every Christian reading, such preunderstanding holds the constant danger of inhibiting, rather than enabling, fresh encounter with the text and with the totality of its witness. Attempts to formulate the Bible's essential message tend to silence dissident voices within the canon and suppress the dialogical character of its witness. Debate is a constituent feature

2. In articulating my own position, I do not wish to argue for a single normative approach or construction — either as dictated by tradition or as demanded by present needs. The option I have chosen takes its clues primarily from the Bible itself and locates the authoritative word of God in the dialogue between ancient and modern witnesses, rather than in the sacred page.

of the biblical canon, reflecting its origins in the conversation of a community over time.[3]

What holds the Scriptures together is the community that created, preserved, and transmitted the writings, Israel and its daughter, the church.[4] United in canonical form, the Scriptures present an overarching story that moves from the beginning of creation to a vision of new creation and, within that framework, the conversation of the community about the implications of that story for its life. That conversation spans a millennium in its recorded memory, but it does not end with the last canonical writing; it continues today, as the story itself continues. I will not rehearse that story here or attempt to characterize the distinct voices that contribute to the dialogue, except to emphasize that they are many.

One voice requires special note, however, for its absence. As many of us have become painfully aware in recent times, the voices we hear in Scripture and through whom we claim to hear the word of God do not represent the full testimony or experience of the people of God, but rather that of its male members, and an elite among them. Thus the conversation of Scripture is both incomplete and biased. This means, I believe, that the testimony of Scripture may not be absolutized, or viewed as final revelation. It does not mean that the Scriptures lack authority; rather it makes unavoidably clear that the authority of Scripture is the authority of historical witness. Standing in time, the Scriptures point beyond time, but always and only as a product of the cultures out of which they speak. The word of God in Scripture is always an incarnate word, and therefore limited.[5]

Although I find the Bible's limits most serious in its inadequate and distorted representation of women's experience, I believe its testimony is true in its essential message, and sufficient both to direct us in the way we must travel and to provide sustenance for the journey. The Bible's message of God's creating power, redeeming grace, and demand for righteousness, together with its proclamation of God's suffering and reconciling love in Jesus Christ that

3. For a fuller statement of my understanding, see Phyllis A. Bird, "The Authority of the Bible," in *The New Interpreters Bible,* ed. Leander Keck (Nashville: Abingdon, 1994), 1:31-64.

4. I stress the continuity here while recognizing two distinct communities, each internally diverse. The problem of unity is posed within each Testament as well as in their union.

5. The relative absence of women in the text serves as a pointer to the more fundamental character of the texts and the culture as governed by patriarchal and androcentric norms — features of direct consequence for all questions of sexual identity, activity, and roles.

breaks the bonds of sin, has made it possible — and necessary — within the biblical period and beyond, to redefine the boundaries of the community that lives by that message and reformulate the rules for participation. In my lifetime it has meant a fundamental change in the roles of women in the church and a revolution in theology — changes that are still in process and are leading us into new perceptions and questions we could not have known or anticipated in an earlier age.

Today the question of homosexuality presents the church with another case that calls it to reexamine its understanding of the boundaries of the community, the terms of membership, and the forms of leadership and service to which it calls members. I do not intend to suggest a parallel to the case of women except in a very general way. There are distinctive factors in the biblical tradition and in the current phenomenon that demand individual and differentiated treatment. One of these, which makes deliberation so difficult, is that homosexuality is not a single question and there is no consensus concerning the nature of the phenomenon, or phenomena, identified by this term. Thus the first problem that confronts us in seeking biblical guidance is the question of where to look and what to look for.

Old Testament Texts with Explicit References to Homosexual Behavior

I begin with the texts that have traditionally been understood to relate to homosexuality, although these are not the texts to which I would appeal in constructing ethical guidelines for church policy today. This starting point is dictated by the course of debate in the church and the need for biblical scholars in the service of the church to engage that debate with corrections as well as alternatives. I limit my treatment to Old Testament texts, recognizing that they cannot stand alone. Biblical references to homosexual behavior are rare in both Testaments, exclusively negative, and commonly associated with other types of immoral or excluded behavior. They treat only acts, not relationships,[6] and with the exception of Romans 1:26 speak only of acts between

6. Jonathan's love for David (1 Sam. 18:1) does not belong to the OT's understanding of homosexual relations, which is interested only in acts, not affections. Similar disinterest in affections also characterizes rules governing heterosexual relations. Sex, love, and marriage are not correlated in the same manner in ancient Israel as in contemporary Western society. It is precisely the OT's disinterest in affective bonds and the quality of relationships that makes the Bible's pronouncements on prohibited sexual unions problematic as

males. Richard Hays rightly observes that "in terms of emphasis, it [homosexuality] is a minor concern, in contrast, for example, to economic injustice."[7] Why that is the case is less obvious, however, and paucity of reference may not simply be equated either with ignorance or tolerance.[8]

Narrative Texts: Genesis 19:1-29 and Judges 19:22-24

Hays comments that the notorious account of the men of Sodom (Gen. 19:1-29) is "actually irrelevant to the topic [of consensual homosexual intercourse]," since the men's intent was apparently gang rape of Lot's two visitors.[9] I believe he is right in insisting that this text does not address the cases under consideration today, but I do not think it can be dismissed as testimony to the OT's attitude toward homosexual activity. In both the Sodom account and the story of the Judean Levite and his concubine among the Benjaminites of Gibeah (Judg. 19, a story modeled on Gen. 19), "foreigners" or outsiders are depicted as exhibiting moral depravity in their inhospitality toward visitors.[10] The honor due a guest is violated (at least by threat) in the most objectionable way conceivable, by sexual humiliation.

In both texts the request for sexual favors by the men of the city uses language employed elsewhere for normal (hetero)sexual relations, "to know."[11] The verb itself contains no sense of coercion, which is supplied by the context — the demand that the host "bring out" his male guest(s) (Gen. 19:5; Judg. 19:22) and the depiction of the threatening crowd. The response of the host,

---

guides to contemporary sexual ethics. Nissinen (p. 17) uses the term "homosociability" to describe interaction between people of the same sex where the erotic-sexual aspect is not emphasized or essential. See Nissinen, pp. 53-56.

7. Richard B. Hays, "Awaiting the Redemption of Our Bodies: The Witness of Scripture concerning Homosexuality," in *Homosexuality in the Church: Both Sides of the Debate,* ed. Jeffrey S. Siker (Louisville: Westminster/John Knox, 1994), p. 5.

8. See Thomas B. Dozeman, "Creation and Procreation in the Biblical Teaching on Homosexuality," *USQR* 49 (1995): 172.

9. Hays, p. 5. See also Choon-Leong Seow, "A Heterotextual Perspective," in *Homosexuality and Christian Community,* ed. C. L. Seow (Louisville: Westminster/John Knox, 1996), pp. 15-16; Nissinen, p. 46.

10. The issue of foreign mores is clear in Gen. 19:9 when the men of Sodom dismiss Lot's protest as that of an "alien." Although the Judges account deals with an intertribal conflict, the Benjaminites are presented here as acting like the wicked Sodomites, i.e., like "foreigners."

11. See, e.g., Gen. 4:1, 17, 25, and 1 Sam. 1:19 of sexual relations as a prelude to conception. Cf. Gen. 38:26 (NRSV, "lie with") and 1 Kings 1:4.

who pleads with his "brothers" not to act wickedly (*'al-nā' 'aḥay tārē'û* [Gen. 19:7; similarly Judg. 19:23]) and offers female substitutes, confirms the view that it is the male object that makes the action offensive — so that it is branded a *nĕbālâ* (outrage)[12] in Judges 19:23. The analogy is clearly with rape, as exhibited by the language used in reference to the female substitute. In Judges 19:23-24 the old man offers his virgin daughter and his guest's concubine in place of his male guest, inviting the men to "ravish them" *(wĕ'annû 'ôtām).*[13] Thus desire for a male sexual partner, represented as a "simple" request, is countered by an invitation to violate a woman, and her sexual honor, in its most prized and protected state — an offer made by the male charged with protecting that honor, whose own honor must suffer from the invited action.[14]

The account carries the clear message that male honor is threatened by homosexual intercourse and that it is valued even above a daughter's virginity. The parallel and contrasting language of "ordinary" sexual intercourse (with a male) and abusive sex (with a female) equates homoerotic relations with rape, and the portrayal of the request as a threat suggests that the Israelite authors could only conceive of participation in male homoerotic acts as forced. It is not clear whether they viewed homoerotic activity among the inhabitants of these wicked cities as consensual and habitual or only as perverse sport with visitors. They do appear to suggest, however, that no Israelite male would consent to engage in homoerotic relations — at least not as the passive partner. In these accounts we catch glimpses of an undergirding code of sexual behavior governed by views of gender roles and sexual honor that are rarely, if ever, spelled out, but only exemplified. Inferring the unarticulated norms from the biblical narratives and laws is an essential, if uncertain, task of biblical ethics.

These two texts strongly suggest that the ancient Israelites had no experience or conception of male homoerotic relations as consensual or expressive of a committed relationship. They appear to view the "use" of a male in

12. NRSV, "vile thing." The term is translated variously as "senselessness" (in disregard of moral or religious claims [BDB]), "wanton crime," "disgrace," "vile outrage," and "folly." It is not specifically related to sexual outrages, although it is used to characterize the rape of Dinah in Gen. 34:7 — and the outrage against the Levite's concubine (together with the threat to the Levite himself?) as reported in Judg. 20:6, 10. It describes a violation of a community norm or taboo and is used in the older narrative sources with much the same sense as *tô'ēbâ* (abomination) in later sources.

13. Cf. Gen. 19:8: "do to them as you please." The reported action in Judg. 19:25 combines the term *YD'* with the verb *yit'allĕlû,* "act wantonly," to give the sense of "wanton intercourse."

14. Cf. Gen. 34:7, 31.

sexual relations (initiated by a male) as a violation of male honor, more serious than the worst violation of female honor. This interpretation is corroborated by Martti Nissinen's cross-cultural study of homoerotic activity in the ancient Near Eastern and Mediterranean world, in which a distinction of active and passive partners is seen to be fundamental and universal, and in which the passive role is always defined as feminine. Hence involvement in homosexual acts in the passive role involves a threat to male identity. Sexual acts, whether heterosexual or homosexual, were not conceived as a relationship between equals.[15]

Legal Texts: Leviticus 18:22 and 20:13

The OT contains two explicit prohibitions of homosexual activity, both in the larger collection of laws known as the "Holiness Code" (Lev. 17:1–26:46) for the governing idea that informs its demands: "You shall be holy, for I YHWH your God am holy" (Lev. 19:2). The two texts occur in parallel series of prohibitions and are essentially duplicate statements, employing the same terms and differing only in style, as dictated by the individual series. They are positioned differently, however, in the two series, creating different contexts of interpretation. Both have entered the growing corpus of priestly law at a relatively late stage and are closely related to the theological perspectives of the final document.[16]

Leviticus 18:22

Leviticus 18 has been shaped into a literary and rhetorical whole by a theological framework in verses 2b-5 and 24-30, which begins and ends with the declaration "I am YHWH your God." In both opening and closing exhortations, Israel is enjoined not to follow the practices of the Canaanites who preceded them in the land, but to observe YHWH's statutes and ordinances,

15. Nissinen, p. 26; see below.

16. I assume an exilic date for the final work, although both chapters show stages of growth. Individual laws and collections of laws may go back to much earlier times, while additions continued to accrue to the already completed work. Cf. Karl Elliger, *Leviticus* (Tübingen: J. C. B. Mohr, 1966), pp. 14-20, 229-35, 263-72; Martin Noth, *Leviticus,* trans. J. E. Anderson (Philadelphia: Westminster, 1965), pp. 127-28, 134, 146-47. Nissinen (p. 37) assumes a postexilic setting, while Jan Joosten, *People and Land in the Holiness Code: An Exegetical Study of the Ideational Framework of the Law in Leviticus 17–26,* VTSup 67 (Leiden: Brill, 1996), pp. 202-7, argues for a preexilic dating of the Holiness Code as a whole.

which assure life to those who do them. With this hortatory framework, legal custom is proclaimed as divine law. The concluding exhortation spells out the consequences of disobedience with a lesson from history, cast in cultic terms: the previous inhabitants, through their "defiling" actions, caused the land to become defiled so that God punished the land, making it vomit out its inhabitants. I note this theological framework to highlight two fundamental differences in reasoning from our own: (1) issues of prohibited sexual relations are presented here in essentially cultic rather than ethical terms: they defile, and therefore endanger, the community; and (2) historical process and divine agency are understood in terms that are foreign, and unacceptable, to most modern American readers. Any contemporary appeal to these texts must consider these differences.

Within the hortatory framework of Leviticus 18 is a collection of laws whose core (vv. 7-16) is a unified series of ten prohibited classes of sexual relations with relatives, (re)interpreted as marriage prohibitions (v. 6). Both the apodictic form of the series (direct and absolute prohibition, as in the Decalogue, without specification of punishment) and the nature of the protected relationships, which describe a circle of persons living together in a three-generational extended family, point to an early period of Israel's history, marked by kinship-based organization. The laws forbid promiscuity within this family circle constituted by marriage as well as "blood" relationships, and all are addressed to adult males.[17] This older series of prohibited sexual relations with female family members, which lacks any religious language, has been extended in verses 17-23 by further sexual (and in one case, cultic) prohibitions of quite disparate nature, couched in cultic terminology. This has the effect of creating a more comprehensive list of proscribed sexual practices, but it also shifts the emphasis of the whole from family ethos to concern for ritual purity.

Verses 17-18 are closely linked to the preceding series, but concern marriage rather than sexual relations. Verses 19-23 form a block distinguished by language of (ritual) uncleanness or defilement (*tom'â*, vv. 19, 20, 23). This language links it to the concluding paranesis, which begins with the summary statement, "You shall not defile yourselves *('al-tiṭṭammĕ'û)* in any of these ways" (v. 24), and concludes with the admonition not to commit any of "these abominations *(ḥuqqôt hattô'ēbôt)* that were done before you," and not to "defile yourselves *(wĕlō'-tiṭṭammĕ'û)* by them" (v. 30). The appendix is a

17. On the significance of the male address, see Sarah Melcher, "The Holiness Code and Human Sexuality," in *Biblical Ethics and Homosexuality: Listening to Scripture,* ed. Robert L. Brawley (Louisville: Westminster/John Knox, 1996), esp. pp. 91-93.

miscellany of defiling practices, including intercourse with a menstruating woman (v. 19), sexual relations with a kinsman's (or neighbor's) wife (*'ēšet ʿămîtĕkâ*, v. 20), sacrificing offspring to Molech (v. 21), sexual relations with a male "as with a woman" (v. 22), and sexual relations with an animal (v. 23). The Molech prohibition appears as an exception to the common subject matter of sexual violations, but it has the effect of identifying the supplementary prohibitions with alien cultic practice, and perhaps more specifically with alien gods.[18] Standing at the center of the appendix, it characterizes the act as "profan[ing] *(ḤLL)* the name of your God," following this with the declaration "I am YHWH," which connects it to the opening and closing words of the chapter. Thus it serves to link the appendix as a whole to the governing ideas of the chapter in its final edition.

The prohibition of homosexual relations is formulated as follows: "With a male you shall not lie (as) lyings with a woman; it is an abomination" (*wĕ'et-zākār lō' tiškab miškĕbê 'iššâ tôʿēbâ hī[w]'*, v. 22). The formulation emphasizes the inappropriateness of a male as the object of the (male-initiated) sexual act, which is defined by reference to a woman. The use of the term "male" *(zākār)* is not coupled here with the corresponding biological term "female" *(nĕqēbâ)*, as in Genesis 1:27-28, but simply "woman" *('iššâ)*. Thus it does not appear to echo the creation account or emphasize procreative function, but simply describes the normative pattern of sexual relations.[19] The prohibition is accompanied by the declaration, "it is an abomination *(tôʿēbâ)*."

The term *tôʿēbâ* is concentrated in exilic texts (forty-three times in Ezekiel) and cultic contexts, where it serves to characterize practices as incompatible with Yahwistic practice, or "taboo."[20] It is lacking in the old legal collec-

18. See Noth, p. 136; cf. Elliger, p. 24; Rainer Albertz, *A History of Israelite Religion in the Old Testament Period*, 2 vols. (Louisville: Westminster/John Knox, 1992), 1:190-94; George C. Heider, *The Cult of Molek: A Reassessment* (Sheffield: JSOT, 1985), pp. 248-49; John Day, *Molech: A God of Human Sacrifice in the Old Testament* (Cambridge: Cambridge University Press, 1989), pp. 22-24.

19. Cf. Judg. 21:11, 12. The use of *zākār* (male) is not confined to texts concerned with physical attributes or sexual function, but also appears in texts stressing male gender roles, rights, and obligations (e.g., Exod. 23:17).

20. See Erhard S. Gerstenberger, "*tʿb* pi. verabscheuen," in *Theologisches Handwörterbuch zum Alten Testament* 2, ed. Ernst Jenni and Claus Westermann (Munich: Kaiser; Zürich: Theologischer Verlag, 1979), cols. 1051-55; Paul Humbert, "Le substantif *tôʿēbâ* et le verbe *tʿb* dans l'Ancien Testament," *ZAW* 72 (1960): 217-37; Jean L'Hour, "Les interdits *tôʿēbâ* dans le Deutéronome," *RB* 71 (1964): 481-503. In its basic use and meaning it describes something that is "not done (here)," or is "unthinkable (to us)," i.e., practices unacceptable in Israelite culture. See Seow, p. 14, for examples.

tions, as well as the older narrative traditions (where *nĕbālâ* functions as an equivalent, as in Gen. 34:7 and Judg. 19:23), but is common in late Deuteronomic texts (seventeen times in Deuteronomy), where it carries connotations of foreign/pagan cultic practice.[21] In Leviticus it occurs only in the duplicate prohibitions of homosexual acts and the epilogue of chapter 18 (four times). It is not an ethical term, but a term of boundary marking. In its basic sense of taboo it describes a feeling of abhorrence or revulsion that requires or admits no rational explanation. It may be given a theological grounding by reference to the deity: "X is an abomination/abhorrent to YHWH."[22] The attachment of the *tôʿēbâ* declaration to the homosexual prohibition serves in Leviticus 18 not only to characterize this act, but to link the prohibition to the concluding parenesis with its fourfold repetition of *tôʿēbâ* (vv. 26, 27, 29, 30), closely associated with the idea of defilement. It belongs to the language of separation and distinctness from the nations that came to expression during the exile and was applied retroactively to earlier stages of Israelite history.

The prohibition of homoerotic relations, like all of the prohibitions in the chapter, addresses males, and thus only considers relations with another male. In view of the fundamental orientation of the OT laws toward the rights and responsibilities of males, primarily in relation to other males, I do not think we can conclude anything from this formulation about the incidence or acceptance of lesbian relations, except that sexual relations confined to the realm of female activity were apparently not considered threatening to the male-dominated community. If the primary issue in the condemnation of homosexual acts is male honor, then female homoeroticism is of no interest or concern.[23]

Leviticus 20:13

Leviticus 20 appears in its present form to be a later composition than chapter 18 and to draw upon both chapters 18 and 19. Although it covers many of the same cases as chapter 18, the arrangement is different and the core series of sexual prohibitions appears to have arisen separately.[24] The chapter opens

21. E.g., Deut. 13:14 (Heb. 15) and 27:15. The term has no specific associations with "fertility rites," and is only associated with cult-related sex in Deut. 23:17-18 (Heb. 18-19; see appendix A).

22. *tôʿăbat yhwh,* esp. in Deuteronomy and Proverbs. Cf. KAI 13.6 (a sixth century B.C.E. Phoenician grave inscription forbidding damaging of the grave as an "abomination to Astarte").

23. See Nissinen, pp. 35-36, 43.

24. Elliger, pp. 25-72; Noth, p. 146.

with an extended treatment of the Molech sacrifice (vv. 1-5), followed by "turn[ing] to mediums and 'wizards'" (v. 6).[25] These religious practices are described in terms of idolatry, employing the language of harlotry *(ZNH)*, rather than defilement, as the key interpretive term.[26] The opening section concludes with an exhortation to be holy, and a new series of capital crimes begins in verse 9.

Verses 10-21 detail sexual offenses, but these are introduced in verse 9 by a case of "curs[ing] father or mother." The curious inclusion of this case suggests that the chapter has been constructed on the pattern of the Decalogue: cases involving the violation of YHWH's honor (by worship of other gods) are placed first, while the dishonoring of parents serves as a transition to the second division of laws concerning the violation of a neighbor's or kinsman's honor. The primary concern in this series is with relations within the larger community and the immediate family — not the extended family, as in Leviticus 18:1-16.[27] Thus homoerotic acts (v. 13)[28] and bestiality (vv. 15-16) are included in the primary series of sexual offenses, with adultery (v. 10) heading the list. Verses 17-21 (together with v. 14) have the character of an appendix, exhibiting a mixture of styles and sentences and evidence of internal accretions. The *môt yûmat* ("he shall certainly be put to death") formula is applied to all of the cases in verses 1-16, but is lacking in the appendix, suggesting less serious infractions. The main series of capital offenses appears to be graded, with the most serious placed first.

The chapter concludes with an extended paranesis (vv. 22-26) introducing themes picked up from chapter 18, including the themes of separation

25. Heb. *'ōbōt* and *yiddĕʿōnîm,* which Heider (pp. 249-50) convincingly identifies with the practice of necromancy, establishing a connection with the Molech cult in a common association with the cult of the dead (pp. 250-51).

26. The metaphorical character of the "whoring" language is especially clear here, since neither of the two cases suggests any association with "sacred prostitution" or a fertility cult.

27. The cases treated are as follows: sexual relations with a neighbor's wife (v. 10, using the specific language of adultery, *N'P*), a father's wife (v. 11), a daughter-in-law (v. 12), a male (v. 13), (marriage to) a woman and her mother (v. 14), an animal (by a man or a woman, vv. 15-16), a sister (v. 17), a menstruating woman (v. 18), a mother's or father's sister (v. 19, in apodictic form), an uncle's wife (v. 20), and (marriage to) a brother's wife (v. 21).

28. The prohibition here is formulated in the same terms as in chap. 18, but in the casuistic style of the series and with an additional declaration of guilt: "A man who lies with a male (as) lyings with a woman: the two of them have committed an abomination; they shall surely be put to death; their blood is upon them" (*wĕ'îš 'ăšer yiškab 'et-zākār miškĕbê 'iššâ tôʿēbâ ʿāśû šĕnêhem môt yûmātû dĕmêhem bām,* v. 13). The guilt of both parties is also emphasized, in keeping with the series.

from the nations (vv. 23-24, 26b), the land's vomiting out its inhabitants (v. 22b), and possession of the land (v. 24), here expanded. It closes with an exhortation to be holy, as YHWH is holy (v. 26; cf. 19:2). Thus, as in chapter 18, an interpretive framework has been supplied to the laws, which stresses holiness as the governing theological principle and links the demand for holiness with separation from the peoples. Here, however, these themes lack linguistic connections with the individual laws. In chapter 20 the homosexual prohibition is simply another sexual taboo, without clear cultic associations, and its characterization as an "abomination" finds no echo in the paranesis.

The inclusion of the homosexual prohibition in the main series of sexual offenses raises the question whether this represents an understanding of (male) homosexual acts in primarily ethical terms, in contrast to chapter 18, where ritual/cultic associations predominate.[29] There does appear to be an attempt in both Leviticus 18 and 20 to create comprehensive lists of sexual acts that undermine community and family relations, with the list in chapter 20 presenting a more integrated conception. But neither is complete and neither has any place for circumstantial considerations, such as questions of age, initiative, or consent. This lack of interest in essential ethical criteria is strikingly clear in the assessment of penalties. In all of the cases in chapter 20, both of the sexual partners are subjected to the same punishment, including the animal, who is to be put to death together with the man or woman who has used it sexually. In verse 16 both the woman and the animal are explicitly declared "guilty," in the same terms applied to those who engage in homoerotic activity ("their blood is upon them"). Thus the fundamental character of the prohibitions in both chapters as boundary defining, as well as their judgment of sexual acts in purely objective terms, their interpretive framework based in cultic notions of purity and defilement, and their exclusively male orientation, limit their usefulness for contemporary sexual ethics.

Neither the OT nor the NT offers a comprehensive approach to sexual ethics, but these two chapters of Leviticus mark an important step on the way toward bringing the "private" and "secular" realm of sexual relations into the sphere of religious concerns and lay groundwork for the development of a theological ethics of sexual relations. What is lacking here, in addition to the deficits and biases already noted, is an articulation of the underlying principles and examples of how the judgments were applied.

29. Cf. Rom. 1:26-27, which places homosexual conduct in the context of pagan practice and impurity, rather than with other sexual offenses such as adultery, rape, or incest.

Conclusions and Implications for Contemporary Use

1. The OT prohibitions of homosexual relations may not be understood as timeless decrees that can be applied to contemporary situations on the assumption of one-to-one correspondences. The language and contexts of these formulations betray a worldview and a theology that is both inconceivable and unacceptable to most Western Christians. The theological issues that govern the introduction of the homosexual prohibition into the biblical canon are purity and defilement, of people and land — notions that place sexual relations with a menstruating woman (including a man's own wife) and child sacrifice in the same category of offenses as homosexual relations (Lev. 18:19, 21-22).

2. Although the prohibitions are presented as absolute and unconditioned decrees in first-person divine speech, the two series of laws in their settings within the Holiness Code and in the larger canonical context witness to a more dynamic and historically conditioned understanding of divine law than the individual compositions suggest or the historical literalism of modern readers commonly recognizes.[30] The difference between the two occurrences of the prohibition is not simply a matter of spelling out the penalties in chapter 20. It involves a fundamental reordering of the categories, eliminating some cases and rearranging others to indicate different orders of seriousness and different types of infractions. The second series (chap. 20) moves in the direction of more distinctly ethical reasoning — though it still leaves that reasoning unarticulated.

The two lists of sexual prohibitions within the Holiness Code point to *changing* views of sexual relations in response to changing social, political, and religious conditions. Urban society and a more cosmopolitan milieu, including perhaps the experience of foreign domination under Assyrian and/or Babylonian rule and concomitant exposure to other peoples and practices, have required a rethinking of categories and a reordering of priorities relating to sexual practices, even within the relatively homogeneous theological tradition represented by the Holiness Code.[31] Even more striking differences and

30. When the ancient writer spoke of the need for Israel to separate itself from the nations that YHWH was driving out before them, his seventh or sixth century B.C.E. audience understood this as a transparent reference to their own need to maintain, or redefine, their identity as a people distinct from the peoples among whom they were living.

31. It is not essential to my argument to determine precisely the date of the Holiness Code or the individual collections of laws within it, which have been dated from late preexilic to postexilic times. While greater precision would help to clarify the particular dynamics at work in the formulation and reformulation of these two series, it is sufficient

changes in perspectives, issues, and emphases are evident, however, when the Holiness Code is compared with other collections of laws within the larger OT legal tradition.

3. The absence of the prohibition in any of the older law codes and its first appearance in a context characterized by themes of purity and separation from the nations/peoples point to the emergence of the issue of homosexual practice as a theological concern in the context of an attempt to redefine the boundaries of the community in terms of praxis rather than in geographical or ethnic terms, a praxis governed by a cultically derived notion of holiness, extended from ritual practice to personal relations. The "Israel" of these laws is no longer a geographical entity, and the geographically based and kinship-ordered agricultural village is no longer the controlling social organization. Homosexual practice belongs to the behavior that is understood to break community solidarity at a time when the community is under stress and the old kinship-based mechanisms of social control are threatened or no longer operative. The first move of Leviticus 18 is to appeal to old family law controlling sexual relations, redefining it as incest prohibitions; the second is to prohibit "pagan" sexual practices as defiling.

4. From the position of the prohibition in Leviticus 18, where it stands apart from the family-oriented law, it appears that male homoerotic activity was not viewed as threatening to male interests within the family. Prior to Leviticus it also does not appear to have been recognized as a threat to community norms, in contrast to bestiality, which is treated in both of the older law codes (Exod. 22:19; Deut. 27:21). If we consider the narratives of Genesis 19 and Judges 19, homoerotic activity seems to have been considered a threat only in "foreign" cities — where the threat is to male honor and clearly not to marriage, since a spouse and marriageable daughters are offered as a substitute! I believe we must conclude from this evidence that male homosexual relations were rare, and abhorrent, in the tightly knit patriarchal village life of ancient Israel.

5. The language of "abomination" that attaches to the prohibition in both chapters of Leviticus reinforces the view of a history of abhorrence, rather than tolerance. The term appears nowhere else in Leviticus apart from the parallel law in 20:13 and the epilogue of chapter 18, where it serves to associate the prohibited practices (as a whole) with foreign/pagan practice. The fact that the same declaration is found in 20:13, without the editorial connec-

---

for my purposes to argue that the essential features of the context in which they have emerged are a breakdown of an older, unwritten consensus and increased exposure to and/or involvement with alternative practices.

tion, strongly suggests that it antedates both collections, or that its appearance in chapter 20 is dependent on chapter 18. Thus the testimony of the laws corresponds to that of the narratives.

The designation "abomination" is instructive, I believe, for our attempts to discover the underlying reasons for the prohibition. It points to a nonrational and preethical judgment, a sense of revulsion toward a practice that is "not done here." The abhorrence may be rationalized or theologized in various ways, e.g., by association with "foreigners" or as divinely repudiated,[32] but such interpretations do not explain the socially grounded root response. It appears most likely in the patriarchal ethos of ancient Israel that homosexual activity carried a sense of male shame for the partner "forced" to assume the "female" role (or shamelessness for the male who assumed it voluntarily), a judgment corroborated by Mesopotamian evidence.[33] There is nothing to suggest that it was viewed as threatening the survival of the species — despite the fact that such an argument would have had far greater cogency in ancient Israel than it does today. There is no indication that homosexual relations in ancient Israel, or anywhere in the ancient Near East, were ever an exclusive option, and eunuchs played an important role in both Egyptian and Mesopotamian royal service as well as in Israel's own royal bureaucracy.[34] Behind the prohibition is, I think, a fear of deviation from the socially dominant pattern of male-female intercourse, a biologically favored pattern grounded in reproductive needs but by no means limited to them — as the toleration of prostitution evidences. In the final analysis it is a matter of gender identity and roles, not sexuality — which must conform to the socially approved gender patterns. Nor is it a matter of misuse of male "seed,"[35] a judgment relevant only to circum-

32. It is noteworthy that the "unnatural" argument is not found in the OT, nor in any of the ancient Near Eastern texts that disparage or condemn homosexual relations (see appendix B). The language of "abomination" and the associations with defilement in Lev. 18 contrast with the language used in condemning sexual relations with an animal (Lev. 18:23), which characterizes the act as *tebel,* "perversion" (from the root *BLL,* "to mix, confuse"). Attitudes toward homoerotic acts appear to relate primarily to issues of social order, not natural order.

33. That the fundamental issue is a transgression of gender roles is suggested by the prohibition of wearing apparel of the opposite sex (Deut. 22:5), which is also branded an "abomination" *(tôʿăbat yhwh ʾĕlōhêkā).*

34. See A. Kirk Grayson, "Eunuchs in Power: Their Role in the Assyrian Bureaucracy," in *Vom Alten Orient zum Alten Testament,* ed. Manfried Dietrich and Oswald Loretz, Festschrift for W. von Soden, AOAT 240 (Kevelaer: Butzon & Bercker; Neukirchen-Vluyn: Neukirchener Verlag, 1995), pp. 85-97; and Nissinen, p. 31.

35. Cf. Dozeman, pp. 175-76; see below.

stances where a male has a duty to produce offspring (as in Gen. 38:9-10) — and not applied to relations with prostitutes.

6. The suggestion that the prohibition of male homoerotic activity received explicit formulation in a context in which Israelite sexual norms were being defined over against those of other peoples requires a word of caution concerning attempts to locate and assess the practice against which it was aimed. It is possible that the breakdown of the old village culture, increased mobility (including forced migrations), and the anonymity and heterogeneity of city life were sufficient to permit or encourage the homoerotic encounters that are condemned in our texts, without positing significant foreign influence. The identification of abhorrent practices as "foreign" is a common polemical ploy and may be entirely baseless, or grounded in highly evolved "myths" whose origins can no longer be traced or confirmed.

a. Evidence for same-sex erotic interaction from the ancient Near East is meager and ambiguous, but supports the view that sexual relations (of all types) were defined and judged according to gender-role prescriptions that identified the male as the active partner and the female as the passive.[36] No clear reference to homoeroticism is found in the Ugaritic or Hittite texts,[37] and only two Egyptian texts speak unambiguously of sexual acts between males. One suggests disapproval of pedophilia, while the other describes a case of anal intercourse as an act of sexual aggression intended to humiliate and demonstrate superior power.[38] Mesopotamian evidence, though fragmentary and scattered, offers instructive parallels to OT attitudes, but its contribution to the question of cultic sex as the source of the Levitical prohibitions is disputed.[39]

(1) Assyrian law decrees harsh sanctions (including rape and castration) for a male who "lays" a "comrade" (i.e., an equal), and it also punishes a man

36. Nissinen, p. 19. Cf. Jean Bottéro and H. Petschow, "Homosexualität," in *Reallexikon der Assyriology* 4, ed. Dietz Otto Edzard (Berlin and New York: De Gruyter, 1972-75), pp. 459-68. See appendix B for details.

37. Nissinen, p. 20.

38. Nissinen, p. 19. See appendix B.

39. Excluded from consideration here is the relationship between Gilgamesh and Enkidu, which Nissinen describes as a prime example of homosocial-type bonding in an "equal relationship between the men, with no clear social or sexual role division" (p. 24). In Nissinen's words, "They experience unity and share each other's worlds — unlike a man and a woman, who lived in separate worlds" (p. 24; see further pp. 20-24; cf. Gwendolyn Leick, *Sex and Eroticism in Mesopotamian Literature* [London and New York: Routledge, 1994], pp. 254-69). Although this represents the bonding of two superheroes, it has analogies in the male friendships that are formed in patriarchal societies, best illustrated in the OT by the friendship of David and Jonathan (n. 6 above).

who slanders a comrade with a false accusation of inviting, or consenting to, repeated sexual advances by other males.[40] Omens, myths, and proverbs suggest that occasional homoerotic contacts were tolerated, on a consensual or contractual basis. Unlike the laws, these sources are not concerned with enforcing community norms; hence their references contain no moral judgments. They suggest nevertheless that the male who played the female role suffered social deprecation or belonged to a lower social class.[41] No examples of female-female sexual relations are known from Mesopotamian texts.[42]

(2) In addition to texts that speak directly of sexual relations between males, Mesopotamian sources attest a number of classes of male cult personnel *(assinnu, kurgarrû, kulu'u,* and *sinnišānu)* that have frequently been described as male prostitutes,[43] although their role in homoerotic encounters is disputed and evidence for their sexual activity is almost exclusively inferential. As devotees of the goddess Inanna/Ishtar, they reflect her androgynous nature as the Venus star and her control of sexuality, including her power to "change men into women." Their role in the cult was characteristically asexual rather than homosexual, according to Nissinen, frequently (though not necessarily) involving castration, and marked by female dress and symbols or a combination of male and female attributes (e.g., swords and spindles).[44] Since the *assinnu's* prescribed cultic role required him to renounce the distinctive attributes of the male role, he would appear to provide an ideal passive partner for male homosexual encounters. There is no clear evidence, however, that such practice was a part of the cult, although one might say that wherever the *assinnu* practiced this trade, he did so as a votary of the goddess.

40. Nissinen, pp. 24-27; Bottéro and Petschow, p. 462.

41. Nissinen, pp. 27-28; Bottéro and Petschow, pp. 460-63. Nissinen's statement (p. 28) that "men could sometimes find amusement in taking the role of the opposite sex" would appear to apply primarily to partners of equal status.

42. Bottéro and Petschow, p. 468. The lack of documentary evidence appears, as in the OT, to reflect the male-oriented interest of the texts and society, which focused on the problem of a male assuming a "female" role. Thus the silence of the texts concerning lesbian relations is insufficient evidence to rule out the practice, though it could scarcely have been common. Nissinen (pp. 35-36) underscores its rarity by observing that the one possible reference to lesbian relations (an omen apodosis) parallels it to the curiosity of two male dogs copulating.

43. Bottéro and Petschow (p. 463) refer to them as "professionals of passive homosexuality."

44. Nissinen, pp. 30-31, 34. While Nissinen (p. 34) suggests that men of homosexual orientation (to use modern categories) may have sought out this role, as well as transsexuals or those born intersexed, he emphasizes that the role requirements determined the behavior and the sexual identity, not sexual impulse.

It is difficult to estimate the incidence of male prostitution (only one text speaks of "hire") since prostitution (both male and female) lies within the sphere of tolerated liminal activity and is not treated in laws or admonitions relating to infraction of sexual norms. There does not appear to be a "secular" term for a male prostitute corresponding to *ḫarimtu* (the "ordinary" female prostitute).[45] If the *assinnus* and/or related classes supported themselves as male prostitutes, they had a cultic role to fall back on, unlike the *ḫarimtu.* This did not spare them, however, from the social denigration and ostracism that attached to their aberrant gender role.[46]

b. The frequently suggested association of the homosexual prohibition in the OT with Canaanite religion must be rejected for a number of reasons.

(1) Identification of homosexual activity with what is generally characterized as a "fertility cult" makes no sense — and finds no documentation in Canaanite sources. The "sacred marriage" model used to explain the phenomenon of female "sacred prostitution" cannot be extended to transgendered or asexual male cult personnel such as the *assinnu,* and the model itself is now seriously questioned as an explanation for cult ritual in ancient Syria-Palestine or Mesopotamia.[47] Generalizations about the sexual "deprav-

45. Unless it is the *sinnišānu* (lit. "man-woman"), mentioned in one text in connection with an inn or brothel (Nissinen, p. 33; cf. Wilfried G. Lambert, *Babylonian Wisdom Literature* [Oxford: Oxford University Press, 1960], pp. 218-19; Leick, p. 160). See appendix B. Nissinen (p. 28) includes this term with the other cult-related classes. None of the *assinnu* or *kurgarrû* texts that he cites contain references to a brothel or hire, and he does not use the term "prostitute" to describe the roles or activities of these classes. Nor does he treat the question of remuneration, either as a source of temple income or as a means of livelihood.

46. A passage in the Erra Epic describes *kurgarrû*s and *assinnu*s as men "whose masculinity Ishtar changed into femininity to strike horror into the people" and as "bearers of daggers, razors, pruning-knives and flint blades who frequently do abominable acts [i.e., deeds under a taboo, forbidden to ordinary people] to please the heart of Ishtar" (Nissinen, pp. 30, 148-49 nn. 63 and 64). The sense of fear and abhorrence expressed in this text is close to the sentiment of Leviticus. The text pairs this reference with a reference to prostitutes and female devotees of the goddess (*kezertu*s, *šamḫatu*s, and *ḫarimtu*s) "whom Ishtar deprived of husbands and kept in her power." Both references reflect anxiety concerning transgression of gender roles and boundaries. As the *assinnu* transgresses the normative male gender role (dominance in sexual relations), so the (female) prostitute or devotee of Ishtar transgresses the normative female gender role (sex confined to marriage). Cf. Ereshkigal's curse of the *assinnu* (*kurgarrû* in the Sumerian version) in Ishtar's Descent to the Underworld (Nissinen, p. 32), which is virtually identical to Enkidu's curse of the prostitute Shamhat in the Gilgamesh Epic. Both curses are etiologies for a marginal and despised class, living on the borders of the city and subjected to insults and abuse.

47. See Phyllis A. Bird, "The End of the Male Cult Prostitute," in *Congress Volume*

ity" of the Canaanites that indiscriminately combine all forms of nonmarital sexual activity do not help to explain the particular attention given to male homosexual acts in the Hebrew Bible — or Assyrian law.

(2) The *assinnus* and other male devotees of Inanna/Ishtar who assumed female or androgynous roles in their identification with the goddess do not provide a model for the homosexual practice condemned in the Hebrew Bible. No clear evidence for this class of personnel or the cult to which they belonged has been demonstrated for the OT period.[48] Moreover, cult-related sex, either as a sideline of cultic personnel or as "ordinary" sexual commerce dedicated to temple service, is treated separately in the Hebrew Bible from the texts condemning (male) homosexual activity — and focuses on female, rather than male, practitioners.[49]

(3) The attempt to link male homosexual practice to Canaanite religion or culture through the language of "abomination" fails to distinguish homosexual relations from a host of other rejected practices and fails to recognize the identification as a rhetorical weapon of an age when Canaanites had long since disappeared. It belongs to the language of Israelite polemic that stigmatizes practices deemed unacceptable by identifying them with the "nations" that YHWH drove out before the Israelites — with much the same intention and effect as the terms "Communist" or "un-American" have had at times in American political and religious rhetoric.[50]

7. Despite the cultural differences (including theological understand-

---

Cambridge 1995, ed. J. A. Emerton, VTSup 66 (Leiden: Brill, 1997), pp. 37-43; Tikva Frymer-Kensky, *In the Wake of the Goddesses: Women, Culture, and the Biblical Transformation of Pagan Myth* (New York: Free Press, 1992), pp. 199-202; Johannes Renger, "Heilige Hochzeit. A. Philologisch," in *Reallexikon der Assyriology* 4, pp. 251-59; cf. Karel van der Toorn, "Cultic Prostitution," in *ABD*, 5:510.

48. See appendix A for assessment of attempts to identify the OT *qĕdēšîm* with these classes. The cult of Cybele in Asia Minor and that of the Syrian Atargatis had a similar class of male devotees (the *galli*) who castrated themselves in honor of the goddess. Because Nissinen's main evidence comes from the Mesopotamian sources, I have focused on them. The Syrian evidence, though closer geographically, is later and derives largely from outside observers. Nissinen (p. 32) suggests a connection with the Mesopotamian *assinnus*, citing Will Roscoe, "Priests of the High Goddess: Gender Transgression in Ancient Religion," *History of Religions* 35 (1996): 195-230.

49. See appendix A, pp. 170-73 below.

50. If this language is understood to target practices introduced by Israel's conquerors or neighbors in the period of the nation's collapse or restoration, it is remarkably lacking in specificity — and in associations with identifiable foreign practices, such as divination, the Tammuz cult, and the cult of the Queen of Heaven (the Judean form of Assyrian Ishtar). Moreover, it also lacks associations with the Canaanite/Hebrew goddess Asherah — the clearest example of persisting "Canaanite" religion.

ings) that separate these texts from us and make it impossible for us to appropriate their words directly, they may still contribute to our current deliberation. The branding of male homosexual acts as an "abomination" suggests close correspondence to contemporary attitudes. What is shared, I think, is a deep sense of revulsion and/or ambivalence toward a practice that is perceived as "unnatural" or contrary to the fundamental order of society — conceived on a patriarchal model. The "reasons" given are secondary and culturally variable. Thus, while Israel's attempt to associate homosexual practice with foreign/pagan peoples *may* reflect something of its encounter with surrounding cultures, it is no more adequate an explanation of the taboo than modern arguments that seek to ground it in the consequences of AIDS or the threat of genocide.

8. The context of the present debate is similar to that in which the subject of homosexual practice emerged as an issue of theological interest in ancient Israel and the biblical canon. The prohibition received "canonical" formation in a period of transition and breakdown of older community boundaries and norms, when the question of communal identity had become the central theological question. The answer provided by the Holiness Code applies a cultic concept to the community as a whole and creates legislation that redefines the boundaries of the community, interpreting them in cultic terms of purity and separation from defilement. Although the demand for holiness is spelled out elsewhere in this legislation in ethical commands that link reverence for God and respect for neighbor (with special provisions for protecting the weak neighbor in Lev. 25), in the sexual realm its interest is solely in defining appropriate partners, not in the ethics of sexual relations and relationships.

The Levitical response to the challenges of a changing political, social, and religious order is not the only biblical model. Deuteronomy exhibits a different response — which may have been in part contemporaneous. The Deuteronomic move is toward restriction in cultic expression but greater inclusiveness in defining the cultic community. Women, slaves, and resident aliens are now explicitly brought within the provisions of the law and are the object of both cultic and ethical legislation.[51] The canon also witnesses attempts to define the identity and boundaries of the community in the writings of Ezra and Nehemiah — focused on the role of Torah and the problem

51. See, e.g., the recasting of the old law of the Hebrew slave (Exod. 20:2-6) to include women in Deut. 15:12-18, and the new legislation for the annual harvest pilgrim feasts in Deut. 16:11, 14 which specifies inclusion of all of the landless classes: slaves, Levites, resident aliens, widows, and orphans. See Norbert Lohfink, "Poverty in the Laws of the Ancient Near East and of the Bible," *TS* 52 (1991): 43-47.

of intermarriage with foreigners[52] — and various NT writings attest to the struggle of early Christian communities to define themselves over against their Jewish and pagan ancestors and neighbors.

9. Today the issue of Christian identity and the boundaries of Christian community is once more a critical issue, with its attendant concerns over rights and obligations of members. In the debate over these issues, the status of homosexual acts and persons has emerged as perhaps the most important case for testing our understanding of Christian identity and community. In this new situation none of the old answers will suffice, and those that are reaffirmed will be reinterpreted. But while the specific terms of the Holiness Code cannot serve our present needs, the legal tradition of the OT exemplified in the Covenant Code, the Deuteronomic Code, and the Holiness Code offers precedent and models in its attempts to create — and re-create — representative but encompassing statements of the principles and values that define community for a people that understands itself as the people of God.

a. The OT contributes to Christian ethics the conviction that the demands of love of God and neighbor must find expression in concrete acts and specific principles. Thus the OT legal tradition contains efforts to formulate general norms, as in the Decalogue, together with specific cases that are both expressions and tests of the general norms. Both are essential and both are subject to change as they are brought into new interpretive contexts. The successive, and in part competing, law codes contained in the Hebrew Bible testify to an ongoing process of community deliberation concerning the rules that will govern its life, a process that continues today. Today cases relating to homosexual identity and practice are helping us clarify fundamental principles of Christian ethics.

b. The concept of holiness as embracing all of life and distinguishing life in Christ from life apart from Christ (to translate into Christian terms) is, in my view, a concept of continuing validity for Christian ethics, which requires reformulation. It is in many ways a revolutionary concept when applied to the realm of sexual relations.

c. The attempt of Leviticus 18 and 19 to bring sexual relations into the realm of theological interest, however limited, is an invitation to further theological reflection. It represents a step beyond the older collections of OT laws that show virtually no interest in relations, sexual or otherwise, within the private, male-dominated sphere of the family — or outside the family insofar

52. Ezra 9–10 (which solves the problem by excluding foreign wives and their children) and Neh. 13:23-30.

as they do not affect the rights and/or honor of male citizens. From this point on, sex is not simply a "private" matter, nor a purely social concern.

d. The inclusion of the homosexual prohibitions within a larger collection of laws provides a model for contemporary deliberation. The question of homosexual ethics is properly situated in a broader consideration of the demands of Christian community that place sexual ethics alongside demands for social and economic justice. To isolate the question of homosexual practice from the other demands violates the biblical model.

10. While Leviticus 18 and 20 establish a claim of theological interest in sexual relations, the sphere of interest they define and the factors they identify as relevant are far too limited in their exclusive concern with categories of sexual partners or defiling conditions (menstruation), both objectively defined. Because the laws are meant to establish boundaries, they do not address the more fundamental issue of sexuality and its appropriate uses and expression. That is true of the whole OT — and of the Bible as a whole. Just as gender is not a recognized concept or subject of debate in the biblical world, neither is sexuality, with all of its biological, psychological, and sociological aspects that must figure in any modern discussion. Sexuality and sexual ethics represent new concepts and arenas of discourse and discovery, to which we must attempt to relate the biblical testimony.

11. The OT laws, taken by themselves, are insufficient guides, even for the situations they address explicitly. They serve primarily to indicate areas of interest, principles of justice, and underlying social and religious values. Thus the death penalty attached to the sexual prohibitions shows the intense level of interest in (male-defined) sexual rights and boundaries. But the prohibitions and judgments do not tell us how particular cases were handled or reveal the moral reasoning behind decisions. Here narrative texts may offer illumination, and qualification. The story of Judah and Tamar (Gen. 38) provides an instructive example of a violation of sexual norms in which the condemned woman receives not only a reprieve, but a judgment of "right(eous)" conduct — in view of the circumstances. It warns against absolutizing any of the sexual laws. Circumstances matter and so do motives — even when they are not explicitly articulated. This account reminds us that the laws do not stand alone. They function within a social and canonical context to which the OT narrative, prophetic, and wisdom texts give limited but essential witness.

Extralegal Texts as Sources for OT Ethical Deliberation concerning Homosexuality

The OT legal texts may not be dismissed as sources for Christian theological and ethical reflection by appeal to Christ as the end of the law or because of their particular historical and cultic associations. The laws of the Christian OT do not bind, but instruct, and their power to instruct is not diminished. But the law is only one mode of revelation in the OT canon, and one of the most commonly abused — by isolating individual sentences and absolutizing them as timeless decrees. The canonical context of OT law demands that it be read in the light of the Bible's full testimony to God's saving and revealing presence, and that it must be understood first of all as embedded in a gospel story of God's gracious deliverance, leading, and instructing of a people invited into a covenant relationship and called to be witnesses to that divine action and self-disclosure.

In this larger canonical witness, where does one seek illumination and guidance for the new questions of sexual ethics facing us today, and in particular for the questions relating to homosexual persons and practice? The move from a small number of texts that make explicit, or implied, reference to homosexual activity to the larger canonical witness constitutes a major challenge, since these paths are neither as obvious or as well explored. Recent discussion has turned increasingly to the creation texts as the primary source for a biblical understanding of sexuality and sexual relations against which to view the homosexual prohibition and contemporary issues of homosexuality. I believe that this move is both essential and problematic: essential because the Genesis creation accounts are foundational for all biblical reflection on the meaning of our common humanity and our sexuality; problematic because such appeals often fail to recognize the androcentric shaping and cultural presuppositions of these texts. The creation texts, no less than the laws, are products of an ancient patriarchal society and may not be absolutized. Moreover, their own interests are much more limited than we have traditionally recognized.

The Genesis Creation Accounts

Hays's appeal to the creation accounts may be taken as representative of current arguments in the homosexual debate. In his sketch of a wider biblical framework for the explicit references to homosexual practice, he begins with Genesis 1, under the heading "God's Creative Intention for Human Sexuality." "From Genesis 1 onwards," he writes, "scripture affirms repeatedly that God has made man and woman for one another and that our sexual desires rightly find fulfillment within heterosexual marriage." He continues by citing Mark 10:2-9; 1 Thessalonians 4:3-8; 1 Corinthians 7:1-9; Ephesians 5:21-33; and Hebrews 13:4, concluding that "this picture of marriage provides the positive backdrop against which the Bible's few emphatic negations of homosexuality must be read."[53] Hays's understanding does indeed reflect the history of interpretation in both NT and rabbinic exegesis, but it does not describe the intention of the Genesis creation texts. Moreover, the identification of marriage as the backdrop against which the homosexual prohibitions are to be understood reflects a contemporary understanding of the issues at stake, not an OT view. Homosexual relations in the OT are not viewed as an alternative or a threat to marriage, and the creation texts are neither prescriptions nor models for heterosexual marriage as the context in which "sexual desires rightly find fulfillment." The creation texts are not concerned with right or wrong sexual behavior at all, and the notion of "fulfillment of sexual desire" is alien to these texts — and to OT understanding of marriage.

It is impossible to detail here arguments I have laid out elsewhere on the meaning of these texts in their ancient contexts and their implications for a

53. Hays, p. 10. Surprisingly, he does not treat either of the creation accounts, but appears to interpret them through the NT texts. Cf. Ulrich W. Mauser, "Creation, Sexuality, and Homosexuality in the New Testament," in *Homosexuality and Christian Community*, pp. 47-49, for the NT interpretation of Gen. 1–2. A different approach to the creation texts is taken by Thomas Dozeman, who points to an intercanonical change in understanding of creation (from P to Paul) as consequential for biblical and contemporary theologies of sexuality (p. 184). I am in fundamental agreement with his argument that the topic of sexuality belongs under the rubric of creation theology (pp. 170-71), and commend his attention to changing views within the canon as significant for current debate, but I differ with his interpretation of Gen. 1 in relation to Lev. 18 and 20. My analysis of the OT texts has convinced me that the cosmological underpinnings of the Levitical prohibitions are to be found in the notion of gender identity and boundaries (cf. Tikva Frymer-Kensky, "Sex and Sexuality," in *ABD*, 5:1145-46), not in the theme of procreation articulated in Gen. 1, and interpreted as a life/death option (Dozeman, pp. 175-76). Thus I cannot agree that the prohibition rests in the rejection of a "sexual act devoid of the possibility of reproduction" (p. 176). While the exact relationship of the Holiness Code to P remains disputed in terms of date and authorship, the characteristic concepts of the Holiness Code are recognizably distinct from those of P elsewhere in the Pentateuch, including Gen. 1 (Joosten, p. 193; cf. pp. 13-14, 194-207). Drawing these texts together may serve the needs of contemporary theology, but it misleads, I believe, when Gen. 1 is viewed as the historical matrix in which the homosexual prohibitions arose.

contemporary theology of sexuality.[54] I can only offer a few summary comments related to common arguments in current debate, but they remain inadequate without a fuller discussion of the texts and their larger OT and ancient Near Eastern context. The main point that must be highlighted is that these texts *assume* the common pattern of sexual relations between male and female as the basis for the reproduction of the human species — as of the animal species (Gen. 1:22, 27-28) — and interpret this gift of reproductive capability as God's good design; they further *assume* that the sexual drive that unites man and woman is the basis for marriage (Gen. 2:24). They do not *prescribe* any behavior or institution. They are etiologies, explaining why things are the way they are — and in Genesis 3 explaining why the woman *is* subordinate to the man (in ancient Israelite society), not why she *should* be.[55] They are uninterested in variations of or deviations from the dominant pattern. The theological problem posed by variations in nature, together with the related ethical questions of appropriate social responses, is not adequately treated, or even recognized, in the canonical literature.[56]

The more important reason we cannot expect help from the creation texts on the question of appropriate expressions and constraints of sexuality

54. See esp. Phyllis A. Bird, "Genesis 1–3 as a Source for a Theological Understanding of Sexuality," *Ex Auditu* 3 (1987): 31-44; for the exegetical foundations, see Phyllis A. Bird, "'Male and Female He Created Them': Gen 1:27b in the Context of the Priestly Creation Account," *HTR* 74 (1981): 129-59; Phyllis A. Bird, "Sexual Differentiation and Divine Image in the Genesis Creation Texts," in *Image of God and Gender Models in Judaeo-Christian Tradition,* ed. Kari E. Børresen (Oslo: Solum, 1991), pp. 11-34, republished under the title *Image of God: Gender Models in Judaeo-Christian Tradition* (Minneapolis: Augsburg Fortress, 1995), pp. 5-28; Bird, "Authority of the Bible." Cf. Richard E. Whitaker, "Creation and Human Sexuality," in *Homosexuality and Christian Community,* pp. 3-13; and Gerald T. Sheppard, "The Use of Scripture within the Christian Ethical Debate concerning Same-Sex Oriented Persons," *USQR* 40 (1985): 13-35.

55. The regulation of sexual relations and marriage belongs to the realm of law and custom. A noteworthy feature of the laws and traditions that did serve to regulate sexual relations and marriage in ancient Israel (at least those preserved in the OT canon) is that they never refer to the creation texts as models. See, e.g., the marriage blessing given to Ruth, which invokes the example of Rachel and Leah (Ruth 4:11), not Eve.

56. Mesopotamian tradition preserves an attempt to account for abnormalities in creation — and to provide a constructive social response. In the Sumerian myth of "Enki and Ninmah," the midwife goddess Ninmah, who has assisted Enki in creating humankind, continues to create in a drunken challenge to Enki, now forming misshapen creatures: a giant, a woman unable to bear, and a creature with neither male nor female organs. In each case, however, Enki is able to find a place in society for her creation and ensure it a living (Samuel Noah Kramer, *Sumerian Mythology,* rev. ed. [New York, Evanston, and London: Harper & Row, 1961], pp. 68-72, esp. p. 71; and Thorkild Jacobsen, *The Treasures of Darkness* [New Haven: Yale University Press, 1976], pp. 113-14).

is that sexuality as we understand it today is not addressed in the Bible. It is a modern concept. The Bible treats sexuality only in limited forms of actualization. We can learn a great deal from the experience of Israel and the church in their attempts to comprehend and control sex as a divine endowment and as a human capacity subject to the distorting and alienating power of sin. But we cannot get a ready-made sexual ethic or even an adequate foundation for it from the Bible. The terms of Israel's culturally shaped understanding will not satisfy our present need. In this field we must look to the ongoing revelation of science and of newly emerging voices of experience. That is to follow the pattern exhibited in the Bible itself. But the Bible also gives a more explicit mandate for the appeal to experience and science.

The Wisdom Tradition in the Old Testament

Appeal to experience is given theoretical undergirding by the wisdom literature, which affirms wisdom as a path to piety and observes creation (as mundane world and as cosmic wonder) for signs of the nature and designs of God.[57] In this literature and the intellectual tradition that it represents (including not only Proverbs, Psalms, and Job, as well as the skeptic Qohelet, but also the creation account of Gen. 1), we find biblical authorization for the appeal to science to inform our understanding and judgment of homosexual orientation and practice. I will limit my comments on this underutilized tradition and its implications for our current debate to the following brief points.

1. Contemporary science, in all its ambiguity and fallibility, is a means of revelation of the nature of creation and the mind of the Creator. It may not be contrasted to the science employed by the biblical writers (e.g., the cosmology of Gen. 1) in a manner that privileges biblical science as revealed knowledge.

2. Science is open-ended and characterized by multiple voices, achieving impressive consensuses in some areas and characterized by unresolved tensions in others. The existence within the biblical canon of conflicting voices within the wisdom tradition is an authorization to keep open the debate today, and to give it a place within the witness of the community of believers.

3. Experience is irreducible. It is subject to distortion and error and is always culturally framed, but no other source, and no other's experience, may

57. See Seow, pp. 19-25, for a development of this argument.

cancel or substitute for the experience of any individual or group. The book of Job offers a model for affirming the integrity of individual experience as it affirms Job's integrity in maintaining his innocence against his friends' pious interpretations of his predicament. It also provides a model in suggesting that particular attention must be given to those whose experience does not fit the reigning norms, including theological norms. Qohelet also demonstrates the Bible's openness to the skeptic. With respect to the current debate, I believe this means that the testimony of homosexual or bisexual persons to their experience of sexual need and fulfillment in same-sex relationships is testimony that may not be dismissed as deformed by social or ideological pressure or as incompatible with Christian identity and silenced within the Christian community. Experience must be allowed to speak, and it must be heard — which means that it must be aided in gaining a hearing when it is unpopular, unorthodox, or has been suppressed. Speaking and hearing are the first ethical requirements in the attempt to comprehend homosexual nature and practice and devise guidelines for action.

4. Experience must be tested. Our problem today concerns the criteria for testing. My preference is for criteria that weigh personal and communal consequences in favor of options that conduce to health and wholeness, healing and the upbuilding of community, honor of God, and freeing for the work of the kingdom — tests that should apply equally to heterosexual as well as homosexual acts and relationships.

Implications for Present Action

Because we are currently in a situation where neither science nor experience has achieved a consensus concerning the nature of homosexuality and its individual and social consequences, the first ethical question that confronts us is how to make ethical decisions in a situation where experts do not agree. Although the analogy to the wilderness wanderings proposed by Kathryn Greene-McCreight is not as fitting as she first thought, it is nevertheless suggestive to an OT exegete. We are not yet ready to settle the new land and build houses — at least not as united "tribes." But wilderness is a time of preparation, and an essential part of that preparation is trying out new options. The herding tribes in the biblical account requested and received permission to settle before their "brothers," in the pasturelands of the Transjordan that were suited to their lifestyle (Num. 32), and even after the united settlement, not all lived in the same manner. So one question that Israel's history and the complex testimony of the biblical canon place before us is, How much unity is necessary on this issue? and further, What type and degree of disagreement can be tolerated within the household of faith? In the wilderness, conversation and debate must continue, but it has to be informed by practice. Moving from the known land to the unknown, the preference in situations of uncertainty and conflict will always be to return to the security of the old ways — as evidenced by the Israelites who preferred bondage in Egypt to the uncertainties and hardships of the awful wilderness (Exod. 14:12) and by the spies who preferred not to claim the Promised Land when confronted by its intimidating inhabitants (Num. 13:30–14:4). Those individuals and church bodies today who are willing to challenge the intimidating defenders of tradition perform an essential service to the church by making available a new body of experience to be weighed in reformulating our codes of sexual ethics and our regulations concerning church membership and service. Thus, while I agree with Greene-McCreight that we need a moratorium on legislative action designed to bind all members to a common position, I believe we need to encourage responsible experiments with alternative practices. We need spies in the new land who are not afraid to set up colonies there, even if they must continue to live for a time in tents and booths.

Appendix A: Deuteronomy 23:17-18 (Hebrew 18-19) and "Sacred Prostitution"

The key text linking sex and cult in the OT, and the only text in which this link includes explicit reference to male practitioners, is Deuteronomy 23:17-18 (Heb. 18-19), a text that pairs masculine and feminine terms for personnel in a manner that subordinates the masculine to the feminine. Two prohibitions are linked in these verses, but their meaning and manner of union remain disputed.[58]

The older law, in verse 18 (Heb. 19), prohibits bringing the wages of a prostitute *(zônâ)* or the "hire of a dog" *(mĕḥîr keleb)* into the house of YHWH in payment of any vow. The term "dog" has traditionally been understood to designate a male (homosexual) prostitute.[59] The prohibition is not

58. For a detailed analysis of this text and all texts containing the terms *qādēš/qĕdēšîm,* see Bird, "Male Cult Prostitute."

59. Although some have maintained that a canine is intended here (cf. Larry E. Stager,

directed at these two classes themselves, but at use of the income derived from their practice; sexual commerce, which may have been common around temples as places of pilgrimage (cf. modern convention centers), is not to be a source of temple income. Consorting with (female) prostitutes is not prohibited in the OT, nor penalized by law — and is presented in Proverbs as a safer alternative to adultery.[60] But what of male prostitutes? If *keleb* represents a male counterpart of *zônâ,* it is the only reference to a male prostitute in the Hebrew Bible. The position of the term in the prohibition suggests that the phenomenon was relatively infrequent or unimportant, since it follows the term for the female prostitute — in contrast to the normal male-female order in gender pairs. This passage offers no evidence for identifying male homosexual practice as a distinctive feature of the Canaanite cult, or any foreign cult (the prohibition pertains to the temple of YHWH). If it provides evidence for an accepted (or at least tolerated) form of homosexual practice, then it is instructive that it is in the form of prostitution, a commercial form of sex that in its better-attested female form typically takes place away from home, among strangers, in taverns or traveler's lodges. If the prohibition of homoerotic relations is primarily concerned with the violation of male honor, as suggested above, then the male prostitute, like his female counterpart, provides a safe, though despised, object as one who stands outside the normal system of sexual honor.

In its present context the prohibition of verse 18 (Heb. 19) has been prefaced by a proscription in verse 17 (Heb. 18) of a class of persons identified by the term *qĕdēšâ/qādēš* (consecrated woman/man), and a concluding pronouncement in verse 19 declares the combined classes or activities an "abomination." The term *qdš(h)* is found only in polemical contexts in the OT, with the feminine form always paralleled by *zônâ* (prostitute) (Gen. 38:21-22 and Hos. 4:14 in addition to this text). The feminine noun appears to describe a class of cult-related women whose activity is stigmatized by Israelite authors, who associate them with prostitutes — leading modern interpreters to describe them as

---

Ashkelon Discovered [Washington, D.C.: Biblical Archaeology Society, 1991], chap. 2, "Why Were Hundreds of Dogs Buried at Ashkelon?" esp. p. 36; Mayer I. Gruber, "Hebrew *qedēšāh* and Her Canaanite and Akkadian Cognates," *UF* 18 [1986]: 133 n. 1), the parallelism of female-male pairs in vv. 18 and 19 makes it clear that the author/redactor of the paired verses thought of a male counterpart to the *zônâ.* This identification is strengthened by Akkadian evidence for the *assinnu,* which is written with the cuneiform sign UR.SAL "dog-woman," in which "dog" represents the male element in a combination of genders (Nissinen, pp. 28, 147 n. 45).

60. Prov. 6:26 contrasts a prostitute's fee (as cheap) with the cost of adultery (death).

"sacred/cultic prostitutes."[61] The masculine term follows the feminine in this verse, its first occurrence in the OT, and appears to be literarily dependent upon it. Despite persistent references to male cult prostitutes in modern textbooks, which describe them as a characteristic feature of Canaanite religion and a symbol of its sexual depravity, no such institution or practice is known from any Canaanite texts, and the masculine term is found only in Deuteronomistic sources (all interdependent and all later than the independently occurring feminine forms).[62] The masculine cognate at Ugarit describes a class of married cult personnel subordinate to priests, having no documented associations with sexual activity, heterosexual or homosexual.[63]

Attempts to interpret OT references to *qādēš/qědēšîm* by appeal to the *assinnu* or *galli* rest on inadequate foundations and faulty assumptions concerning gender roles in ancient Near Eastern society. The mimicking language and female-male word order point to the artificial nature of the male class in Deuteronomy 23:18, which must be interpreted as a counterpart of the female class. This violates the pattern of gender-differentiated roles and nomenclature that is the rule for ancient Near Eastern and Israelite cultic offices and professions — as illustrated here by the terms for male and female

61. The expression "sacred prostitute" is a nineteenth-century invention by anthropologists and historians of religion who drew upon a variety of classical and patristic references to premarital and extramarital sexual activity by *women,* associated with various cults of Mesopotamia, Asia Minor, Cyprus, and the Levant, as well as the biblical sources treated here (Marie-Theres Wacker, "Kosmisches Sakrament oder Verpfändung des Körpers? 'Kultprostitution' im biblischen Israel und im hinduistischen Indien: Religionsgeschichtliche Überlegung im Interesse feministischer Theologie," *BN* 61 [1992]: 51-52; Bird, "Male Cult Prostitute," pp. 37-40). No combination of terms for prostitution and the sacred is found in any ancient text, and all of the ancient sources that characterize cult-related activity as "prostitution" are the descriptions of outsiders. For an analysis of the extrabiblical sources and the history of the idea, see Robert A. Oden, Jr., "Religious Identity and the Sacred Prostitution Accusation," in *The Bible without Theology: The Theological Tradition and Alternatives to It* (San Francisco: Harper & Row, 1987), pp. 138-52, and Gernot Wilhelm, "Marginalien zu Herodot Klio 199," in *Lingering over Words: Studies in Ancient Near Eastern Literature in Honor of William L. Moran,* ed. I. Tzvi Abusch, John Huehnergard, and Piotr Steinkeller, HSS 37 (Atlanta: Scholars Press, 1990), pp. 505-24. Cf. van der Toorn, "Cultic Prostitution."

62. 1 Kings 14:24; 15:12; 22:46 (Heb. 47); and 2 Kings 23:7. All lack contextual associations with prostitution or sex and are dependent on Deut. 23:18 for their interpretation. All of the references in the Deuteronomistic History (DH) are collective and appear to function as a summary term for "Canaanite" cult personnel banished by reforming Judean kings. For detailed analysis, see Bird, "Male Cult Prostitute," pp. 51-75. On a possible reference in Job 36:14, see Bird, "Male Cult Prostitute," pp. 75-77.

63. Wolfram von Soden, "Zur Stellung des 'Geweihten' *(qdš)* in Ugarit," *UF* 2 (1970): 329-30; cf. Gruber, p. 147.

prostitutes.[64] Akkadian *qadištu* (the cognate of Heb. *qĕdēšâ*, attested in more than seventy references) has no masculine counterpart, and Ugaritic *qdš* is not attested in a feminine form.[65] The Mesopotamian *assinnu* is not associated with the *qadištu*, who is never identified with Ishtar but is always dedicated to a male deity (usually Adad). And none of the biblical references to *qĕdēšîm* associate them with the "Queen of Heaven," the seventh/sixth-century Judean manifestation of Assyrian Ishtar. Moreover, no class of devotees comparable to the Mesopotamian *assinnu* is attested in Canaanite myths or cultic texts.[66] The interpretation of *qādēš/qĕdēšîm* in DH as a class of male homosexual prostitutes misinterprets religious polemic as social history, creating a class that corresponds neither to the Mesopotamian *assinnu*s nor to attested classes or associations of prostitutes. The biblical references are polemical constructs that exhibit no firsthand knowledge of the institution they condemn — and insist that it was banished by the reign of Jehoshaphat (mid ninth century B.C.E.).[67]

Appendix B: Homoeroticism in the Ancient Near East

Evidence is limited to two references from Egypt and a scattering of Mesopotamian texts from different literary genres, with different purposes and perspectives, and covering a span of more than two millennia.

Egypt. A confession in the Book of the Dead contains the twice-repeated statement, "I have not had sexual relations with a boy," suggesting that

64. The exception is the "charismatic" offices, specifically prophets (Heb. *nābî'/nĕbî'â;* Akk. *āpilu/āpiltu, qabbā'u/qabbātu, šā'ilu/šā'iltu*), whose "office" or profession depends on their ability to transmit and interpret messages from the gods, rather than on specialized training; they are "chosen" by the god, rather than inducted into a gender-specific role through training or apprenticeship in a guild.

65. As a generic term for one "consecrated/dedicated (to a deity or temple)," it may be applied to different classes with distinct roles and duties in different places and periods.

66. The *assinnu*s are not devotees of a "mother goddess," and their cultic role cannot be extended to the service of Asherah, the dominant goddess of the biblical text, who was also prominent at Ugarit. Nor is there evidence of a comparable class associated with Anat, the Canaanite goddess who most closely resembles Ishtar.

67. On the indirect reference in 2 Kings 23:7, see Bird, "Male Cult Prostitute," pp. 64-74. If the references to the *qĕdēšîm* in DH are understood as a reflex of practices introduced by Assyrian or Babylonian rule, such as the cult of Tammuz (Ezek. 8:14) or the worship of the Queen of Heaven (Jer. 7:18; 44:15-19), then the DH insistence on their early eradication and failure to identify them with other foreign abominations are difficult to explain.

homoerotic relations between men (or more specifically pedophilia) were regarded as morally suspect.[68] More significant in revealing attitudes is an episode in the myth describing the power struggle between Horus and Seth, in which Seth abuses Horus sexually, by anal intercourse, while Horus is asleep. Seth's purpose, Nissinen comments, is to "show his superiority by forcing Horus into the position of a defeated and raped enemy." "This story," he concludes, "obviously deals not with same-sex desire but with sexual aggression used in exercising power."[69]

Mesopotamia. The Middle Assyrian Laws contain two cases treating sexual acts between males.[70] Paragraph 19 concerns a man who spreads an unsubstantiated rumor concerning a "comrade" (*tappāšu* = his equal), saying, "Everyone (m.) 'lays' him *(ittinikkūš).*"[71] The case is parallel in construction to paragraph 18, in which the accusation is, "Everyone 'lays' your wife." The punishments in the two cases are identical except for the number of blows the accuser is to receive: forty for the defamation of the woman, but fifty for defamation of the man.[72] This differential reflects values similar to those expressed in the OT narrative accounts where the violation of a woman is represented as a lesser offense than the parallel action with a man. The issue here is not forced, but willing, submission to the receptive role, with an emphasis (in both of the parallel accusations) on habitual promiscuity which amounts to a charge of prostitution.

Paragraph 20 concerns a substantiated charge that a man has "laid" a comrade *(tappāšu inīk).* The punishment applies the rule of talion ("they shall have sex with him" [*inikkūš*]) and adds castration (*ana ša rēšēn utarrūš:* "they shall turn him into a eunuch") — a punishment that not only deprives the offender of his sexual "weapon," but creates a permanent change in his

68. Nissinen, p. 19.

69. Nissinen, p. 19. For additional Egyptian sources that may allude to some kind of same-sex interaction, see Nissinen, p. 144 n. 2; cf. David F. Greenberg, *The Construction of Homosexuality* (Chicago: University of Chicago Press, 1988), pp. 129-30.

70. *Middle Assyrian Laws* §§ 19-20 (KAV 1 ii 82-96), cited by Nissinen, p. 25. They follow a series of cases concerning adultery (§§ 12-18) and form part of a collection of laws known as the "Laws of the Woman" (Bottéro and Petschow, p. 462).

71. The verb *niāku,* which Nissinen translates "have sex with," always has the active and dominant party as its subject, but does not in itself imply force or violence (Nissinen, pp. 25-26).

72. The punishment also included performing the king's service for a month, payment of one talent of lead, and some type of symbolic action *(igaddimu)* whose meaning is not clear (Nissinen, p. 25). It must indicate some form of shaming (cutting off the beard or hair?), though not castration (§ 20) (Nissinen, p. 146 n. 27; p. 26; cf. Greenberg, p. 125 n. 4).

gender role.[73] This example makes clear that the offense was understood as dishonoring another man by forcing him into the role of a woman,[74] a view corroborated by neo-Assyrian curses that threaten a disobedient (male) vassal with becoming a prostitute *(ḫarimtu)*[75] or liken a man to a raped captive, a slave girl, or a woman.[76]

Male-to-male sexual acts are occasionally mentioned in dream omens, a genre concerned with exceptional phenomena and lacking any moral interest — in contrast to the laws, which seek to articulate and enforce community values.[77] The only clear examples come from the omen series *Šumma ālu,* which lists four cases of intercourse with a male in a series of thirty-eight dealing with various aspects of sex life. In the first (CT 39: 44:13), the partner is identified as an equal and anal penetration is specified: "If a man approaches [for copulation] *(iteḫḫe)* his equal *(meḫrīšu)* from the rear, he becomes the leader among his peers and brothers."[78] The following three cases (CT 39: 45:32-34) involve social inferiors and appear to be associated with negative consequences.[79] They identify, in descending order of status, an *assinnu,* a *gerseqqû* ("courtier," a member of the household, possibly a eunuch), and a house-born slave *(dušmu)* as the sexual partner. "Consensual," or contractual, relations seem to be assumed.

These cases suggest that male subordinates or members of special classes might provide a passive partner for homosexual encounters, in addition to occasional "exchange" of roles among equals. They do not fundamentally qualify the underlying assumptions concerning gender roles observed in the laws, which view sexual relations as inherently unequal and identify the

73. Nissinen, p. 25.

74. Although the same verb is used here as in the two preceding laws, the case appears to be treated as an incidence of rape, since only the man who is the active subject of the verb is punished. Cf. §12, where the woman who is raped incurs no punishment in contrast to the cases in which the woman is a consenting partner. In contrast, the accusation of §19 focuses on the shame of the receptive partner, who, analogous to a promiscuous wife, invites sexual advances.

75. Treaty of Ashur-nerari V of Assyria with Mati'-ilu of Arpad (SAA 3 30:1-4, 7), quoted by Nissinen, pp. 26-27; cf. p. 146 n. 33.

76. Nissinen, pp. 26-27. Nissinen cites these as examples of "many other texts [that] take the raping of a man as an ultimate act of disgrace."

77. Nissinen, pp. 27-28; Bottéro and Petschow, pp. 460-61.

78. The omen apodoses often pronounce quite startling, and even conflicting, "consequences," and cannot be understood as "logical" results according to modern notions of causality.

79. The meaning of the apodosis in the case of the *assinnu* is not clear. See Nissinen, p. 27, 147 n. 39; cf. Bottéro and Petschow, p. 461.

active and superior role with the male and the passive with the female.[80] While a series of incantations refers to a man's love *(râmu)* for another man in the same terms as parallel references to a man's love for a woman, and a woman's love for a man,[81] this suggestion of common sentiment in different types of relationships remains in tension with the hierarchy of socially prescribed roles and actions. It is noteworthy that this triad of love relationships does not include love of a woman for another woman.

Although sexual allusions attend many of the references to the male devotees of Inanna/Ishtar known variously by the names *assinnu, kurgarrû, kulu'u,* and *sinnišānu,*[82] there is no clear evidence for sexual activity as a part of their cultic role.[83] The single reference to an *assinnu* in a text treating male-to-male sexual relations gives no information about the circumstances that would allow us to determine whether the contact was part of a cultic action and/or involved payment.[84] The one text that appears to speak of male prostitution is a proverb concerning a *sinnišānu.* On entering the "brothel" *(bīt aštammi),* he "raised his hands [gesture of prayer?] and said: 'My hire goes to the promoter[?] *(anzinnu).* You [Ishtar?] are wealth *(mešrû),* I am half *(mešlu).*'"[85] The meaning of this statement is uncertain, as is the identity of the addressee. Sexual encounters (with men and women) seem to have taken place in the *bīt aštammi* (variously translated "tavern," "hostel," and "brothel"),[86] which was apparently attached to some temples, under the patronage of Ishtar.

80. Nissinen, p. 27; cf. Bottéro and Petschow, p. 462; Clemens Locher, *Die Ehre einer Frau in Israel. Exegetische und rechtsvergleichende Studien zum Deutereonomium 22,13-21,* OBO 70 (Freiburg: Universitätsverlag; Göttingen: Vandenhoeck & Ruprecht, 1986), pp. 369-71. All the verbs used for sexual contacts are one-directional, with the active partner as subject; there is no Mesopotamian vocabulary for mutual and equal sexual relationships (Nissinen, p. 146 n. 31).

81. Bottéro and Petschow, pp. 467-68, citing the "Almanac of Incantations" (BRM 4, 20); cf. Nissinen, p. 35.

82. Nissinen cites only one text referring to a *sinnišānu* (lit. "man-woman") (treated below). He notes (p. 28) that the group sometimes included the *kalû* lamentation priests.

83. On these classes, see Nissinen, pp. 28-35; Bottéro and Petschow, pp. 463-67; Leick, pp. 157-69; cf. Greenberg, pp. 96-97. Richard A. Henshaw, *Female and Male: The Cultic Personnel: The Bible and the Rest of the Ancient Near East* (Allison Park, Pa.: Pickwick, 1994), pp. 284-311, offers an expanded list of titles.

84. The omen text CT 39: 45:32, cited above.

85. Nissinen, p. 33, citing Lambert, pp. 218-19; cf. Leick, p. 160.

86. See Henshaw, pp. 312-23.

CHAPTER 6

Sexuality and Scripture's Plain Sense: The Christian Community and the Law of God

CHRISTOPHER SEITZ

I

This essay assumes that Scripture is the authority that guides the church's reflection on human sexual behavior. It also assumes that the problem with the present debate is that both sides are appealing to Scripture, in some measure, in order to ground what are diametrically opposing views. The thesis argued here is that we have lost the ability to hear a *connected* Old and New Testament witness to God in Christ and have substituted for it a model that isolates texts from their specific canonical context in order to place them in earlier, discrete, historically reconstructed ("original") circumstances. A contest then ensues as to what individual texts "really mean," by appeal to the correct historical context, to the specific cultural circumstances out of which the text is said to have emerged, or to learned lexicographical analysis. This is fine so far as it goes, but it has failed to achieve any consensus in the present debate. Book after book is written, with a mixture of scholarly and popular essays, and the stalemate actually stimulates rather than dampens new publishing efforts.

The thesis argued here is that both sides in the debate are in some measure "biblicistic" — that is, there has been a failure on both sides to relate the exegesis and interpretation of individual texts to the church's understanding of how the two-Testament canon of Scripture is to be heard, interbiblically, according to the rule of faith. This rule constrains the church to bring into relationship distinct portions of Scripture, especially across the Testaments. The pattern for this is found in the church's reflection on the separatedness, but also the essential unity, of the persons of the Trinity. A Christian discussion of human sexual behavior entails a discussion of the law of God as this is revealed to Israel in the Old Testament; radically reconsidered in and by Jesus Christ; and retained with reference to God's work in him, by virtue of the church's decision to hear the word of God through Israel's witness in the Old Testament, in conjunction with the apostolic witness to Jesus Christ in the New.

In the course of the discussion that follows, older understandings of Christian interpretation of Old Testament law are briefly considered. Then texts other than the usual "proof texts" are discussed, with an eye toward understanding the place of the Christian before God's law. These include Romans 3:31; 7:13-25; Matthew 5:17-48; Galatians 5:16-24; John 8:1-11; 19:30; Deuteronomy 22:23-24; Leviticus 20:13; Hebrews 10:1-31; and Mark 7:1-23. Older distinctions among "moral" and "ritual" and "ceremonial" law are reconsidered in the light of the present debate over homosexuality. There is no lengthy engagement with recent secondary literature, but only an occasional reference. This literature has put on display much historical-critical heavy lifting, but only here and there does this particular slant on interpretation produce results that can be reconnected with the church's chief task: faithful hearing of the witness to God in Christ from the two-Testament Christian Scripture.

What the homosexuality debate has exposed is a deep crisis within the church and the academic settings related to its life and mission. Whatever we might think about the appropriateness of homosexual acts, in culture and in the church, yet more widely divergent are our assumptions about how Scripture functions normatively. It is no revelation that the assumptions grounding historical-critical endeavor are under massive reappraisal, and so it should come as no surprise that on the fault line separating the older critical consensus and newer postliberal approaches sits a debate tailor-made to expose our differences.

On the one side, there is maintained an insistence on the *pluriformity* of the scriptural witness, both within the Old Testament and the New. Related to this, though not identical with it, are those tendencies within Christian circles to privilege, often in very subtle and sophisticated ways, the New Testament witness(es) over against the Old Testament, even though in this case and in others there may in fact be very little difference between them. Nevertheless, the homosexuality debate is tailor-made for this because it works, implicitly or explicitly, with a theory of development or progress. That is, there is some general consensus — John Boswell's more recent efforts notwithstanding — that in the modern homosexual phenomenon we are confronting something truly without precedent, within the life of the church if not also within culture. This dovetails nicely with a notion that we move toward gradual enlightenment as we cross from one Testament to the other. This sense of movement, then, informs and enhances a similar feeling about the way the church is confronting a new thing, perhaps on analogy with Gentile inclusion, and so must formulate a new position on a topic which may have been on the relative periphery in the biblical witness but is at the dead center of our concerns today.

Here one sees how historical thinking has the potential to flatten the complex *literary and theological* interrelatedness of Scripture — for all the apparent pluriformity that is gained — by simply getting it to conform to a way of thinking in vogue in the West for the past two hundred years, geared to linear development and change.[1] Since it is in the Old Testament where gender differentiation is grounded theologically and homosexual acts (anal intercourse) are proscribed, one can see how an issue like the modern homosexual phenomenon needs only to highlight the element of development and change that exists within a literary corpus of two parts, one "old" and one "new," and thereby catalyze a sentiment in favor of seeing this issue as truly new and in need of new and enlightened thinking.

Finally, the lasting hallmark of historical-critical endeavor, and the thing that gave it an academic potential in connection with, or divorced from, church life, was its interest in cultural and social contextualization *as truly indispensable for the task of reading and appropriating Scripture "correctly."* The appeal of this sort of objectivism has been enormous. It has energized generation after generation of critical readerships, who have expended enormous amounts of effort setting a text's plain literary sense in the proper time and space category. On the matter at hand, however, it looked like those in favor of churchly endorsement of homosexual behavior had run into a fire wall even historical-critical endeavor could not remove. This was one of those places where the plain sense of the text did not appear to be materially affected by efforts to recover original authorial intention or clearer sociohistorical circumstances. At a minimum, there is no positive statement backing same-sex physical unions in Scripture, occasional or lifelong and committed. And Leviticus and Romans had always been taken as proscribing homosexual behavior, offering one of those instances when Old Testament and New Testament teaching were in basic agreement. Yet over time, greater efforts at critical analysis at last presented a more complex picture, and the older consensus about the plain sense of Scripture on this issue began to collapse.

1. See Hans Frei's *The Eclipse of Biblical Narrative* (New Haven: Yale University Press, 1974).

The relevant question to ask historical-critical endeavor at this juncture is whether it is driven, for all practical purposes, by the necessary requirement to uncover the novel, the different, the complex. That is, historical criticism is *obliged* by its own character to make sure no plain-sense consensus, binding Old and New Testament witnesses, emerges, because to do so would be to admit that the plain sense had a certain priority, in a great many cases, over reconstructions of an "original," historical sense argued to be at odds with it. It would also be to suggest that the way Scripture actually functions normatively — especially on the matter of homosexual activity — is a good deal less complex and less needful of academic reconstructions than one might have thought, as one views the energy expended in the present debate. Deconstruction has presented historical-critical method with two very different faces: one that outflanks its claims to objective meaning gained through historical reconstruction, and one that contests any notion of authority residing in texts to begin with that is not put there by interpreters — precritical and critical alike.

Given this sea change in attitude toward historical-critical method, the debate over homosexual behavior could not be more significantly timed. At stake is not whether the Bible proscribes or does not proscribe homosexual behavior, but just what *proscription* might in fact mean today. Historical criticism may have cut the rug out from under itself with its appeal to objective truth gained through historical analogizing, for now it has been around long enough to cast its own historical shadow, and suddenly the possibility that it too must be examined as a historical phenomenon of the "modern" age looms large. What if, after all, "Holy Scripture" plainly does proscribe homosexual behavior? The question then to be asked is how or if historical criticism pursues its goals in connection with church life. The old enemy was "dogmaticism," but there is little vestige of that in the form it was first denounced by historical criticism, at least in circles where homosexual behavior is being advocated. So what is historical criticism's mandate in such an instance? It would be curious if where once it stood against the stifling influence of church teaching, now it is its greatest ally, in the name of new church teaching on this old issue. I introduce my fairly traditional reassertion of the church's proscription of homosexual acts in this way in order to candidly confess a misgiving and to point to what I believe is a real hypocrisy in this debate. My misgiving is that it does not seem to me that the church was ever in much real doubt about this issue. If it were not for massive changes in sexual behavior over the past decades, I doubt that we would be considering this issue on the grounds that *it is one contested within Scripture itself.* What I judge to be hypocrisy, and probably worth a treatment of its own, is the ongoing appeal to new findings and new learning that will presumably take place if people on opposite sides of this issue, listening hard to the hard work of others, stay "in dialogue" long enough. I may be wrong, but what I see is a hardening of resolve on both sides and greater conviction that one's own side is right after all. This is what is being produced by the appeal to "stay in dialogue." What seems hypocritical, then, at this juncture, is to say that one has wrestled hard to come to some clear conscience on this matter, but that perhaps over time we will all agree. How can that possibly happen?

I think it is better for us to witness to the truth and to clarify how it is we come to it, than to assume that what is confused are our sources of authority and that with just more historical-critical work we will succeed in eliminating the confusion and persuading the other side. Isaiah knew full well that the word of God closed ears as well as opened them, and that for some verdicts to be established it would take the judgment of God in history and the emergence of a new generation with ears opened by God himself. When Jeremiah confronted Hananiah, he simply appealed to the tradition in which prophets stand, and from which Hananiah departed. God rendered the verdict, in that instance quicker than Jeremiah probably thought. Sometimes opposing sides are *not* brought closer together, and both Testaments witness to this tragic reality *within* the people of God. I fear that in this instance, where the church is being asked to change a teaching it has held for its entire existence, we must frankly admit that we are in schism and that God will judge the appeal to his word being made by both sides. In the meantime both sides are obliged to testify to the truth and clarify how they have come to it, without any assumption that a consensus will emerge this side of the judgment of God himself.

II

If it could be shown that Scripture plainly forbids homosexual acts as an offense to God in Christ, would that be sufficient to constrain the church to proscribe homosexual behavior among its members today?[2]

2. That this immediately raises the question of appropriate pastoral care is obvious and reminds one how allergic the church has become to dealing with matters of the flesh in general, as central to the disciplined Christian life. In other words, to answer the question yes would oblige the church to think much more seriously about its responsibility in the "cure of souls" than it may at present be doing. The failure to address the difficult pastoral dimensions of appropriate sexual conduct fits hand in glove with a sense that the proper answer to the question is no longer self-evident. One gets a sense that the proper pastoral stance is now one of lifting sexual taboos, raising cultural consciousness, encouraging "outed" lifestyles, and so forth.

The question is important because a distinction can be made between (1) recognizing the Bible's plain sense on this issue and saying that it does not matter, over against (2) arguing that no such thing is said in Scripture that plainly and directly. Obviously there are modern people engaged in homosexual acts who understand that their behavior is clearly forbidden in the Old Testament and the New, by Moses, Jesus, and Paul, but who do not regard this as relevant. Some may even believe in notions like "holiness" or "offense" or "God" or "Christ" — but they also believe homosexual acts and relationships cannot be wrong if they are said to be "loving" and "caring" or "committed" relationships.

One modern problem is that the "church" now consists of people on both sides of such a distinction, where in the past the church consisted of only one of these groups, namely, those who granted the Bible's authority but who may not have agreed on its plain sense. At the same time, it is increasingly the case that those who favor revision — especially within mainline Protestant or liberal Catholic circles — wish to do so on the basis of an appeal to Scripture, if that is possible. This raises a question as to the relationship between Scripture and its history of interpretation in church and synagogue, without obvious analogy. For all the issues that divided the church in the past — over which Anabaptists, Lutherans, the Reformed, Anglicans, Methodists, Roman Catholics, Pentecostals, and others might have disagreed — tolerance or blessing of homosexual acts was never one of them.[3] Apparently Scripture's plain sense was simply too plain when it came to homosexual behavior. The history of interpretation, Jewish and Christian, bears witness to the "plainness" of Scripture on this matter.

One ought not move too quickly past this fact, since Scripture's plain sense is contained in a wide range of texts, thus leaving open the possibility of disagreement over which texts are to interpret others and offer the controlling context and perspective. It has long been possible to set the Testaments in opposition or disagreement (is tithing required or the Sabbath to be observed?), to distinguish between canonical and deuterocanonical or apocry-

3. The analogy to slavery does not hold up, on closer scrutiny, in spite of its rhetorical appeal. First, there is a failure to distinguish between forms of debt service in antiquity — some of them arguably a social good and dealt with in unique ways within Israel and the early church — and kidnapping, that is, the capture and forced servitude of populations in war or other situations of economic power, harshly displayed. In the American South, the latter form of slavery sought approval from Christian interpreters on the grounds of a Scripture at fundamental odds with it and was finally defeated on those very grounds. Homosexual activity, incidentally, was intimately tied up with various forms of slavery in the Greco-Roman world.

phal books (purgatory, prayers for the dead), Paul or Moses in tension with Jesus (divorce and remarriage), or even the magisterium or the Spirit or tradition over against Scripture itself (on ministry and authority in the church).

An example from an earlier day may serve to illustrate the problem. It is obvious that debates over Scripture's plain sense are not new and that especially problematic has been the relationship between the Old Testament and the New. Luther was unhappy with the citing of Old Testament law by "the enthusiasts" as binding on the Christian community, reinforced with the assertion "God says." He made a distinction between *what* God said and *to whom* he said it (Israel or the church). Yet even Luther understood that at a large number of points there was considerable overlap between what God prescribed as binding on Israel and subsequently, in Christ, on the church. In his zeal to curb "enthusiasm" or "legality," Luther did not reject divine law per se, which might positively constrain the church; rather, he focused instead on the Lawgiver, Christ, in relationship to such constraint. There could well be a great measure of continuity on matters enjoined in the Old and in the New, and certainly sexual behavior between a man and a woman in marriage was one of them. To point out the law's capacity to drive one to despair (Rom. 7:13-25) did not mean for even Luther's extraordinarily dialectical mind a rejection of the law, but an acknowledgment of the law as good and holy and tutor to Christ (Rom. 3:31; 7:7-12), who is the law's telos.

A less dialectical way of putting this can be found in the Thirty-nine Articles of sixteenth-century Anglicanism. After asserting the continuity between Old Testament and New as grounded in Christ, it takes up two areas of possible discontinuity. First, the promises to the fathers, that is, the old people of Israel: such promises did not involve transitory matters only, but truly anticipated the gospel, as Christians would later confess this. Second, the law: "Although the Law given from God by Moses, as touching Ceremonies and Rites, do not bind Christian men, nor the Civil precepts thereof ought of necessity to be received in any commonwealth" — here is Luther's concern with "enthusiasts" — "yet notwithstanding, no Christian man whatsoever is free from the obedience of the Commandments which are called Moral" (Article VII).

That Luther or Cranmer agreed that "no Christian man whatsoever is free from the obedience of the Commandments which are called Moral" did not mean that they simply equated the Christian life with obedience to the law's demands as an end unto itself. Above all, the relationship to God's will for the individual Christian was understood christologically. We relate to God's law *in Christ, through Christ.* To say that Christ has utterly abolished the law revealed in the Old Testament and that Christians have no law but "love" would be to move beyond the plain sense of the New Testament into the realm of "principles" or spiritual abstractions. The New Testament understands the Christian relationship to the law much more dialectically. In some respects, the New Testament witness suggests that the law of God as revealed in the Old, while holy and good and to be retained, is however insufficient in detailing the extent of God's total claim on the sinful human heart (Matt. 5:17-48). To say that Jesus or Paul is "critical" of the law, or that they see the law refracted in a certain way, is true — but this may move in precisely the opposite direction from laxity or abolition.

For this reason, the epistle that most stresses the Christian's freedom from the law *as the means of access to God or the righteousness of God in Christ,* the letter to the Galatians, is also the letter that concludes with a litany on how the Christian under the Spirit — as against the law *qua* law — is enjoined to behaviors the law once attempted to regulate (5:16-24). The criticism is therefore not directed toward the law's content, but toward the law's incapacity to engender the good and the holy, as God requires. The Christian is free from the law only insofar as she or he is a slave to Christ, "and those who belong to Christ Jesus have crucified the flesh with its passions and desires" (Gal. 5:24 NRSV). In Christ the content of the law is revealed for what it truly is: God's own holy will, which, without Christ, cannot be obeyed. In sum, to say that Paul or Jesus has "abolished" the law of God would be to misunderstand the distinction both make between the *content* and the *bestowal* of righteousness, the latter clearing room for obedience to the former.

It is for this reason that the Thirty-nine Articles are fully representative of Christian thought when, reflecting on the ongoing authority of the Old Testament, they conclude that "no Christian man whatsoever is free from the obedience of the Commandments which are called Moral." This article draws a distinction between matters moral and matters cultic or ceremonial, and in so doing introduces a *discrimens* to be applied to the *content* of the Old Testament law. We will take up this distinction in further detail in a moment. It should be clear, however, that such a distinction attempts to comprehend the Christian relationship to the law as this is set forth in the New Testament, where the content is not abolished but released through Christ and in Christ toward God's desired righteousness of life. What one sees enjoined of the Christian, crucified in the flesh with Christ, are certain specific virtues and behaviors whose compatibility with Old Testament "moral" law should be clear.

On the basis of this, it seems clear that reflecting on Scripture's plain sense in order to describe proper sexual behavior for the Christian community is not a foreign or "legalistic" concept in the church's life in the past. The roots of such reflection lie in the New Testament itself, where Jesus is the telos of the law as this was revealed in Israel's Scriptures.

An example of the dialectical and christological character of the law for the Israel of God, the church, is perfectly illustrated in John's narrative of the woman caught in adultery (John 8:1-11).[4] The woman is brought before Jesus. The law of Moses is clear, whether she is married (Lev. 20:10) or a "betrothed virgin" (Deut. 22:23-24), though one might well ask about the male offender, since in both texts his role is addressed as well. The Deuteronomy text stipulates stoning as the means by which the death penalty is to be executed. This is the penalty referred to by the scribes and Pharisees (John 8:5).

Jesus' famous response, "Let him who is without sin among you be the first to throw a stone at her," is not in the first instance a rejection of the law's content regarding adulterous behavior. It is a response directed at what the law attempts to regulate: human sin. This extends to the scribes and Pharisees in such measure that they refuse to exact the penalty prescribed by the law. Jesus has successfully linked the execution of the law's demand to human sinfulness, generally speaking. The question, however, remains: How then is the holy demand of the law to be satisfied, since no one is sufficiently free of sin to execute its penalties as prescribed? Is the content of the law now to be dispensed with, along with the penalty? The obvious answer to the first question is: it would require someone without sin to enforce the law. No one has condemned her, and neither does Jesus, who alone is in a position to do so. As the "one among them without sin," he still does not pick up a stone. On the other hand, he reiterates the content of the law: "Go and sin no more." Adultery is sin. Continuity exists over the law's content. Discontinuity exists over how that content is approached and obeyed: through Jesus.

Yet one might ask, what of the due punishment for the crime committed, since adultery offended against God's holiness and against one within the covenant assembly? And what if the woman does not obey the "statute" of Jesus and instead goes and sins again? How can Jesus take on the role of dispensing justice and relaxing the demand of the law, if its content is regarded

4. For an insightful discussion of the pericope and of the difficulty surrounding text-critical conclusions in regard to it, see Gail R. O'Day, "John 7:53–8:11: A Study in Misreading," *JBL* 111 (1992): 631-40. The impact of the history of interpretation of the text on its proper text-critical evaluation (that is, "[t]he canonical instability of John 7:53–8:11," p. 639) is taken up by O'Day at the close of her remarks (pp. 638-40). Her conclusion is that text-critical marginality cannot be translated into claims for lack of historicity or similar such dismissals. As is becoming clearer in Old Testament text criticism, so-called "higher" and "lower" critical dimensions of a text turn out to occupy similar terrain for one critical phase of their existence.

as good and holy? This concern is in the foreground in Jesus' confrontations with the custodians of the law, because of the arrogation to himself of interpreting and even enforcing the law, by forgiving sins (John 8:12–11:57). Yet the fullest answer is not given until John 19:30. Jesus himself bears the curse and penalty of the law of God on behalf of all: "It is finished," the law's penalty "has been paid for," by Jesus himself, in his own flesh. This is the scandal of the cross, that the law's demands are now, in Christian confession, matters pertaining to Jesus. The content of the law is understood as binding, in him, through him. As the narrative concerning the adulterous woman makes clear, adultery remains sin, but Jesus is the means by which forgiveness is possible. That such forgiveness may not lead to obedience is precisely the love of God made manifest in Christ. Christ continues to pay the penalty even if the adultery persists, making forgiveness in his name always possible. But never does adultery stop being a sin and an offense to God. Without Christ's healing and intervention, sin still leads to death, now understood less immediately, if not also more eternally.

It has been objected in recent years that Jesus nowhere pronounces on homosexual behavior in the New Testament and that this silence is probative. It could just as easily be concluded that all we learn from this silence is that adultery was a more prevalent sin in Israel than homosexual behavior among men; this would explain its more frequent discussion in both the Old Testament and the New. That the prohibition against adultery, together with the death penalty, appears in the same context in Leviticus as the prohibition against homosexual behavior (Lev. 20:13) might lead one to conclude that Jesus would have reacted in exactly the same way if the scribes had brought to him the unusual case of a man accused of "lying with a male as with a woman." In such an account, Jesus would become the means of the accused man's forgiveness, the sinless one who refuses to cast the first stone. Yet then we would have to expect the same final "statute" of Christ: "Go and sin no more." That Jesus does more than simply pay the penalty in obedience to the Father's will entails his capacity both to forgive and to heal, which is amply described in the New Testament. The relationship to Christ is not only one that satisfies the demands of the law juridically, but also one that opens up an entirely new way of living in relationship to God that sets free from sin and death.

The Thirty-nine Articles distinguished between "ceremonial" or "ritual" commandments in the Old Testament and "those called Moral," from which no Christian was free. This represented an effort to comprehend the profound distinction introduced in the New Testament, and illustrated in the encounter between the adulterous woman, Jesus, and the law of Moses, or in the theological reflections of Paul, regarding the content and purpose and ongoing validity of the law as "holy and just and good" (Rom. 7:12). Sexual behavior is not regarded as a "cultic" or ritual matter, in spite of what some recent interpreters have argued, but as a central existential category of ongoing concern and godly purpose.

A different sort of relationship exists between the Christian and the law in respect of matters "ritual" or "ceremonial," as these also exist in the Old Testament. The older rites and ceremonies are summed up in Christ, who reveals what those rites and ceremonies were truly about. For those outside Israel, brought near in Christ, those rites and ceremonies are now experienced as completed *in him,* both high priest and sacrificial victim. They are seen to be shadows of a Reality by whose light their true form is recognized and comprehended in the first place, and hence they have no binding character in any independent sense (Heb. 10:1-31). We know this because the New Testament has specifically addressed them on these terms. In a similar way, explicit handling of ritual laws in the New Testament has made clear their provisional character and judged them no longer binding on Christian men and women (Mark 7:1-23). In other words, the status of the law for the "Israel of God," the church, is wholly governed by the New Testament's plain-sense treatment of the law's content and purpose, and it is here that distinctions of various sorts have been introduced. To point out the flaws in those terms chosen for comprehending these distinctions ("moral," "ritual," "ceremonial") would not be the same thing as saying that no such distinctions exist or that the law is evenhandedly dispensed with in the church, with a New Lawgiver, High Priest, and Perfect Offering.

Even in texts in the New Testament that address ritual and ceremonial aspects of the law, there is no suggestion that Jesus' chief concern is with correction or criticism according to some new enlightened standard (e.g., the laws of Leviticus are too "harsh").[5] In Mark 7, where the narrator understands Jesus as "declaring all foods clean" (v. 19), the form of the discussion is not so straightforward as basic revision or updating due to inherent "Jewish parochialism" or "harshness" or some other such criterion, before which the law itself is judged deficient. The opening exchange (vv. 1-13) introduces a distinction between "traditions" and "the tradition of the elders," on the one side, and "the commandment of God," on the other. Jesus even uses the

5. See, e.g., John S. Spong, *Living in Sin? A Bishop Rethinks Human Sexuality* (San Francisco: Harper & Row, 1988). The Old Testament, and much of the New, is judged by the Episcopal bishop according to standards imported from modern culture. "Harshness" and "ignorance" are at obvious odds with his moral and intellectual horizon.

prophet Isaiah (no foe of "harshness") as support against the Pharisees. The charge is not overzealous or rigid attention to a harsh law, but exchanging for God's law "the precepts of men." The corban illustration (vv. 9-13) provides further evidence of Jesus' concern: "making void the word of God through your tradition which you hand on" (v. 13).[6]

The problem with the ritual laws is not that they are ungodly. Rather, they can be manipulated or rationalized into a system that diverts from their true purpose. And further: they do not reach into the place where clean and unclean originate, "from within" (v. 21). The dietary laws of Leviticus are not "traditions of men" or "clear examples of premodern ignorance."[7] The whole point of the distinctions introduced in Mark 7:1-13 is to make this clear. These laws fall short *because of the nature of the problem they are addressing,* not because they were wrong in and of themselves. They fail to get at the problem; they are not the problem. One might have expected Mark's Jesus, based upon some recent interpretations of the status of the law in the New Testament, to have been chiefly about throwing out distinctions such as clean and unclean altogether. Instead, Jesus begins his ministry with exorcisms! The battle over clean and unclean is more, not less, decisive, even as it is fought on a new front, by the One whom Matthew quotes as saying: "Think not that I have come to abolish the law and the prophets; I have come not to abolish them but to fulfill them. . . . Whoever then relaxes one of the least of these commandments and teaches men so, shall be called the least in the kingdom of heaven" (Matt. 5:17, 19 RSV). The righteousness of Jesus' disciples is to *exceed* that of the scribes and Pharisees in respect of the law (5:20). Harshness or premodern ignorance are irrelevant to the issue at hand.

A similar assessment of the law for Christians can be seen in Hebrews, whose concern is more directly with "ceremonial" laws. These are "but a shadow of the good things to come" (10:1). Sacrificial offerings failed to achieve what Jesus' offering of himself achieved. It would have been far simpler to say that these offerings were too harsh or were examples of premodern ignorance. Jesus' response was "Lo, I have come to do thy will" (10:9 RSV). Jesus has given Christians access, by his blood, to confident entry into the sanctuary (10:19) — something the continual offering, year after year, of the blood of bulls and goats could not do (10:1-4).

6. See Markus Bockmuehl, "Halakhah and Ethics in the Jesus Tradition," in *Early Christian Thought in Its Jewish Context,* ed. J. Barclay and J. Sweet (Cambridge: Cambridge University Press, 1996), pp. 264-78.

7. Spong, p. 146. Spong's arrogance toward the past could be described as "imperialism of the modern" were it not that he is speaking out of an already postmodern Western context.

Here the author makes clear the provisional character of the law of Moses, seen from the perspective of Christ's onetime offering of himself. Christians have no temple in Jerusalem, no Levitical priests, no ark, no mercy seat, and no ceremonial life drawn directly from Leviticus. But the point and purpose of these remains, *in Christ.* At this point, then, the author must contend with a factor the first covenant could regulate but, because it is now taken up into Christ, cannot in the same way. What of deliberate sin "after receiving the knowledge of the truth"? That is, the bold claim by Christians about the status of the law fulfilled in Christ comes with its own provisions, which again exceed in their own way the righteousness enjoined by obedience to the law within the Old Covenant. "It is a fearful thing to fall into the hands of the living God" (Heb. 10:31 NRSV). How much simpler it would be if we were dealing with premodern ignorance or a harshness now tempered by kindly sentiment.

I will bring these various remarks on the law of God, intertextually considered, to conclusion by examining one phenomenon both Testaments of Christian Scripture hold in common.

It has been pointed out that the Bible is not particularly obsessed with the topic of homosexuality — not nearly as obsessed, at any rate, as are church and culture in the late modern West. This may of course point to the relative infrequency of homosexual conduct within Israel, or in the frame of reference of the church's confessed Messiah of Israel, as was earlier suggested. The singular treatments of Scripture (Gen. 18; Rom. 1) are indeed rare, and now they too are being subjected to revisionist interpretations, over against the time-honored ones in church and synagogue. It does not follow from this, however, that the sin of homosexuality is just one among others, of equal character, in the Old Testament. To range the offense of "lying with another man as with a woman" together with incest, bestiality, and adultery and to stipulate the penalty for infringement as capital punishment (Lev. 20:10-16), distinguishes this particular sin from others and suggests a seriousness of concern with which even other "abominations" are not treated. One must take this seriousness into account in any discussion of homosexuality in the modern period, whether from a historical-critical perspective or an interbiblical perspective.

The variety and degree of offenses against God's holiness in the Old Testament is recognized at points in the New, and yet all are caught up within Christ's final sacrifice on behalf of God's creation. At the same time, the "bundling" and "leveling" of offenses and their collective treatment with all other sins is a characteristic of the New Testament that has radicalized and not lessened the force of Old Testament law. Richard Hays has argued convincingly that the rhetorical force of Romans 1 entails linking the specific depravity of homosexual acts (1:24-27) to all manner of human offense against God's holiness (1:28-32).[8] To pass judgment on others is to condemn oneself (2:1) only if the extent and character of all human sinfulness is of like nature, seen from the aspect of God's work in Christ. One is therefore right to say that homosexual conduct is seen as no worse a sin than greed, drunkenness, robbery, and so forth (1 Cor. 6:9).

The conclusion to be drawn from this seems to me the opposite of what is now frequently argued. First, it is clear that members of the body of Christ are enjoined to standards of conduct every bit as stringent as that enjoined on the Old Covenant community, if not more so. The grounding for and facilitation of that enjoining are what have changed. What is truly radical about the love of God in Christ is not that all manner of sinfulness is leveled and dispensed with, but that the distance God is prepared to go to bring creation into fellowship with him *extends even to offenses held by him to demand the death penalty.* That penalty is paid by God's own Son. This is the mystery Paul is pondering in Romans 1. But there it is a matter of reflection because of the obligation it places all creation under: the knowledge that the wrath of God is poured out on all offense, and yet our recourse is the love of the same God made manifest in Christ. It is for this reason that offenses of different character and degree from the Old can be bundled in the way they are in the New.

It follows from this, not that homosexual behavior is less offensive than anger or greed and ought therefore to be permitted, but that it partakes of the selfsame character for which the love of God in Christ was and is the only saving force, set in motion by the one who gave the holy law to his people Israel. To join "love" with "lying with a man as with a woman" would be to ask one sensitive to this dynamic in the New Testament to consider as well "blessed greed" or "holy drunkenness." The bundling has gone on in a very different direction and toward a very different purpose: to show the extent to which God obliterated all distinctions of offense in the sacrifice of his Son, so that "those who belong to Christ Jesus have crucified the flesh with its passions and desires" (Gal. 5:24 NRSV). Paul is stating a fact about the Christian life, achieved by the work of Christ, that grounds his appeal to "live by the Spirit . . . and . . . not gratify the desires of the flesh" (5:16 NRSV). One could no more "bless" homosexual unions than one could bless anger or adultery, for there is no clear warrant for this in the work of Christ as the New Testament understands it. The logic of its bundling has gone in precisely the opposite direction.

8. Richard B. Hays, "Relations Natural and Unnatural: A Response to John Boswell's Exegesis of Romans 1," *Journal of Religious Ethics* 14 (1986): 184-215.

It is the conclusion of this essay that the church is constrained on the basis of Scripture's plain sense to proscribe homosexual behavior among its members. It must, however, carefully distinguish this from "passing judgment" in the manner Paul warns against in Romans 2:1. The proscription flows from an understanding of the holiness of the law and the work of God in Christ. The church has no authority to "bless" gay unions because there is no warrant for this in Scripture. Instead one finds there a specific reminder that along with innumerable other sins, such behavior is inconsistent with the kingdom of God. The proper response of the church remains not condemnation, but the address of the gospel, as this is set forth in the two-Testament Christian Scripture.

III

I want to make two concluding observations. The first has to do with the topic in question, the plain sense of Scripture and homosexual practice in the modern church. The second involves the question of how appropriate New Testament methodology is to be deployed in the exegesis of Romans 1–2.

1. It seems to me the place where the Testaments display their most obvious plain-sense conformity on the matter of human sexuality involves appeal to God's action in creation. Mark 10 makes this clear. When asked about divorce and remarriage, Jesus offers no private opinion but appeals to Scripture. And even though Scripture itself witnesses to some obvious tension ("What did Moses command you?" [v. 3 NRSV]), this is linked to human sinfulness, not to fresh revelation or shifts in the mind of God. Jesus assembles texts from Genesis 1–2 to establish God's will for sexuality, "From the beginning of creation, 'God made them male and female.' 'For this reason a man shall leave his father and mother and be joined to his wife, and the two shall become one flesh'" (Mark 10:6-8 NRSV). How could any departure from this teaching, for the purposes of endorsing other forms of human sexual intercourse, be anything less than a similar instance of human hard-heartedness? If what God revealed to Moses was an accommodation to human sinfulness and not what God fully intended — and Christ alone speaks with the authority to reveal this, and dies on the basis of that authority — then how could the church depart from this will of God and speak not of hardened hearts, but of actual blessing and positive endorsement? This flies in the face of the logic of Jesus as revealed in its apostolic witness. To say this is not to offer a condemnation of divorce or same-

sex physical relationships but to point to the problem of the human heart the gospel is fundamentally concerned to address.

2. What cries out desperately for resolution is the use by New Testament scholarship of source material from the Greco-Roman milieu in an effort to clarify the thought of Paul. Richard Hays's deployment of a term like "echo" reveals the nature of the problem even as it points to a possible model for hermeneutics and modern interpretation. He of course means by "echo" the resonance, not from the Greco-Roman milieu as such, but from texts of the Old Testament and whatever "milieu" they may come to present to Paul.

An alternative understanding, sometimes working in conjunction with the above, posits the influence of milieu differently. Does the resemblance between certain aspects of Paul's thought in Romans 1 and that of Greek and Roman sources point to a material and substantive comparative base? Or is the resemblance more oblique and essentially adventitious, making appeals to such material for the purposes of clarification insufficiently controlled? How acquainted with his milieu and its reflections on sexuality was Paul, and perhaps more importantly, how probative would such reflections have been for Paul?

These questions prove relevant precisely when one reckons with a clear epistemological distinction that runs throughout the Epistle to the Romans. This distinction is derived from Israel's Scriptures, which as a *single,* epistemologically privileged witness nevertheless serves to reveal *two* distinctive categories for knowing God and relating to him, through the law of Moses and prior to and apart from that revelation. Adam and Abraham are examples from Israel's Scriptures of life prior to and apart from God's revelation to Moses. Both led "commanded lives," to be sure (Rom. 4:1-25; 5:15-20), but because they lived apart from the law as revealed to Moses, and because Paul takes that distinction as meaningful for him and for the present church, they remain typologically or figurally representative of life as it is lived in the world more generally.

This means that when Paul seeks to understand how God is at work in the world more broadly, his version of "natural law" is one fundamentally rooted in Israel's privileged witness. To seek to understand how God relates to the created order apart from his specific relationship to Israel, Paul studies Israel's Scripture. This is not to say that he lives in a cave or never picks up a copy of the *Athenian Times,* with its reflections of the "milieu" morality, but that his categories of knowing and his reflections on knowing are fundamentally stamped by the Scriptures of Israel. They "echo" in ways that are not always easy to track down, in strict exegetical terms — in much the same way that MS-DOS is indispensable to my writing this piece, even though it remains invisible. Here the analogy is broken, of course, because Scripture is not invisible in Paul but intrudes itself explicitly as well as implicitly, or yet more subtly. The MS-DOS of Scripture is fully available for independent study and investigation.

As one who lives exegetically as much or more in the Old Testament as in the New, I am struck by the resonances that appear to surface in Romans 1. Many of these are noted by interpreters. Before looking at these, consider the logic of Paul's argument more generally. At verse 18 Paul is most concerned to demonstrate how all humanity — that is, humanity apart from Israel — is without excuse in the same way that Israel is without excuse (2:1). The latter has God's revealed law and is therefore without excuse before God. The former is likewise without excuse, but for different reasons.

Now where does Paul get this understanding of the natural person? One governing assumption tracks the flow of the argument and sees the eventual appeal to the self-evidently immoral and idolatrous character of same-sex relationships (vv. 24-27) as evidence of widely held views to this effect in Paul's milieu. Paul's appeal here serves to catch his own religious compatriots in their judgmental conceit (chap. 2). God shows no partiality (2:11). The law does not give one higher moral ground, but ground for God's judgment as "without excuse."

How would Paul's Jewish listeners know for sure that God's judgment had been so manifestly poured out on Gentile idolaters?[9] The argument runs that Greco-Roman literature reveals a sort of natural law logic on the depravity or inappropriateness of same-sex physical relationships as examples of unrestrained sexual desire. Moderation and temperance overthrown in the name of desire brings its own punishment. The self-evidence of these claims is thrown in the face of Paul's Jewish listeners to the rhetorical purpose of exposing their own sinfulness before God's holiness. The scholarly task of collating sources from the Greco-Roman milieu is vindicated by demonstrating their utility and the indispensability of their observations, as these now function in the movement from Romans 1 to Romans 2.

But would such an appeal to God's judgment on same-sex relationships, as this is grounded in Greco-Roman sources, have proven probative to Paul's Jewish listeners/readers? Would the *theology* of these sources and their

9. I adopt the general view here that the force of Paul's argument in Rom. 1–2 is ultimately aimed at Christians who have lived under the law as Jews. They constitute the "implied audience" if not the real audience of Paul's initial argument in these opening chapters. The Jew-Greek distinction and its reorientation by God in Christ frames the argument (1:16; 2:9-10). For a provocative effort to see it otherwise, derived from an analysis of the problem of "audience" in the letter, see Stanley K. Stowers, *A Rereading of Romans: Justice, Jews, and Gentiles* (New Haven: Yale University Press, 1994).

theological account of moral law in creation have been adequate to serve the purpose of persuading Paul's listeners about God's judgment? Could Paul entertain the notion of a general "godly judgment" and a correlative "moral law" displayed in creation, apart from the specific judgment of the God of Israel, whose will against homosexual activity is revealed in the Old Testament? Critical for Paul's argument at this point is the citing of evidence of judgment upon those *outside the covenant community,* thereby establishing them as "without excuse" before God in a manner convincing to his Jewish audience.

It might be objected that Paul is appealing to judgments on same-sex behavior only subsequently described in Greco-Roman sources, and therefore has in mind the behavior itself, as he observes it and its consequences, and not the logic associated with its impropriety in the source material. This may well be true. But it seems to me likely that if Paul were aware of same-sex behavior in his "milieu" and the self-evidence of God's judgment on it, the source for his information in this regard would be the "oracles of God entrusted to the Jews" (see Rom. 3:2). Their "echo" would override any logic about divine judgment available in the "milieu." Appeal to the wrongfulness of such behavior, as such and as rhetorically useful, given his audience, would best be grounded by appeal to Israel's witness to God's will in the Old Testament.

With this perspective in view, how does the word of the Old Testament about God's judgment in creation make itself felt in Romans 1? The whole discussion is preceded in 1:17 by a quote from Habakkuk 2:4, "The one who is righteous will live by faith" (NRSV), as if to signal Paul's main "source" for commending what God has done and is doing in Jesus Christ, that is, the Scriptures entrusted to Israel. The present judgment to which appeal is eventually made (Rom. 1:24-27) is grounded in a past record: "ever since the creation of the world" (v. 20 NRSV). When idolatry is concretely described as the outcome of foolish minds (1:23), the categories into which it is poured are those of Genesis 1: "a mortal human being or birds or four-footed animals or reptiles" (NRSV). The "claiming to be wise" of Romans 1:22 evokes the challenge of the serpent (Gen. 3:5) and the description of the narrator in the story of the garden (Gen. 3:6). Striking in this regard is the use of the definite article in Romans 1:25: "they exchanged the truth about God for *the* lie" (RSV adapted) which has been noted by commentators as traceable to the same Genesis account.[10] Worshiping the creature instead of the Creator has a

10. In his essay in this volume (p. 227 below), Robert Jewett speaks of "the fundamental ploy of humans to replace God with themselves, visible from the Fall to the crucifixion of Christ." J. Fitzmyer (*Romans: A New Translation with Introduction and Commentary* [New York: Doubleday, 1993], pp. 284f.) refers to the "big lie . . . the deception that smothers the truth."

certain rhetorical generality (1:25), but in the context of Genesis "the creature" who moves human beings away from God by means of "the lie" is none other than the serpent.

When Paul goes on to describe the "degrading passions" that inflame those given up by God to their darkened minds (v. 26), is he speaking about homosexual activity in his milieu, of which he and his audience are aware and whose inappropriateness is confirmed in Greco-Roman sources? The first part of this is of course quite possible. But the past-tense description would allow a further dimension to come into play: Paul and his audience share knowledge of God's judgment on homosexual activity on the basis of the Old Testament. He has introduced his argument with reference to "the wrath of God . . . revealed from heaven against all ungodliness and wickedness" (1:18 NRSV) and has spoken about the obvious way that God has made known his character, "his eternal power and divine nature" (1:20 NRSV). In my judgment, Paul assumes here a continuity between the judgments visited on natural man in the Old Testament, apart from the law, and those that could be evidenced in the present period.

It is one thing to argue in the modern period that the story about the outcry and grave sin (Gen. 18:20) of the citizens of Sodom did not entail homosexuality between consenting adults. It is another thing to ask how Paul himself might have heard the story of God's wrath from heaven being poured out on that city (Gen. 19:24) and the blindness with which God struck those whose inhospitality included the demand, "Where are the men who came to you tonight? Bring them out to us, so that we may know them" (19:5 NRSV). Given the flow of Paul's argument, beginning at Romans 1:18 and running into chapter 2, it would seem reasonable to assume that Paul was searching for an example of God's wrath being made immediately and unequivocally manifest upon natural man, one known to his Jewish audience and testified to in "the oracles of God" (3:2). He chooses an example appropriate to his rhetorical context and capable of recognition and correlation in the example of that homosexual activity known to him, in his "milieu."

If this reading is correct, then Paul chooses homosexual behavior not because he regards it as a worse sin than others, but because the judgment of God on it was such a visible manifestation of his wrath against ungodliness, patent and deserving of attention by natural man. If one thought that the ways of God with the natural world were subtle enough to leave the latter "with excuse," Paul reminds his readers of instances from the Old Testament that prove otherwise, and that do so with particular urgency. It could be the case that God's judgment against homosexual behavior opened up in a particularly potent way the possibility for feelings of superiority on the part of

Paul's audience, which are then roundly rejected in Romans 2. But in my judgment the example is not chosen for that reason, but rather because it illustrated an instance when the wrath of God was so visibly displayed against natural man, apart from the law or any special revelation from God to his people Israel. Whether Greco-Roman sources confirm or deny Paul's logic from the Old Testament in the case of contemporaneous homosexual activity — including that of women (Rom. 1:26) — is an interesting question from the perspective of intellectual history. But such an inquiry could prove distracting in coming to terms with Paul's logic in Romans 1–2.

CHAPTER 7

Natural and Unnatural Use in Romans 1:24-27: Paul and the Philosophic Critique of Eros

DAVID E. FREDRICKSON

> *Wherefore God delivered them to the desires of their hearts for the purpose of impurity, for their bodies to be dishonored among them — they who exchanged the truth of God for a lie and reverenced and worshiped the creation rather than the creator, who is blessed for ever, amen. Because of this, God delivered them to dishonoring passions. Their females exchanged natural use for that which is beyond nature. Likewise, the males left off the natural use of the female and were inflamed for one another in their appetite, males among males producing disgrace and receiving back in themselves the punishment which was necessary from their error.*
>
> Romans 1:24-27

> *Or do you not know that the unjust will not inherit the kingly rule of God? Do not be led astray. Neither fornicators, nor idolaters, nor adulterers, nor those who lack self-control, nor the arrogant who penetrate boys, nor thieves, nor those who get more than their fair share, nor dissolute and rowdy drinkers, nor revilers, nor robbers will inherit the kingly rule of God.*
>
> 1 Corinthians 6:9-10

A. Introduction

To say there is no uniformity in the ways of studying the topic of sex in ancient texts is an understatement. Some scholars have insisted on the transhistorical validity of homosexuality and heterosexuality. They believe that ancient texts share the modern interest in knowing, classifying, and evaluating sexual orientation.[1] Other scholars have amplified and refined the basic insights of Kenneth Dover and Michel Foucault, summarized by Mark Golden, "that forms of sexual activity were not a major concern, that homosexual and heterosexual desire were regarded as identical, that excess (failing to control oneself) and passivity (falling under another's control) were the main forms of sexual immorality for men."[2]

The Dover/Foucault framework informs this paper, which first treats Romans 1:24-27 at considerable length, moving at the end to a brief examination of 1 Corinthians 6:9.[3] My guiding question is this: How do the ways of

1. Authors with divergent opinions about the morality of same-sex love still share these assumptions. For example, it is interesting to compare the work of J. Boswell with J. De Young, "The Source and NT Meaning of ARSENOKOITAI, with Implications for Christian Ethics and Ministry," *Master's Seminary Journal* 3 (1992): 191-215.

2. Mark Golden, "Thirteen Years of Homosexuality (and Other Recent Work on Sex, Gender and the Body in Ancient Greece)," *Echos du Monde Classique* 35 (1991): 334. For a statement of the Dover/Foucault trajectory by one of its best representatives, see D. Halperin, "Historicizing the Sexual Body: Sexual Preferences and Erotic Identities in the Pseudo-Lucianic *Erôtes*," in *Discourses of Sexuality: From Aristotle to AIDS*, ed. D. Stanton (Ann Arbor: University of Michigan Press, 1992), pp. 236-61. The most significant refinements are found in D. Cohen, *Law, Sexuality, and Society: The Enforcement of Morals in Classical Athens* (Cambridge: Cambridge University Press, 1991); Cohen, "Sexuality, Violence, and the Athenian Law of Hubris," *Greece and Rome* 38 (1991): 171-88; and A. Richlin, "Not before Homosexuality: The Materiality of the *Cinaedus* and the Roman Law against Love between Men," *Journal of the History of Sexuality* 3 (1993): 523-73. They raise doubts about the first point, that the form of sexual activity was not a matter of concern. Given the accuracy of the third point, the first had inevitably to come under scrutiny. The second point (the unity of desire) was recognized early on by J. Henderson (*The Maculate Muse: Obscene Language in Attic Comedy* [New York: Yale University Press, 1975], pp. 52-53) and has stood the test of time.

3. D. Martin ("Heterosexism and the Interpretation of Romans 1:18-32," *Biblical Interpretation* 3 [1995]: 332-55) has anticipated some of the arguments below. Martin's legitimate concern for "ideological analysis of modern scholarship on Rom. 1:18-32" does not, however, allow him the opportunity to develop the philosophic background in as great detail as offered here. Nevertheless, his critique (pp. 333-39) of the traditional interpretation that the creation story in Genesis is the proper background of Paul's argument is brilliant and complements my attempt to place Paul in his contemporary intellectual environment. J. Fitzmyer (*Romans*, Anchor Bible 33 [New York: Doubleday,

conceptualizing sexual matters in Paul's philosophic and literary environment help us make sense of his argument? I will conclude that these Pauline texts are not about the condemnation of homosexuality. Rather, in Romans 1:24-27 Paul points to the problem of passion without introducing the modern dichotomy of homo/heterosexuality. In 1 Corinthians 6:9 the term "soft" refers to lack of self-control (not the boy prostitute) and ἀρσενοκοίτης is the hybristic pederast whose vice is not misplaced desire but injustice. Obviously, these are not new conclusions about these texts. What I hope to offer are additional reasons to believe that they are true.

B. What Does "Natural Use" Mean?

My guiding question presumes that Paul's language about sex has much in common with the erotic discourse of his contemporaries and that interpreters must take this overlap seriously. One important point of contact between Paul and his intellectual environment is the notion of sexual activity as use (χρῆσις).[4] Interpreters of Romans 1:24-27 have been remarkably incurious about this term. Most assume that it means "relation" or "intercourse" and quickly pass it by on the way to more interesting terminology such as "nature." This is unfortunate, because "relation" imports the modern notion that sex is (or should be) a matter of mutuality. The texts collected and discussed below will demonstrate that χρῆσις does not refer to a relation carried out in the medium of sexual pleasure but the activity of the desiring subject, usually male, performed on the desired object, female or male.[5]

The fact that sexual desire and hunger were thought to be analogous alerts us to the way that the very concept of relation distorts Paul's argu-

---

1993], pp. 274-77) is also critical of reading too much of Genesis into Rom. 1:18-32, but he fails to carry through on this insight and makes the mistake of regarding 1:24-27 as the reason for God's wrath.

4. Sex as use is a building block in Foucault's description of the Greek "moral problematization of sexual conduct." See *The History of Sexuality,* vol. 2, *The Use of Pleasure* (New York: Pantheon, 1985), pp. 53-62.

5. The only exception I have been able to discover is Chariton, *Chareas and Callirhoe* 2.8.4. For the new idea in the romances of both partners enjoying sex, see D. Konstan, *Sexual Symmetry: Love in the Ancient Novel and Related Genres* (Princeton: Princeton University Press, 1994). For enjoyment (ἀπόλαυσις) — a term sometimes coordinated with χρῆσις — shared between male and female lovers and asserted not to be possible in pederasty, see Ps.-Lucian, *Affairs of the Heart* 27.

ment.[6] This analogy becomes even more significant when texts are taken into account which assert a similarity between the use of sex and the use of food.[7] Aristippus, whose sexual activity with Laïs occurred without her loving (φιλούσης) him, is paraphrased by Plutarch: "He didn't imagine, he said, that wine or fish loved him either, yet he used both with pleasure (ἡδέως ἑκατέρῳ χρῆται)."[8] This remark reflects more than an errant philosopher's machismo. In it we see the pervasive interpretation of sexual activity as use.[9] The analogy of sex with food furthermore helped to define sexual norms, since the pleasure of sex, it was argued, needs to be limited by satisfaction just as a full stomach limits eating.[10]

In order to distinguish modern and ancient ways of thinking about sex, it is worth underscoring that neither the gender of the subject nor that of the object is material to the concept of use. Frequently, as in the case of Romans 1:27, the term refers to the husband's sexual activity with respect to the wife,[11] though this does not mean that χρῆσις is invariably associated with a husband/wife or, for that matter, a male/female pairing.[12] Epictetus's advice

6. For ἔρως as an appetite like hunger or thirst, see D. Halperin, "Platonic *Erôs* and What Men Call Love," *Ancient Philosophy* 5 (1985): 164-66, and D. Brown, *Lucretius on Love and Sex: A Commentary on "De Rerum Natura" IV, with Prolegomena, Text, and Translation* (Leiden: Brill, 1987), pp. 231-33.

7. Henderson, p. 47.

8. Plutarch, *Amatorius* 750D-E. (Unless otherwise indicated, translations are from the Loeb Classical Library; translation modified in this instance). For the concept of use in Aristippus's treatment of pleasure, see Stobaeus, *Anthology* 3.17.17; Diogenes Laertius, *Lives of Eminent Philosophers* 2.75.

9. For the correlation of using food and using sex, see Stobaeus, *Anthology* 3.9.46; Musonius Rufus, *Fragment* 16; Epictetus, *Discourse* 2.8.12; Galen, *On the Doctrines of Hippocrates and Plato* 5.7.21-25.

10. Clement of Alexandria, *Paedagogus* 2.10.90.2-3 (translation is S. P. Wood, *Clement of Alexandria: Christ the Educator,* FC 23 [New York: Fathers of the Church, 1954], p. 169): "We should consider boys as our sons, and the wives of other men as our daughters. We must keep a firm control over the pleasures of the stomach, and an absolutely uncompromising control over the organs beneath the stomach. . . . In lawful wedlock, as with eating, nature permits whatever is conformable to nature and helpful and decent; it allows us to desire the act of procreation. However, whoever is guilty of excess (ὑβερβολήν) sins against nature and, by violating the laws regulating intercourse, harms himself." Cf. Xenophon, *Symposium* 8.15; Philo, *Special Laws* 3.9; Plutarch, *Advice about Keeping Well* 124E-125A; *On the Eating of Flesh, II,* 997B.

11. Clement of Alexandria, *Stromateis* 3.11.71.4: σωφρόνως ἐβούλετο ταῖς γαμεταῖς χρῆσθαι τοὺς ἄνδρας ὁ νόμος καὶ ἐπὶ μόνῃ παιδοποιίᾳ; Justin Martyr, *Dialogus cum Tryphone Judaeo* 110: μόνῃ τῇ γαμετῇ γυναικὶ ἕκαστος χρώμενοι; Athenagoras, *Legatio* 32.1: γυναικὶ δὲ τῇ ἰδίᾳ ἀδελφῇ χρώμενον.

12. K. Preston, *Studies in the Diction of the Sermo Amatorius in Roman Comedy*

about casual affairs illustrates male use of the female outside of marriage: "In your sex-life preserve purity, as far as you can, before marriage, and, if you indulge, take only those privileges which are lawful. However, do not make yourself offensive, or censorious, to those who do indulge (χρωμένοις), and do not make frequent mention of the fact that you yourself do not indulge (χρῇ)."[13] Rarer than the male's use of the female are instances of the wife's use of the husband,[14] to which Paul most likely alludes in Romans 1:26: "their females exchanged natural use for that which is against nature (τὴν φυσικὴν χρῆσιν εἰς τὴν παρά φύσιν)."[15] The paucity of examples of the female's use of the male can be explained in part by the lack of attention paid by male authors to female sexual experience and also by their reluctance to think of women as users, a male social role.

The metaphor of use in sexual matters does not in itself raise the issue of the gender of the persons involved. Thus, parallel to the husband's use of the wife, we find that pederasty was routinely conceptualized in terms of the use to which ὁ ἐραστής (the lover) put ὁ ἐρώμενος (the boy loved).[16] Peder-

---

(Chicago: University of Chicago Libraries, 1916), p. 30: "These two verbs [*utor* and *fruor*] are practically interchangeable, as are their Greek equivalents [χρῶμαι and ἀπολάυω], though in the case of fruor and ἀπολαύω more zest is perhaps implied. Utor is in effect rather neutral, formal, and reminiscent of legal phraseology." Cf. Seneca, *On the Happy Life* 10.3. See also J. N. Adams, *The Latin Sexual Vocabulary* (Baltimore: Johns Hopkins University Press, 1982), pp. 189, 198; Brown, pp. 219, 234, 239. For the sexual sense of χρῆσις in medical writers, see L. Dean-Jones, "The Politics of Pleasure: Female Sexual Appetite in the Hippocratic Corpus," in *Discourses of Sexuality,* p. 57.

13. Epictetus, *Encheiridion* 33.8. Cf. Diogenes Laertius, *Lives of Eminent Philosophers* 2.74; 7.131; Dio Cassius, *Roman History* 54.16.3-5; Plutarch, *Amatorius* 751B; *Gnomologium Vaticanum* 376; Ps.-Lucian, *The Ass* 51.

14. Plutarch, *Advice to Bride and Groom* 144B. See also Brown, p. 308.

15. I have been unable to discover any examples of "use" in descriptions of female sexual activity with females. This suggests that Paul is not alluding to lesbianism in 1:26, as many exegetes assume; rather the reference is to inordinate desire within marriage. Other insights confirm this. B. Brooten ("Patristic Interpretations of Romans 1:26," in *Studia Patristica XVIII,* vol. 1 [Kalamazoo: Cistercian Publications, 1985], pp. 287-91) cites patristic readings which do not assume lesbianism, and J. Miller ("The Practices of Romans 1:26: Homosexual or Heterosexual?" *NovT* 37 [1995]: 4-8, 10) argues persuasively that only when the categories of homo/heterosexuality are assumed does 1:26 appear to speak of females having sex with females.

16. Aristippus (in Diogenes Laertius, *Lives of Eminent Philosophers* 2.99): "The wise man will use boys (τοῖς ἐρωμένοις χρήσεσθαι) openly and without any regard to circumstance." On this passage, see G. Gerhard, *Phoinix von Kolophon* (Leipzig: Teubner, 1909), pp. 145-46. Similar terminology is attributed to Zeno at *Stoicorum Veterum Fragmenta* 1.59.30: καὶ τοῖς παιδικοῖς χρῆσθαι ἀκωλύτως. See also Athenaeus, *Deipnosophistae* 13.604D-E; Fronto, *Epist. Graecae* 8.7.

asty was spoken of as "using the male as a woman."[17] This indicates the earlier place of the metaphor in the husband's sexual use of the wife, but such priority did not imply male/female pairing as a norm. Indifference to gender is seen most clearly when χρῆσις (or its cognates) refers in the same passage to the male's use of males and females. Reporting on the dissolute life of Sardanapallus, Diodorus of Sicily points to the king's pursuit of "the delights of love with men as well as with women, for he practiced sexual indulgence of both kinds without restraint (ἐχρῆτο γὰρ ταῖς ἐπ' ἀμφότερα συνουσίαις ἀνέδην)."[18] From Diodorus's perspective, Sardanapallus's fault was not his choice of sexual objects but the unrestrained manner in which he pursued his desires.

So far we have seen that χρῆσις emphasizes the instrumentality of the object of sexual desire and does not draw particular attention to the gender of the persons involved. Where does this conceptualization of sexual activity, so foreign to modern thinking about sex as a relation, originate? We have seen above that the analogy between eating and having sex was widespread. This is one possible source. Another important background is the topic of household management (οἰκονομία).[19] Use of possessions is a practical task for the head of the household.[20] One theorist aligns use with acquiring, preserving, and improving property.[21] The more common division of the topic is simply possession (κτῆσις) and use (χρῆσις) of property.[22] The Pythagorean Callicratidas employs this division: "But of the parts of a family there are two first and greatest divisions: viz. man and possessions (κτᾶσις), the latter of which is a thing governed, and affords utility (χρᾶσιν). Thus, also, the first and greatest parts of an animal are soul and body; and soul, indeed, is that

17. Xenophon, *Memorabilia* 2.1.30: γυναιξὶ τοῖς ἀνδράσι χρωμένη. Cf. Dio Cassius, *Roman History* 62.28.3; Lucian, *A True Story* 1.22.3-4; Ps.-Lucian, *Affairs of the Heart* 27.

18. Diodorus Siculus, *Library of History* 2.23.2. Cf. Xenophon, *Symposium* 8.28-29; Diogenes Laertius, *Lives of Eminent Philosophers* 10.132; Epictetus, *Encheiridion* 10; Ps.-Lucian, *Affairs of the Heart* 25.

19. Foucault has drawn attention to male sexual practice as a problem of household management. See especially *The Use of Pleasure*, pp. 141-84.

20. See, for example, *Stoicorum Veterum Fragmenta* 3.159.6.

21. Ps.-Aristotle, *Oeconomica* 1.6.1: "There are four qualities which the head of a household must possess in dealing with his property . . . acquiring (κτᾶσθαι) . . . preserving (φυλάττειν) . . . how to improve (κοσμητικὸν), and how to make use of it (χρηστικόν)." For the last in this list, see S. Pomeroy, *Xenophon, Oeconomicus: A Social and Historical Commentary* (Oxford: Clarendon, 1994), pp. 219-20.

22. Plato, *Euthydemus* 280E; Clement of Alexandria, *Paedagogus* 2.3.38.4; 3.8.41.3; *Stromateis* 6.12.100.1; Iamblichus, *Protrepticus* 37. For a fuller collection of philosophic texts displaying this organization of the topic, see Gerhard, pp. 113-15.

which governs and uses (χρεόμενον), but the body is that which is governed and imparts utility (χρᾶσιν)."[23] Wives fall within the category of things to be used, though sexual use specifically is not mentioned by these authors.[24]

A significant issue in household management was the matter of correct use (ὀρθὴ χρῆσις).[25] It depended on employing ἀδιάφορα (matters of indifference) without passion, as Clement of Alexandria emphasized in his discussion of the Christian's relation to wealth: "So let a man do away, not with possessions, but rather with the passions of the soul, which do not consent to the better use (τὴν ἀμείνω χρῆσιν) of what he has; in order that, by becoming noble and good, he may be able to use these possessions also in a noble manner (τοῖς κτήμασι χρῆσθαι δυνηθῇ καλῶς)."[26] Control of passions, if not their complete eradication for some authors, is the path to correct use of possessions.[27]

Broadening the investigation beyond the limits of the topos on household management, we discover a drive, particularly among Stoics (by no means limited to them, however), to articulate the correct use of externals in all areas of life. Correct use is a component in the chief doctrine of the philosophers according to Epictetus's understanding of Zeno's maxim: "'To follow the gods is man's end, and the essence of the good is the correct use (χρῆσις οἵα δεῖ) of external impressions.'"[28] In Stoic doctrine the happiness of the

23. Text is H. Thesleff, *The Pythagorean Texts of the Hellenistic Period,* Acta Academiae Aboensis, Ser. A, vol. 30 (Åbo: Åbo Akademi, 1965), 104.7-11. Translation is T. Taylor, *Political Fragments of Archytas, Charondas, Zaleucas, and Other Ancient Pythagoreans* (Chiswick: Taylor, 1822), p. 51.

24. Xenophon, *Oeconomicus* 3.10; *Symposium* 2.10; Philo, *On Virtues* 30.

25. Plato, *Euthydemus* 280E; *Republic* 451C: "right possession and use of children and wives (ὀρθὴ παίδων τε καὶ γυναικῶν κτῆσίς τε καὶ χρεία)." See also Ps.-Plato, *Eryxias* 403B. In a summary of Aristotelian ethical doctrine (Ps.-Aristotle, *De virtutibus et vitiis*) preserved in Stobaeus, one of the "works of prudence" is "to use well all existing goods (τὸ χρῆσθαι καλῶς πᾶσι τοῖς ὑπάρχουσιν ἀγαθοῖς, Stobaeus, *Anthology* 3.140.3-4)." On the other hand, a characteristic work of foolishness is "to use existing goods in a bad way (τὸ χρῆσθαι κακῶς τοῖς παροῦσιν ἀγαθοῖς, Stobaeus, *Anthology* 3.143, 19-20)." See further Stobaeus, *Anthology* 3.264.12–265.4; Iamblichus, *Protrepticus* 25-28. For "just use (δικαία χρῆσις)," see Theano, *Epistle* 6.2 (Thesleff, 197.34).

26. Clement of Alexandria, *Quis dives salvetur* 14. Cf. *Stromateis* 3.1.4.2; *Paedagogus* 2.1.9.2; Seneca, *Epistle* 74.18.

27. Clement of Alexandria, *Quis dives salvetur* 15: "A man must say good-bye, then, to the injurious things he has, not to those that can actually contribute to his advantage if he knows the right use of them (τὴν ὀρθὴν χρῆσιν); and advantage comes from those that are managed (οἰκονομούμενα) with wisdom, moderation and piety."

28. Epictetus, *Discourse* 1.20.15-16. For Zeno on χρῆσις, see also *Stoicorum Veterum Fragmenta* 1.57.17-24. For Epictetus's sustained interest in the moral problem of using externals, see *Discourses* 1.28.6-7, 12; 2.16.28; 4.5.23; *Fragment* 4; *Encheiridion* 6.

sage could be attributed to the use of matters of indifference for benefit — not for pleasure.[29] While the sage "consistently uses (χρώμενος συνεχῶς)" the experiences of life "prudently, with self-control, decently, and orderly (φρονίμως καὶ ἐγκρατῶς καὶ κοσμίως καὶ εὐτάκτως)," the bad person fails to understand ὀρθὴ χρῆσις and necessarily lives a life of regret.[30] Correct use of any object requires the control of passion. The wise man will "feel no attraction or confusion in treating (χρήσεται) the things from which the passions spring, like wealth and poverty, glory and ingloriousness, health and disease, life and death, trouble and pleasure. To use indifferently things which are matters of ethical indifference (ἀδιαφόρως τοῖς ἀδιαφόραις χρησώμεθα) we need considerable powers of discrimination. . . ."[31] Correct use is measured use of objects necessary for life and the strict avoidance of luxury.[32] The use of sexual objects was similarly evaluated in terms of control of passion.[33] Using sex sparingly was the ideal.[34]

We have now come to the point where the philosophic view of correct use points the way to an interpretation of Romans 1:26-27. The philosophers had one more synonym of correct use; it was the very phrase which Paul employs — natural use (φυσικὴ χρῆσις). Natural use is characterized by an avoidance of luxury and the control of passion.[35] According to Epictetus, "the

29. Diogenes Laertius, *Lives of Eminent Philosophers* 7.104. Note here the Stoic formula εὖ καὶ κακῶς χρῆσθαι; good use makes something indifferent good: see *Stoicorum Veterum Fragmenta* 3.20.6; 3.29.28; 3.29.41-42; 3.49.23-29. This notion is reflected in Epictetus (*Discourse* 2.6.2): "Although life is a matter of indifference, the use which you make of it is not a matter of indifference (οὕτως τὸ ζῆν ἀδιάφορον, ἡ χρῆσις οὐκ ἀδιάφορος)." Cf. 3.3.2. For use aiming in benefit rather than in pleasure, see Galen, *On the Doctrines of Hippocrates and Plato* 4.2.42 (text and translation is P. De Lacy, *Galen on the Doctrines of Hippocrates and Plato,* 2nd ed. [Berlin: Akademie-Verlag, 1981], pp. 246-47): "When a person is led by reason alone to the experience (χρῆσιν) of pleasant things, such a person is called temperate (σώφρων), for he has made his aim in choosing them not the enjoyment (ἀπόλαυσιν) but the benefit (ὠφέλιαν)."

30. Stobaeus, *Anthology* 2.102.20-25. Cf. Ps.-Crates, *Epistle* 10; Plutarch, *On Tranquility of Mind* 466C.

31. Clement of Alexandria, *Stromateis* 2.109.3-4 (translation is J. Ferguson, *Clement of Alexandria: "Stromateis" Books One to Three,* FC 85 [Washington, D.C.: Catholic University of America Press, 1991], p. 229). Cf. *Paedagogus* 2.12.121.1: χωρίς προσπαθείας καὶ διαφορᾶς χρώμεθα αὐτοῖς.

32. Stobaeus, *Anthology* 2.127.11-25; 135.5-10; 136.3-8; Musonius Rufus, *Fragment* 18B; Clement of Alexandria, *Paedagogus* 2.1.12.1; 2.12.120.5-6.

33. Stobaeus, *Anthology* 3.360.6-21.

34. Clement of Alexandria, *Stromateis* 4.23.147.1; Ocellus, *On the Nature of the Universe* 54-55; Aristoxenus (in Stobaeus, *Anthology* 4.879.8).

35. Seneca, *On the Happy Life* 17.2: *naturalis usus.*

function of the good and excellent man is to deal with his impressions in accordance with nature (τὸ χρῆσθαι ταῖς φαντασίαις κατὰ φύσιν)."[36] On the other hand, careless use of externals, that is, when passion is present, is παρὰ φύσιν.[37]

So far we have located the Pauline argument within the ethical problem of the correct, or natural, use of externals. Paul is not condemning homosexual relations as such; the notion of sexual relation is itself foreign to his way of thinking. We have seen that χρῆσις, properly understood as use, entails a completely different moral problem than the one implied by χρῆσις mistakenly translated as relation. χρῆσις does not make gender thematic. Rather, the problem becomes the psychological significance of the act for the subject of sexual desire. We are able to confirm this interpretation when we turn from an analysis of use and explore further the concept of nature in the philosophic treatments of passion in general and sexual desire in particular. We will find a connection between "against nature" and the notion of the normal, acquisitive aspect of the self's relation to the world given over to excess.

On this point I am in agreement with Dale Martin, who has suggested that what Paul meant by παρὰ φύσιν was not "*disoriented* desire" but "*inordinate* desire."[38] Martin's work has made it clear that we need a more differentiated sense of what "according to nature" meant in the ancient world when it came to matters of sex. Natural sex was understood in three distinct ways: sex for the sake of procreation (thus only male with female);[39] sex which symbolizes and preserves male social superiority to the female (males penetrate/females are penetrated);[40] and sex in which passion is absent or at least held to a

36. Epictetus, *Discourse* 3.3.2. Cf. *Discourses* 3.16.15; 4.5.23; 4.10.26; *Fragment* 4; *Encheiridion* 6.

37. Epictetus, *Discourse* 3.3.2, 3, 6, 24.

38. Martin, p. 342 (emphasis Martin's).

39. Plato, *Laws* 838D-839A; Ocellus, *On the Nature of the Universe* 44-45, 55; Musonius Rufus, *Fragment* 12; Philo, *Special Laws* 3.34-36; Dio Chrysostom, *Discourse* 7.136; Clement of Alexandria, *Paedagogus* 2.10.87.1-4. The naturalness of sex for procreation is rejected in Ps.-Diogenes, *Epistle* 21. For an attempt to read "against nature" as nonvaginal sex into Rom. 1:24-27, see Miller, pp. 8-11.

40. Philo, *Abraham* 135-36; *Special Laws* 1.325; 2.50; 3.39; *On the Contemplative Life* 59; Dio Chrysostom, *Discourse* 7.149; Plutarch, *Amatorius* 750D-E; 751C-D; Ps.-Lucian, *Affairs of the Heart* 19-20 (on which see S. Goldhill, *Foucault's Virginity: Ancient Erotic Fiction and the History of Sexuality* [Cambridge: Cambridge University Press, 1995], p. 105); Clement of Alexandria, *Paedagogus* 2.10.90.2-3; 3.3.23.1; *Greek Anthology* 11.272; Seneca, *Epistle* 95.20-21. Discussion of sex as symbolic of social power must begin with K. Dover, *Greek Homosexuality* (Cambridge: Harvard University Press, 1978), pp. 100-109. Artemidorus's dream analysis has been highly prized as a way into Greco-Roman attitudes toward sex. For

minimum. Significant for our interpretation of Romans 1:24-27 is the fact that only the last of these is coordinated in ancient texts with the concept of use.[41] By combining "use" with "natural," Paul follows a pattern established by the moral philosophers whose concern was to make passion and its control the core ethical problem in all matters of life.

The mutual implication of passion and "against nature" is basic to the Stoic evaluation of action. Diogenes Laertius reports that "passion, or emotion, is defined by Zeno as an irrational and unnatural movement in the soul, or again as impulse in excess."[42] What makes an action wrong and against nature is the presence of passion in the agent.[43] Musonius Rufus, Epictetus, and Seneca provide copious references to nature in descriptions of the ideal life spent in pursuing necessities without indulging passion.[44] The association of the unnatural with passion is not limited to Stoics.[45]

---

his understanding of natural sex as symbolic of male domination of the female, see J. Winkler, *The Constraints of Desire: Essays in the Anthropology of Sex and Gender in Ancient Greece* (New York: Routledge, 1989), pp. 36-37. This approach, which highlights the dimension of power in sexuality, has been employed fruitfully in the explanation of Jewish and rabbinic condemnation of male-with-male sexual activity. See M. Satlow, "'They Abused Him Like a Woman': Homoeroticism, Gender Blurring, and the Rabbis in Late Antiquity," *Journal of the History of Sexuality* 5 (1994): 1-25; D. Boyarin, "Are There Any Jews in 'The History of Sexuality'?" *Journal of the History of Sexuality* 5 (1995): 333-55.

41. The only possible exception I have discovered is Athenaeus, *Deipnosophistae* 13.605D: "So beware, you philosophers who indulge in passion contrary to nature (οἱ παρὰ φύσιν τῇ Ἀφροδίτῃ χρώμενοι)." Yet this is a difficult text. The context is certain philosophers' pederastic practice. In 13.605E the philosophers' problem is not knowing that desire is transitory. Similarly, the boy's beauty comes to an end, while the philosophers' passion does not cease. Might "against nature" here mean the impossibility of fulfilling desires?

42. Diogenes Laertius, *Lives of Eminent Philosophers* 7.110. πάθος is by definition against nature. That which makes it so is excess of rational impulse toward objects. See the convenient collection of texts in A. Glibert-Thirry, *Pseudo-Andronicus de Rhodes: ΠΕΡΙ ΠΑΘΩΝ*, Corpus Latinum Commentariorum in Aristotelem Graecorum, Suppl. 2 (Leiden: Brill, 1977), pp. 273-74. For an illuminating discussion of this topic, see B. Inwood, *Ethics and Human Action in Early Stoicism* (Oxford: Clarendon, 1985), pp. 154-73.

43. Representative is Clement of Alexandria, *Stromateis* 2.109.1. See G. B. Kerford, "The Origin of Evil in Stoic Thought," *Bulletin of the John Rylands Library* 60 (1978): 488-92.

44. See, for example, Musonius Rufus, *Fragment* 17; Epictetus, *Discourses* 1.4.15; 3.7.24-28; Seneca, *Epistle* 122.5-19; *On the Happy Life* 13.4-5: natural desires are ones which are neither excessive nor insatiable.

45. Plutarch, *On Moral Virtue* 450E: "But he who permits the better part to follow and be in subjection to the intemperate and irrational part of his soul is called worse than himself and incontinent (ἀκρατής) and in a state contrary to Nature (παρὰ φύσιν)."

Building on the equivalence of "without passion" and "according to nature," a basic distinction between two types of sexual desire took shape, not only among the Stoics but among other philosophical schools, with adaptations in terminology appropriate to each school.[46] The first type is natural desire (φυσικὴ ἐπιθυμία), put forward by Aristotle in analogy with the consumption of food; continuing on with the analogy, the second type of sexual desire is understood as if it were an excess in the quantity consumed.[47] Epicurus proposed a more complex categorization of pleasures: the natural and necessary, the natural but unnecessary, the empty or unnatural and unnecessary. Sexual desire was placed in the second category, yet when this desire becomes excessive it moves into the third.[48] For a broad range of thinkers, since Eros is insatiable, it is "against nature."[49]

C. The Problem of Eros in Romans 1:24-27

Our investigation of the philosophic background of Paul's term χρῆσις leads us to consider the possibility that Romans 1:24-27 highlights the problem of passion and its consequences rather than the violation of a divinely instituted norm of male and female intercourse. Additionally, we have seen that although "the natural" has a range of meaning in ancient writers, the most likely parallel to Paul's usage is the philosophic interest in the problem of self-control in the face of erotic love. Unnatural use, from this perspective, has less to do with the gender of the persons having sex and more with the loss of self-control experienced by the user of another's body.

46. *Stoicorum Veterum Fragmenta* 3.98.20-21: natural needs, including marriage, can be pursued without passion. Panaetius (in Seneca, *Epistle* 116.5) hints at the possibility of the wise man becoming a lover while preserving his rationality because of his prior victory over passion. Cf. Epictetus, *Encheiridion* 34, 41. See G. Luck, "Panaetius and Menander," *American Journal of Philology* 96 (1975): 257-62. For the distinction between passionate love and harmless love, see M. Pohlenz, "Das dritte und vierte Buch der Tusculanen," *Hermes* 41 (1906): 349-51.

47. Aristotle, *Nicomachean Ethics* 3.11.1-3.

48. Brown, p. 105; M. Nussbaum, "Beyond Obsession and Disgust: Lucretius' Genealogy of Love," *Apeiron* 22 (1989): 13; J. Annas, "Epicurean Emotions," *Greek, Roman and Byzantine Studies* 30 (1989): 147-53. Cf. Plutarch, *Beasts Are Rational* 989C-990F; Clement of Alexandria, *Stromateis* 2.20.118.7; 3.1.3.2; *Paedagogus* 2.10.94.2.

49. See S. Lilja, *Homosexuality in Republican and Augustan Rome,* Commentationes Humanarum Litterarum 74 (Helsinki: Societas Scientarum Fennica, 1982), pp. 124-25; Brown, pp. 107, 229-31.

This interpretation is confirmed once the case has been made that key points of Paul's argument are informed by a psychology of erotic love known to the ancient world.[50] Although Paul does not explicitly name ἔρως as the culprit in the human condition described in 1:24-27,[51] a string of terms points in its direction:

ἐπιθυμία (desire, 1:24)
πάθος (passion, 1:26)
ἐκκαίω (inflame, 1:27)
ὄρεξις (appetite, 1:27)
πλάνη (error, 1:27)

Each term by itself can be shown to have a key role in the ancient discussion of erotic love; taken together we have a rough outline of the philosophic critique of ἔρως. Romans 1:24-27 is not an attack on homosexuality as a violation of divine law but a description of the human condition informed by the philosophic rejection of passionate love.

The first indication that Paul is going to build an argument around the topic of ἔρως comes in 1:24: "the desires of their hearts (ταῖς ἐπιθυμίαις τῶν καρδίων αὐτῶν)." Desire (ἐπιθυμία) was one of the four major types of passion, along with grief, fear, and pleasure.[52] Although it is necessary to distinguish ἐπιθυμία and ἔρως, since the latter was a "more exclusive passion involving emotional and psychological commitment beyond the consummation of any desire,"[53] erotic love was nevertheless thought to be a kind of ἐπιθυμία.[54] It began in ἐπιθυμία,[55] and could be characterized as the "runaway movement of the desiderative power (ἐπιθυμητικῆς δυνάμεως)."[56] Love's object was the body of

50. For a concise history of Eros, which correctly emphasizes the issue of self-control, see Konstan, pp. 178-85.

51. For Paul's familiarity with literary conventions pertaining to ἔρως, see C. Smith, "Ἐκκλεῖσαι in Galatians 4:17: The Motif of the Excluded Lover as a Metaphor of Manipulation," *Catholic Biblical Quarterly* 58 (1996): 480-99. Consider also the cliché "love as slavery" in 1 Cor. 6:12; see S. Lilja, *The Roman Elegists' Attitude to Women* (New York: Garland, 1978), pp. 76-89.

52. See the collection of texts in Glibert-Thirry, 223.3-10; pp. 274-76.

53. Dean-Jones, p. 57 n. 18. Cf. Halperin, "Platonic *Erôs,*" pp. 171-76.

54. Glibert-Thirry, 229.76; A. C. van Geytenbeek, *Musonius Rufus and Greek Diatribe* (Assen: Van Gorcum, 1962), p. 76; M. Schofield, *The Stoic Idea of the City* (Cambridge: Cambridge University Press, 1991), p. 30 n. 17.

55. Plato, *Phaedrus* 237D; 238BC; Xenophon, *Memorabilia* 3.9.7; *Stoicorum Veterum Fragmenta* 3.96.43; Plutarch, *Amatorius* 767C.

56. Galen, *On the Doctrines of Hippocrates and Plato* 4.1.16. Cf. Plutarch, *Fragment*

another, with no specification of gender.[57] Also, as in Paul, philosophic and literary discourse associated the heart with matters erotic.[58]

In 1:26 Paul employs another term borrowed from philosophy's treatment of erotic love: "passion" (πάθος).[59] The fact that ἐπιθυμία and πάθος stand in parallel phrases in 1:24 and 26 ("God handed them over . . .") justifies our attempt to interpret them together under the theme of excessive sexual desire.[60] The connection between dishonor and the experience of passion to which Paul's phrase "dishonorable passions (πάθη ἀτιμίας)" alludes will be discussed below. For now it is only necessary to take note of Paul's use of πάθος as a reflection of the discussion of ἔρως in philosophic and literary contexts. We see in these sources that it was the unbridled character of erotic love that was expressed with the help of πάθος.[61] We should also note that in sexual matters πάθος is employed without regard to the gender of either the subject or the object of desire.[62]

---

135. Along these same lines, the Stoics placed two types of excessive sexual passion under the category of ἐπιθυμία: ἔρωτες σφοδροί and ἐρωτομανία. See Preston, pp. 8-9.

57. Xenophon, *Symposium* 8.2, 13.

58. Zeno, for example, placed ἐπιθυμία and θυμός in the heart. See Galen, *On the Doctrines of Hippocrates and Plato* 3.2.7. Cf. 4.1.17 for Chrysippus's similar view. See also Achilles Tatius, *Leucippe and Clitophon* 3.37.6-10. For "hearts on fire," a notion discussed below in connection with Rom. 1:27, see *Greek Anthology* 5.260; 9.627; 12.130. For the heart's place in speech about ἔρως, see Preston, p. 49; D. H. Garrison, *Mild Frenzy: A Reading of the Hellenistic Love Epigram* (Wiesbaden: Steiner, 1978), pp. 75-77.

59. For the definition of πάθος, see n. 42 above.

60. In 1 Thess. 4:5 Paul's exhortation implies the possibility of sex without passion: μὴ ἐν πάθει ἐπιθυμίας. For the notion of passionless sex, see Brown, pp. 216-18. Within the context of marriage, see Philo, *Special Laws* 3.9; Clement of Alexandria, *Paedagogus* 2.10.92.2; Ps.-Phocylides, *Sentences* 193-94; 4 Maccabees 2:11. For discussion of these texts, see I. Heinemann, *Philons griechishe und jüdische Bildung: Kulturvergleichende Untersuchungen zu Philons Darstellung der jüdische Gesetze* (Hildesheim: Olms, 1962), pp. 276-77; van Geytenbeek, pp. 72-73. Passionless sex may also be what Paul has in mind when he exhorts his male readers in 1 Thess. 4:4: τὸ ἑαυτοῦ σκεῦος κτᾶσθαι ἐν ἁγιασμῷ καὶ τιμῇ. For "having a wife in honor" and its connection to the passion of the husband, see M. Foucault, *The History of Sexuality,* vol. 3, *The Care of the Self* (New York: Random House, 1988), p. 174.

61. See Lilja, *Roman Elegists' Attitude,* pp. 89-109; A. Allen, "Propertius I, 1," *Yale Classical Studies* 11 (1950): 258-64; Brown, p. 197. Cf. Ps.-Phocylides, *Sentences* 194: "For 'eros' is not a god, but a passion destructive of all" (translation is P. W. van der Horst, *The Sentences of Pseudo-Phocylides* [Leiden: Brill, 1978], p. 240).

62. Plutarch, *Amatorius* 751F: "Excitement (πάθος) about boys and women is one and the same thing: Love." See also Ps.-Lucian, *Affairs of the Heart* 4. Plutarch's observation is a lesson learned easily from reading erotic epigrams. See *Greek Anthology* 5.19, 65, 116, 278, 302; 12.31, 41, 86, 90.

Paul's familiarity with the literary and philosophical ways of speaking about ἔρως becomes even more evident when we consider the phrase "they were inflamed for one another (ἐξεκαύθησαν εἰς ἀλλήλους)" in 1:27.[63] Fire was the principal metaphor of sexual love in a broad range of literary genres and in philosophy.[64] The metaphor emphasized the misery of the lover, his perpetually unsatisfied state, and the loss of self-control. Fire imagery makes vivid the philosophic description of the perennial battle between reason and passion in sexual matters.[65] Significantly, there is no restriction on the gender of the beloved who has inflamed the lover. One and the same ἔρως inflames males for males, males for females, females for males, and females for females.[66]

The experience of erotic love as fire was given a physiological foundation by some authors. Hot blood in young men causes "desire (τό ἐπιθυμήτικον)" to be "at its height."[67] Heat had a crucial role to play in the production of semen, which, when expelled, quenched the fire of love.[68] It is important to observe that when the fire of love is explained in physiological

63. For Paul's familiarity with fire imagery for excessive sexual desire in 1 Cor. 7:9, see W. Deming, *Paul on Marriage and Celibacy: The Hellenistic Background of 1 Corinthians 7*, SNTS 83 (Cambridge: Cambridge University Press, 1995), pp. 130-31.

64. Henderson, pp. 177-78; E. Fantham, *Comparative Studies in Republican Latin Imagery* (Toronto: University of Toronto Press, 1972), pp. 8-12, 83-88. Fire imagery (with giddiness, distraction, turning pale, and the like) is almost always present in descriptions of persons who have fallen under the spell of ἔρως: Plutarch, *Amatorius* 763A; *Fragment* 137; Philo, *On the Decalogue* 122; Chariton, *Chareas and Callirhoe* 4.2.4-5; Longus, *Daphnis and Chloe* 1.11, 13, 14, 18, 23; 2.7, 8; *Greek Anthology* 5.264.

65. *Stoicorum Veterum Fragmenta* 3.179.20-26; Plutarch, *On Moral Virtue* 448B; 4 Maccabees 3:17. This philosophic cliché shows up in literary contexts as well: Ovid, *Remedies for Love* 115-34; Chariton, *Chareas and Callirhoe* 2.4.4-5.

66. The metaphor's indifference to gender is well illustrated in the opening of the following epigram (*Greek Anthology* 12.90) spoken by a male: "No longer do I love (ἐρῶ). I have wrestled with three passions that burn (ἔκαυσε): one for a courtesan, one for a maiden, and one for a lad." Males on fire for males: *Greek Anthology* 5.6; 12.74; Chariton, *Chareas and Callirhoe* 4.16-17; Maximus of Tyre, *Discourse* 20.5D; males on fire for females: Virgil, *Eclogues* 8.80-83; Ps.-Hippocrates, *Epistle* 17.42; female desire for males: Plutarch, *Amatorius* 753A-B; Ovid, *Remedies for Love* 267, 287-88; Achilles Tatius, *Leucippe and Clitophon* 2.37.9; female for female: Plutarch, *Amatorius* 762F.

67. Ps.-Plutarch, *Desire and Grief* 9; Cf. Clement of Alexandria, *Paedagogus* 2.2.20.3–21.1. For the role of warmth in the generation of desire, see Brown, pp. 182-83. In addition, see Plutarch, *Amatorius* 765B; Philo, *Special Laws* 3.10. The physiological basis of sexual desire did not, however, make it exempt from moral reflection and control. See Diogenes Laertius, *Lives of Eminent Philosophers* 7.17; Stobaeus, *Anthology* 3.428.1–429.8 (Hierocles).

68. Clement of Alexandria, *Stromateis* 3.1.2.1-2.

terms, the causes of the heat are located within the individual's body. This should be contrasted with the overwhelming majority of cases in which fire imagery emphasizes the external source of erotic passion. Here, I believe, is the background for understanding Paul's use of the image. Fire imagery most often reinforced the notion that sexual passion is a force which invades the lover from the outside.[69]

Fire imagery thus accents the passive character of the desiring subject.[70] Paul's use of ἐκκαίω in the passive voice reflects the idea bemoaned by philosophers and reluctantly celebrated by poets that the passion of love invades and overwhelms the individual.[71] Like an arrow dipped in fire, ἔρως penetrates the heart.[72] Erotic madness seizes its victims and sets them on fire.[73] Just how fire is kindled by the beloved may have remained a mystery to some.[74] Yet it was often suggested that the eyes of the lover are the medium to the outside world, and through them fire enters the soul.[75] To see or imagine the beloved kindles fire.[76] One of the most common clichés in the love epigram, that a beautiful form "casts fire" on the lover, expresses well his passive role.[77] Thus, while modern thinking about sexuality posits erotic desire as the externalization of a deep, internal disposition, the imagery of fire employed by the ancients reveals a movement in just the opposite direction. Our interpretation of Paul's use of fire imagery in 1:27 will need to take into account this difference. Paul is not speaking of the externalization of sexual orientation deep in the individual's personality. Rather, he expresses the philosophic view that passion invades from outside and overwhelms the subject. As we will see below, this latter interpretation fits best with the overall rhetorical purpose of Romans 1:18-32.

Fire imagery also communicated ideas of frustration and insatiability.

69. K. Dover, "Classical Greek Attitudes to Sexual Behaviour," *Arethusa* 6 (1973): 272.

70. *Greek Anthology* 5.10, 75; 11.36; 12.46, 48, 63, 79, 99, 178; Alciphron, *Epistle* 3.31; Ovid, *Affairs of the Heart* 1.2.9-17.

71. For the complex meaning of the images which reverse the role of the lover from the one who penetrates to the one penetrated by passion, see Garrison, pp. 26-27.

72. *Greek Anthology* 9.443; 12.76.

73. Plutarch, *Amatorius* 759B-C.

74. *Greek Anthology* 5.131.

75. Xenophon, *Symposium* 4.24-25; Plutarch, *Amatorius* 759C; *Fragment* 138; *Greek Anthology* 12.81, 83, 87, 93, 99, 151; Heliodorus, *Aethiopica* 1.24; Philostratus, *Epistles* 8, 11, 12. On this theme, see A. Walker, "Eros and the Eye in the Love-Letters of Philostratus," *Proceedings of the Cambridge Philological Society* 38 (1992): 132-48.

76. Plutarch, *Advice to Bride and Groom* 138F; Chariton, *Chareas and Callirhoe* 6.4.5-7.

77. *Greek Anthology* 12.81, 82, 86, 87, 109. See also the texts in Brown, p. 195.

With respect to the former, any impediment to the lover's possession of the beloved, whether it be refusal of advances or unforeseen circumstances, inflamed the soul.[78] More significant for our interpretation of the Pauline argument, however, is the association of fire with the perpetuation of erotic desire after the sexual act.[79] As Chariton reminds his readers, ἔρως in its very nature is always looking for something new (φιλόκαινος): "that is why poets and sculptors depict him with bow and arrows and associate him with fire, the most insubstantial, mutable of attributes."[80] Under the influence of erotic desire, the lover is inflamed by consummation of sex itself to seek more and novel loves.[81] Epictetus compares passionate love to a feverish thirst which is intensified by drinking water.[82] Dio Chrysostom's depiction of the person devoted to pleasure brings together the themes of fire, insatiability, and, as in Paul's argument, the resulting movement from females to males as objects of male sexual desire: "He is of many hues and shapes, insatiable (ἀπλήρωτος) as to things that tickle nostril and palate. . . ." Dio continues:

> He is passionately devoted to all these things [pleasures of the five senses], but especially and unrestrainedly to the poignant and burning madness (ὀξεῖαν καὶ διάπυρον μανίαν) of sexual indulgence, through intercourse both with females and with males, and through still other unspeakable and nameless obscenities; after all such indiscriminately he rushes and also leads others, abjuring no form of lust and leaving none untried.[83]

78. Seneca, *On Benefits* 4.14.1; Philo, *On the Contemplative Life* 61; *Greek Anthology* 5.255, 279; Philostratus, *Epistle* 13.

79. Brown, pp. 236, 238-39.

80. Chariton, *Chareas and Callirhoe* 4.7.6. Cf. Ps.-Lucian, *Affairs of the Heart* 2: "For, almost from the time I left off being a boy and was accounted a young man, I have been beguiled by one passion after another. One Love has succeeded another, and almost before I've ended earlier ones later Loves begin. . . . For one flame is not extinguished by another. There dwells in my eyes so nimble a gadfly that it pounces on any and every beauty as its prey and is never sated enough to stop."

81. Philo, *Special Laws* 3.9-10: "Now even natural pleasure (ἡ κατὰ φύσιν ἡδονή) is often greatly to blame when the craving for it is immoderate and insatiable (ἀμέτρως καὶ ἀκορέστως χρῆται τις αὐτῇ), as for instance when it takes the form of voracious gluttony . . . or again the passionate desire for women shewn by those who in their craze for sexual intercourse behave unchastely, not with the wives of others, but with their own. But the blame in most of these cases rests less with the soul than with the body, which contains a great amount of fire and moisture; the fire as it consumes the material set before it quickly demands a second supply. . . ." Cf. Clement of Alexandria, *Paedagogus* 2.10.102.1-2; *Quis dives salvetur* 25.

82. Epictetus, *Discourse* 4.9.3-5. See above, n. 29.

83. Dio Chrysostom, *Discourse* 4.101-102.

The ancient psychology of Eros pictured the fire of love springing up in the ὄρεξις (appetite), a word which Paul employs in Romans 1:27. This was a fundamental term in the Stoic analysis of human action and was often coordinated with πάθος and ἐπιθυμία in broader philosophic discussions of sexual desire. The Stoics defined ὄρεξις as an impulse toward that which the agent thinks is good.[84] Ancient writers sharpened the meaning of ὄρεξις by comparing it with ἐπιθυμία. Clement of Alexandria, for example, alludes to a common distinction: "They who are skilled in such matters distinguish propension (ὄρεξις) from lust (ἐπιθυμία); and assign the latter, as being irrational, to pleasures and licentiousness; and propension, as being a rational movement, they assign to the necessities of nature."[85] Discussions of erotic passion generally assume ὄρεξις as a neutral term, a structured way humans appropriate parts of the external world; ἔρως is ὄρεξις which has become irrational and excessive.[86]

Epictetus is an important source for understanding the role ὄρεξις plays in the Stoic analysis of human action and ultimately in Paul's argument.[87] According to Epictetus, three fields constitute human activity: desire (ὄρεξις), choice (ὁρμή), and assent (συγκατάθεσις).[88] Each has to do with the agent's activity of selecting and acquiring objects in the external world.[89] ὄρεξις depicts the agent's movement toward the object; its opposite is aversion (ἔκκλισις).[90] For Epictetus, ὄρεξις was natural when its object could be ob-

84. M. Reesor, *The Nature of Man in Early Stoic Philosophy* (New York: St. Martin's Press, 1989), pp. 91, 97. Diogenes Laertius, *Lives of Eminent Philosophers* 7.116; *Stoicorum Veterum Fragmenta* 3.42.20; 3.94.10; Stobaeus, *Anthology* 2.97.15–98.6; Galen, *On the Doctrines of Hippocrates and Plato* 4.4.2; 5.7.29. Brad Inwood's paraphrase of the Stoic definitions is helpful: "Any action whose object is the good or what the agent takes to be good will be caused and defined by the form of impulse known as orexis" (Inwood, p. 114). Cf. pp. 115, 227-37.

85. Clement of Alexandria, *Stromateis* 4.18.117.5 (translation is *Ante-Nicene Fathers,* 2:431). For ἐπιθυμία as irrational appetite (ἄλογος ὄρεξις), see texts collected in Glibert-Thirry, 223.16-17; pp. 278-79. For the definition of legitimate sexual practice in terms of this distinction, see Foucault, *Care of the Self,* p. 200. Cf. Ocellus, *On the Nature of the Universe* 44.

86. Plutarch, *Amatorius* 750D. This was emphasized particularly by Epicureans; see *Stoicorum Veterum Fragmenta* 3.181.22, 27-28 and the texts discussed in Brown, pp. 113, 277, and Nussbaum, pp. 11-17. Cf. Clement of Alexandria, *Stromateis* 2.20.118.7–119.6.

87. For Epictetus's teaching on ὄρεξις in relation to the Old Stoa, see Inwood, pp. 116-26.

88. For the three fields of human activity, see P. More, *Hellenistic Philosophies* (Princeton: Princeton University Press, 1923), pp. 108-13. In Epictetus, see *Discourses* 2.8.29; 2.17.15-16; 3.2.1-4; 3.12.1-12; 3.22.42-44; 4.4.14-18; 4.6.18, 26.

89. Epictetus, *Discourse* 4.6.26.

90. Epictetus, *Discourses* 1.17.24; 2.24.19.

tained with certainty and without hindrance.[91] Desire for objects which might not come into the subject's acquisition and yield satisfaction, Epictetus labels "unnatural."[92]

Examination of an individual's ὄρεξις and its objects could reveal whether he was happy or miserable, self-respecting or full of shame, since this analysis discovered whether the person was effectual in his desires or continually wanting things over which he had no control.[93] Now, with respect to this inner connection of ὄρεξις and satiability, we find an illuminating parallel between Paul and Epictetus. Both use fire imagery, which calls forth the idea of insatiability, to depict the ὄρεξις in a bad state. Paul's phrase "they were inflamed in their desire (ἐξεκαύθησαν ἐν τῇ ὀρέξει)" in Romans 1:27 echoes Epictetus's use of fire imagery to depict the impulse toward the perceived good that through passion has oriented itself to objects over which it does not have control.[94] Calling upon the three fields of human activity, Epictetus outlines the philosopher's diagnosis of an individual in such a state: "Your desires are feverish (αἱ ὀρέξεις σου φλεγμαίνουσιν), your attempts to avoid things (ἐκκλίσεις) are humiliating, your purposes (ἐπιβολαί) are inconsistent, your choices (ὁρμαί) are out of harmony with your nature, your conceptions (ὑπολήψεις) are hit-or-miss and false."[95] In-

91. Epictetus, *Discourses* 1.4.1; 1.19.2; 2.8.29; 2.14.8; 2.17.15-18; 3.9.22, 104; 3.23.9, 12; 4.1.1, 4; 4.10.4-7. Cf. *Stoicorum Veterum Fragmenta* 3.88.42-44.

92. Epictetus, *Discourse* 1.21.2. Cf. *Stoicorum Veterum Fragmenta* 3.6.30.

93. Epictetus, *Discourses* 3.22.61; 3.26.14; 4.4.35; 4.5.27; 4.4.6; *Encheiridion* 1.1-3; 2.1-2.

94. "Inflamed desire" designates the sudden transformation of the normal appetite for necessary things and their natural use into πάθος: *Stoicorum Veterum Fragmenta* 3.124.38–125.1: τῆς φλεγμονῆς τῶν παθῶν; Galen, *On the Doctrines of Hippocrates and Plato* 4.7.27-28: παθετικὴ φλεγμονή; Plutarch, *Fragment* 137: φλεγμονὴ ἐπιθυμίας; Philo, *On the Posterity of Cain and His Exile* 71: φλεγούσης τῆς ἐπιθυμίας; *On the Giants* 34-35: "For there are some things which we must *admit,* as, for instance, the actual necessities of life, the use of which (χρώμενοι) will enable us to live in health and free from sickness. But we must reject with scorn the superfluities which kindle the lusts (ἐξαπτόμεναι αἱ ἐπιθυμίαι) that with a single flame burst consume (καταφλέγουσι) every good thing. Let not our appetites (αἱ ὀρέξεις), then, be whetted and incited towards anything dear to the flesh." See also Clement of Alexandria, *Paedagogus* 2.4.42.1; *Quis dives salvetur* 15. See Inwood, p. 152.

95. Epictetus, *Discourse* 2.14.21. Plutarch (*On Moral Virtue* 450E-F) also knows the inflamed ὄρεξις; his Platonism, however, leads him to conceptualize the root problem as the ill effects of embodied existence rather than the Stoic emphasis on erroneous choice: "For, in accordance with Nature, it is proper that reason, which is divine, should lead and rule the irrational, which derives its origin directly from the body to which Nature has designed that it should bear a resemblance and share in the body's passions and be contami-

flammation in the ὄρεξις is desire for an object which does not bring satiation. Again Paul follows the philosophic critique of Eros by highlighting the problem of passion.

Our exploration of the psychology and critique of erotic desire behind Paul's argument moves to its final term in 1:27: πλάνη (error). Here again Paul makes use of a commonplace in literary treatments of ἔρως. The Latin equivalent of πλάνη, *error,* was synonymous with *furor* and *insania,* and for those writers who distinguished between sex with passion and sex without, *error* designated the former.[96] A similar idea is found in Testament of Reuben where the spirit of error marks the transition from sex for the sake of begetting children to sex for pleasure.[97] The source for this image of wandering from the path is most likely the philosophic notion of losing one's way on the road of life.[98] As Seneca testifies, *error* is introduced when natural desire is exceeded and passion enters into the way objects are possessed.[99]

This examination of the philosophic critique of Eros which stands behind Romans 1:24-27 has helped us to confirm the earlier conclusion that it is not Paul's interest to condemn homosexuality but to highlight sexual passion (ἐπιθυμία, πάθος), which is uniform with respect to the gender of the desired object. Paul tells the story of humans who have been overwhelmed by passion. The capacity (ὄρεξις) for acquiring what they believe to be good has been inflamed, and so they are in a constant state of frustration, unable to be sated. Their error (πλάνη) was to exchange normal use for erotic love.

---

nated by it, since it has entered into the body and become merged with it; that this is so is shown by our impulses (αἱ ὁρμαί), which arise and set in motion toward corporeal objects and become violent or relax in keeping with the changes of the body. For this reason young men are swift and impetuous and fiery in their appetites (τάς ὀρέξεις διάπυροι), and stung by madness, as it were, through the abundance of and heat of their blood; but in old men the source of desire (ἀρχὴ τοῦ ἐπιθυμήτικου), which is seated in the liver, is in the process of being extinguished (κατασβέννυται) and becoming small and weak. . . ." Further examples of inflamed ὄρεξις: Clement of Alexandria, *Quis dives salvetur* 25; Heliodorus, *Aethiopica* 1.26.

96. Preston, p. 10. For πλάνη/*error* in erotic contexts, see Plato, *Phaedo* 81A; Plutarch, *On the Eating of Flesh, II,* 997B; Ovid, *Amores* 1.2.35; Virgil, *Eclogues* 8.41. These and other texts are discussed by Lilja (*Roman Elegists' Attitude,* pp. 93, 108, and *Homosexuality,* p. 63 n. 55) and Brown (pp. 221-23, 239).

97. Testament of Reuben 2:1, 8; 3:2; 4:6.

98. *Tabula of Cebes* 5.2–6.6. See the helpful note in J. Fitzgerald and L. White, *The Tabula of Cebes,* Texts and Translations 24, Graeco-Roman Series 7 (Chico, Calif.: Scholars Press, 1983), p. 139 n. 16. See also Epictetus, *Discourse* 1.18.3-6; Stobaeus, *Anthology* 3.233.8-11; 3.235.4-5.

99. Seneca, *Epistle* 16.9.

D. Punishment and the Result of Erotic Passion

We will conclude our study of Romans 1:24-27 by attempting to make clear why Paul highlights passion. According to 1:18-32, passion and the dishonor it brings is the divine punishment for ingratitude and failure to glorify God. The topic of 1:18-32 is the anger of God, its provocation, and its consequences. As for the cause of God's anger, a relation between anger and injustice is established in 1:18: "For the anger of God is being revealed from heaven against all irreverence and injustice of humans who are suppressing the truth of God in injustice." Paul states that God's anger comes from injustice intentionally committed against his person.[100] Irreverence was widely recognized as the form injustice took in the relation of the human to the divine.[101]

In 1:21 we discover the nature of the wrong committed against God. It is the refusal to give God what is God's due: glory and gratitude.[102] This refusal is inexcusable since God's divinity and eternal power can be read off of the arrangement of the universe.[103] Receiving neither honor nor thanksgiving, God is wronged and dishonored.[104] Paul thus treats idolatry as a personal affront to God; it robs him of honor.[105] The consequence of God's anger is punishment of those who have treated him unjustly. This fits well with the definition of anger which sees in it a desire for punishment so that the wrongdoer suffers dishonor on par with the one wronged.[106] How does "handing over" generate dishonor among those who have wronged God?

The commonplace notion that erotic passion brings the lover into dishonor underlies Paul's argument in 1:24-27. In 1:24 we read that God handed idolaters "into impurity in order that their bodies might be dishonored among them (εἰς ἀκαθαρσίαν τοῦ ἀτιμάζεσθαι τὰ σώματα αὐτῶν ἐν αὐτοῖς)."

100. For the definition of anger, see Glibert-Thirry, 231.81-82; p. 290.

101. Glibert-Thirry, 267.37.

102. For gratitude and reverence as types of δικαιοσύνη, see Glibert-Thirry, 255.34-36; 257.43-52; pp. 313-14. For gratitude as the proper response to the divine, see Dio Chrysostom, *Discourse* 12.43.

103. Testament of Naphtali 3:1-5; Dio Chrysostom, *Discourse* 12.27-34, 39. Note especially *Discourse* 12.35 where divine "will and power (γνώμη καὶ δύναμις)" are "very clear (ἐναργής) and evident (πρόδηλος)," and the proper response is to "recognize and honour (τιμᾶν) the god and desire to live according to his ordinance." See also *Discourse* 12.70.

104. Cf. Rom. 2:23: τὸν θεὸν ἀτιμάζεις.

105. Philo (*On Drunkenness* 110) similarly regards idolatry as dishonoring God: "God's honor (θεοῦ τιμῆς) is set at naught by those who deify the mortal." Cf. Dio Chrysostom, *Discourse* 12.36: ὑπερφρονοῦσι τὰ θεῖα.

106. See n. 100 above.

Excessive passion (ἐν ταῖς ἐπιθυμίας τῶν καρδίων) is the means by which this handing over occurred.[107] In 1:26 Paul reiterates the connection between punishment, passion, and dishonor: "God handed them over into passions of dishonor (παρέδωκεν αὐτοὺς ὁ θεὸς εἰς πάθη ἀτιμίας)." Here again punishment consists of being handed over to passion — itself dishonorable to have.[108]

In 1:27 Paul speaks of "the punishment which was necessary from their error (τὴν ἀντιμισθίαν ἣν ἔδει τῆς πλάνης αὐτῶν)." The striking aspect of this formulation is the necessity which links punishment (ἀντιμισθία) to error (πλάνη). Punishment was a central metaphor for the ill effects on the lover of his own passionate love.[109] Punishment following the consummation of erotic desire was part of a larger configuration of ideas in which Eros was a destructive passion, taking its toll on the finances, mental equilibrium, and the honor of the lover.[110]

Finally, in 1:27 the term ἀσχημοσύνη (unseemly conduct) accentuates the theme that erotic passion brings dishonor in its wake.[111] Its antonym,

107. The notion of dishonor is obvious in the term ἀτιμάζεσθαι, but ἀκαθαρσία requires some clarification. For the notion of sexual offenses as "metaphorical moral pollutions" and the connection between degradation and defilement, see R. Parker, *Miasma: Pollution and Purification in Early Greek Religion* (Oxford: Clarendon, 1983), pp. 94-100, 146-53; Adams, pp. 198-99. Other examples are found in Epictetus, *Discourses* 2.8.14; 4.11.5; Dio Chrysostom, *Discourse* 7.134; Ps.-Lucian, *Affairs of the Heart* 22; and especially Plutarch, *Fragment* 47. For this development in Jewish sources, see van der Horst, pp. 258-60. See further Testament of Joseph 4:6; Testament of Benjamin 6:5; 8:2; Epistle of Aristeas 152.

108. For the theme of sexual passion bringing dishonor (ἀτιμία), see N. R. E. Fisher, *Hybris: A Study in the Values of Honour and Shame in Ancient Greece* (Warminster: Aris & Phillips, 1992), p. 14; Lilja, *Roman Elegists' Attitude*, pp. 89-96; van der Horst, pp. 158-59. See also Clement of Alexandria, *Paedagogus* 2.10.100.1; Ps.-Lucian, *Affairs of the Heart* 20: "a little pleasure at the cost of great disgrace (μεγάλην ἀδοξίαν)." Cf. *Affairs of the Heart* 24: "honourable names to dishonourable passions (πάθεσιν αἰσχροῖς)."

109. Brown, pp. 216-19, 227. In addition to the texts cited by Brown, see Philo, *On the Contemplative Life* 61; Clement of Alexandria, *Quis dives salvetur* 25.

110. See Brown, pp. 111-13, 248-51. See also Epictetus, *Discourse* 4.1.15-23; Plutarch, *Fragment* 136; Seneca, *Epistle* 116.5.

111. It is difficult to see this idea in modern translations. NRSV: "Men committed shameless acts with men." NIV: "Men committed indecent acts with other men." The problem here is thinking of ἀσχημοσύνη as an act, since the social dimension (present in a word containing the σχημ- root) is lost. Furthermore, a word ending with -συνη tends not to refer to an act but to a state of being. Thus, "producing dishonor" might better catch the sense. Phrases similar to Paul's do not accentuate the deed so much as the dishonor arising from the passion which propels the deed: Aristotle, *Nicomachean Ethics* 4.6.7: ἀσχημοσύνην φέρῃ; Athenaeus, *Deipnosophistae* 13.607B-C: τὴν πᾶσαν ἀσχημοσύνην ἐπιδείκνυνται; Dio

εὐσχημοσύνη (decorum), denoted the respectable appearance of the person who displayed control over the passions.[112] ἀσχημοσύνη, on the other hand, pointed to the public perception of failure to control passion.[113] Overindulgence in the pleasures which might otherwise be used with moderation produces ἀσχημοσύνη.[114] This is especially true of erotic pleasure.[115]

E. Loss of Self-Control and Hybris in 1 Corinthians 6:9

In the context of a vice list (1 Cor. 6:9-10) meant to amplify the notion of injustice, Paul calls upon the terms μαλακός (soft) and ἀρσενοκοίτης.[116] The meaning of each term has been hotly contested, but there seems to be some agreement on viewing the terms as the passive and active partners in male-with-male sexual activity.[117] Another way to understand these two terms is

---

Chrysostom, *Discourse* 7.110: ἀσχημοσύνην τε καὶ ἀνελευθερίαν ἐντίκτουσι. As for κατεργάζομαι, is it fanciful to think that Paul is punning on a common euphemism for sexual effort, "work (ἔργον)"? For ἔργον in erotic contexts, see Preston, pp. 15-16, 33-34; D. F. Kennedy, *The Arts of Love: Five Studies in the Discourse of Roman Love Elegy* (Cambridge: Cambridge University Press, 1993), pp. 59-60, 62. Achilles Tatius, *Leucippe and Clitophon* 2.37.5; Strabo, *Geographica* 10.4.21: κατεργάζονται τοὺς ἐρωμένους.

112. In Stoicism it is coordinated with the important concept of τὸ πρέπον (that which is fitting). See P. A. Brunt, "Aspects of the Social Thought of Dio Chrysostom and the Stoics," *Proceedings of the Cambridge Philological Society* 19 (1979): 19-20. For good examples of εὐσχημοσύνη as moderation for the sake of public perception, see Musonius Rufus, *Fragments* 8, 18B; Epictetus, *Discourses* 2.5.23; 4.9.9-12. Public perception is important in 1 Thess. 4:12.

113. The public aspect is stressed by Epictetus (*Discourse* 3.22.2, 8, 15, 52); see M. Billerbeck, *Epiktet: Vom Kynismus,* Philosophia Antiqua 34 (Leiden: Brill, 1978), p. 47.

114. Ps.-Crates, *Epistle* 10.2; Diogenes Laertius, *Lives of Eminent Philosophers* 1.103; 3.39.

115. Recognized by Paul; see Deming, pp. 206-7. For εὐσχημοσύνη as self-control in erotic contexts, see Ps.-Musonius, *Epistle* 1.4; Theano, *Epistle* 5.3 (Thesleff, 199.14). For ἀσχημοσύνη in erotic contexts, see Musonius Rufus, *Fragment* 12 (cf. Clement of Alexandria, *Paedagogus* 2.10.97.2); Epictetus, *Discourse* 4.9.5; Philo, *On the Decalogue* 168-69; Ps.-Phocylides, *Sentences* 67; Plutarch, *Amatorius* 751E; Ps.-Lucian, *Affairs of the Heart* 28.

116. Since translation of ἀρσενοκοίτης *is* its interpretation, I shall leave it untranslated for now.

117. R. Scroggs, *The New Testament and Homosexuality: Contextual Background for Contemporary Debate* (Philadelphia: Fortress, 1983), pp. 40-42, 62-65, 108. This interpretation is anticipated by Origen *(Fragmenta ex commentariis);* text is C. Jenkins, "Documents: The Commentary of Origen on I Corinthians," *Journal of Theological Studies* 9-10 (1908): 369.

possible, however, if we put them in the context of Greco-Roman ethical reflection on the problem of ἀκράτεια (lack of self-control) leading to ὕβρις (outrage).[118]

First, the issue of loss of self-control. Although μαλακός frequently designated the sexually passive, penetrated male (and did so in a highly derogatory way), we should not simply assume that this is the only way a first-century audience could have made sense of the term.[119] Recent investigations of gender markers in the Roman world have emphasized that "softness" includes much more than the passive role in male/male sexual activity.[120] Even men who are too interested in having sex with women, their wives included, were deemed soft, as also were adulterers.[121] So too were males who used males.[122] It is therefore a legitimate question whether Paul's first hearers would necessarily have thought of the passive object of desire when hearing the word μαλακός, especially in a list of *active* deeds of injustice like theft, adultery, and the like listed in verses 9-10. Furthermore, vice lists similar to Paul's which mention μαλακία do not condemn the male allowing himself to be sexually penetrated. Rather, they point more generally to the evils of excess or greed and lack of self-control.[123]

118. ὕβρις, as Fisher, p. 1, has amply documented, is more than an inner attitude; it "is essentially the serious assault on the honour of another, which is likely to cause shame." For ὕβρις mediated through the pleasures of the body, see Fisher, pp. 13-14, 28-33, 109-11.

119. For "soft" as a term of abuse which did its work by making a man (active/penetrating) appear as a woman (passive/penetrated), see M. Gleason, *Making Men: Sophists and Self-Presentation in Ancient Rome* (Princeton: Princeton University Press, 1995), pp. 58-81; Kennedy, pp. 31-34. For historical reconstruction of the men who chose to be penetrated by other men and forced to bear this term of abuse, see Richlin, pp. 523-73. Richlin helps us understand the scorn communicated when this term was applied to the passive sexual partner.

120. The accusation of softness must be understood in a framework broader than sex. See C. Edwards, *The Politics of Immorality in Ancient Rome* (Cambridge: Cambridge University Press, 1993), pp. 68-78; Dean-Jones, p. 53.

121. Edwards, pp. 65, 75, 81-85, 93. In addition to the texts she cites, see Plutarch, *On Moral Virtue* 447B; *Amatorius* 750B.

122. Diodorus Siculus, *Library of History* 2.23.1-4. See Gleason, p. 42.

123. Epictetus, *Discourse* 2.16.45: φιλαργυρία, μαλακία, ἀκρασία. For this and similarly constructed lists, see Preston, pp. 10-11. Paul's list typifies the male who cannot control his desires and who is, in Samuel Goldhill's description of Longus's portrayal of Gnathon, "the negation of the *sophron* citizen" (Goldhill, p. 48). Cf. Lysis, *Epistle to Hipparchus* 4-5 (Thesleff, 113.8-16). Some of the vices are reminiscent of parodies of the Greek symposium (e.g., Philo, *On the Cherubim* 91-93). Drunkenness especially needs to be understood as a metonymy of the dissolute life. See Testament of Judah 16:1; Brown, p. 263. For softness related to avarice and drunkenness, see Edwards, pp. 85 n. 79, 188-90.

The association of μαλακία with lack of self-control had a long history in ancient moral philosophy and widespread acceptance in the schools. Discussing the problem of self-restraint with respect to bodily pleasures (food and sex),[124] Aristotle observes that "men are self-restrained (ἐγκρατεῖς) and enduring (καρτερικοί), unrestrained (ἀκρατεῖς) and soft (μαλακοί), in regard to Pleasures and Pains."[125] He goes on to connect μαλακία with excess or luxury, establishing a pattern of thought for future moralists.[126] This broad sense of μαλακός is the correct background for interpreting 1 Corinthians 6:9. This term, in association with "greedy ones" and "carousers," communicates the notion of lack of self-control. The unjust (ἄδικοι) who run the law courts are anything but the ideal of the temperate citizen who is able to pass out just judgments. Paul thus deconstructs the moral legitimacy of the elite who run the law courts.

So far we have considered the way the vice list speaks about lack of self-control. There is another moral dimension to the list, that of injustice and hybris, and it is against this background that we should understand the other term which figures so prominently in debates concerning Paul's attitude toward homosexuality: ἀρσενοκοίτης. Translation of this term is a notorious problem not only because no occurrence before Paul has been discovered but also because such a lexical void tempts modern readers to import the category of sexual orientation into the text. Another approach, which asserts that Hellenistic Judaism "under marked Levitical inspiration" coined the term, is able to provide only speculation as evidence.[127] That Paul invented the term himself is of course possible but not likely, since it occurs in a vice list whose rhetorical force would have relied on the language of moral failure already known to the audience. We are thus left with an examination of the word's post-Pauline history. From this approach, we learn that ἀρσενοκοίτης means "one who has a boy as an ἐρόμενος."[128] We also see that ἀρσενοκοιτία is

124. For the notion of "necessary pleasure," see n. 48 above.

125. Aristotle, *Nicomachean Ethics* 7.4.2. Cf. 7.4.4. For the continuation of juxtaposing μαλακία to pleasure and pain, see Stobaeus, *Anthology* 3.145.6-12; Glibert-Thirry, pp. 265-67; Hippodamus, *Republic* 4 (Thesleff, 101.2-7); Theano, *Epistle* 1.1 (Thesleff, 196.7); Ps.-Crates, *Epistles* 19, 29; Ps.-Diogenes, *Epistles* 12, 29.2; 36.5.

126. Aristotle, *Nicomachean Ethics* 7.7.4-5. Cf. *Stoicorum Veterum Fragmenta* 1.65.34-39; Dio Chrysostom, *Discourse* 4.101-115; Seneca, *Epistle* 114; Musonius Rufus, *Fragments* 1, 11, 46; Lucian, *Dialogues of the Dead* 10.6.

127. D. Wright, "Homosexuals or Prostitutes? The Meaning of ΑΡΣΕΝΟΚΟΙΤΑΙ (1 Cor 6:9, 1 Tim. 1:10)," *VC* 38 (1984): 138.

128. Hippolytus, *Refutatio omnium haeresium* 5.26.22-23. Cf. Eusebius, *Preparatio evangelica* 6.10.25.

treated as an example of unjust, violent behavior of the person lacking self-control, and it has a hybristic intent.[129]

It seems likely that with this term Paul is picking up a thread of Greek and Jewish tradition which regarded pederasty as an illegitimate form of erotic love not only because of the lover's loss of self-control but also because of the younger male's disgrace in being penetrated.[130] Stock arguments against the practice of pederasty turned inevitably to the ὕβρις inflicted on the boy.[131] Vice lists like Paul's often included violent, hybristic love of boys in association with other unjust acts, such as adultery, theft, slander, and avarice.[132]

129. Wright ("Homosexuals or Prostitutes?") fails to recognize the emphasis on *hybris* in the texts that he cites to dispute Boswell's claim for the meaning of the term as active male prostitutes. Furthermore, he distorts the ancient texts by assuming they speak of the modern concept of homosexuality; for the problem of anachronism in Wright's work, see W. Petersen ("Can ΑΡΣΕΝΟΚΟΙΤΑΙ Be Translated by 'Homosexuals'?" *VC* 40 [1986]: 187-91). For the association of ἀρσενοκοίτης with ἀκράτεια and ἀδικία, see 1 Tim. 1:8-11; *Acta Joannis* 36.7; Theophilus of Antioch, *Ad Autolycum* 1.14; Eusebius, *Demonstratio evangelica* 1.6.67. For the explicit connection to ὕβρις, see Theophilus of Antioch, *Ad Autolycum* 1.2.25. Macarius (*Homiliae spirituales* 49.5.6) treats ἀρσενοκοιτία in Sodom as a bold and reckless act (τόλμημα) against the angels. For the τολμ- root in the condemnation of male sexual designs on males, see Plato, *Laws* 636C; Ps.-Demosthenes, *Eroticus* 20; Musonius Rufus, *Fragment* 12; Ps.-Lucian, *Affairs of the Heart* 16. See further Preston, p. 29; Goldhill, p. 54.

130. For loss of self-control, see Gerhard, pp. 152-53. Recent scholarship has emphasized the public disgrace of being penetrated. See Cohen, "Athenian Law of Hubris," pp. 171-88; E. Fantham, "*Stuprum:* Public Attitudes and Penalties for Sexual Offenses in Republican Rome," *Echos du Monde Classique* 35 (1991): 267-91; Richlin, pp. 561-66. For the *hybris* inflicted upon the penetrated male, see Sibylline Oracles 3.180-187; 4.33; Dionysius of Halicarnassus, *Roman Antiquities* 16.4.1-3; *Greek Anthology* 12.228. In the Greek ethical tradition, a distinction between "just love" and "love with ὕβρις" was often made. See Dover, *Greek Homosexuality,* pp. 45-46; Brown, p. 116.

131. Plutarch, *Amatorius* 768E; Dio Chrysostom, *Discourse* 7.149-152; Ps.-Lucian, *Affairs of the Heart* 27; Achilles Tatius, *Leucippe and Clitophon* 2.37.3; Clement of Alexandria, *Paedagogus* 2.10.89.2. See Konstan, pp. 119-20.

132. Testament of Levi 17:11; Ps.-Phocylides, *Sentences* 3-6; Philo, *Special Laws* 2.49-50; Ps.-Heraclitus, *Epistle* 7.3-8; Ps.-Hippocrates, *Epistle* 17.48; Clement of Alexandria, *Paedagogus* 3.12.89.1. See especially Epictetus, *Discourse* 2.22.26-29: "For it is no judgement of human sort which makes them bite (that is revile [λοιδορεῖσθαι]) one another, and take to the desert (that is, to the market-place) as wild beasts take to the mountains, and in courts of law act the part of brigands; nor is it a judgement of human sort which makes them profligates (ἀκρατεῖς) and adulterers (μοιχούς) and corrupters (φθορεῖς)." Cf. *Discourse* 3.3.12: κλέπτης . . . μοιχός . . . περὶ παιδάρια ἐσπούδακεν. See also Gleason, pp. 41-42.

F. Conclusion

We have seen that in Romans 1:24-27 Paul borrows two things from the philosophic discourse on erotic love:

1. "natural use" as a standard for legitimate sexual practice, and
2. a psychology of erotic love that makes intelligible the detrimental effects of passion.

An important consequence follows from this insight into the overlap of Paul's argument with the erotic discourse of his contemporaries. Neither the standard nor the psychology operates with the modern notions of sexual orientation and sexual relation. Therefore, it is anachronistic and inappropriate to think that Paul condemns homosexuality as unnatural and praises heterosexuality as a reflection of the God-given order of things. Sexual activity between males is not portrayed as the violation of a male-female norm given with creation but as an example of passion into which God has handed over persons who have dishonored him. The immediate problem is passion, not the gender of the persons having sex. The argument of Romans 1:18-27 rests on the conception familiar to Paul's audience that passion itself is dishonorable. Similarly, in 1 Corinthians 6:9 Paul draws from the philosophic tradition's aversion to passion. In this instance he uses the concept of softness to portray persons who lack self-control. He then mentions the figure of the hybristic pederast known in antiquity as one who through loss of self-control demeans others. The moral issue is not sexual orientation but the connection between passion and injustice.

CHAPTER 8

The Social Context and Implications of Homoerotic References in Romans 1:24-27

ROBERT JEWETT

The denunciation of homoerotic relations in Romans 1:24-27 stands at the center of the current debate over sexual ethics. This passage is so troubling to some branches of current thought that extraordinary efforts have been made to reinterpret Paul's words. This paper attempts to clarify the translation and significance of the passage within the context of the Roman letter. In the light of those conclusions, I then wish to turn attention to several resultant issues. Why did Paul apparently feel that his denunciation would be so readily accepted by the audience of Christians in Rome? What was the social context of this audience, and of their attitude toward homoerotic relations? If further light could be shed on these matters, a new resource might be at hand to think through the difficult ethical and theological questions before us.

A brief word of introduction may be in order concerning my approach to Romans, developed in the context of currently writing a commentary. In the light of recent research into the rhetoric and social setting of the letter, I believe it is directed to house and tenement churches that are situated mainly in the slum districts of the city. These groups were marked by separate and competitive development. Paul is attempting in this letter to find common ground between these splintered congregations so that they might be willing and able to participate in the Spanish mission project. The letter is organized with an exordium/introduction (1:1-15), a proposition/thesis statement (1:16-17), four proofs (1:18–4:25; 5:1–8:39; 9:1–11:36; 12:1–15:13), followed by an extensive peroration (15:14–16:23). The purpose of the first proof, in which the same-sex references appear, is to confirm the thesis of 1:16-17, showing that while all persons and groups have sinned and fallen short of the glory God intended for the human race, they are all granted grace through Christ's ministry to the shamed and his atoning death in their behalf. In the second pericope of this first proof, Paul is showing that the distortion of all human relations is a current indication and rationale for divine wrath. He is redefining sin as a distortion of the systems of gaining honor in Greco-Roman society, showing that in the wake of the tendency to seek honor for oneself and one's group, one ceases to worship the Creator and falls into twisted relationships. The purpose of this section is theological, not ethical. Although Paul is working with ethical commonplaces that he feels sure will be accepted by his audience, it is not until the fourth proof that he begins to set forth a systematic ethic.

My translation of Romans 1:24-27 is as follows:

> 24 Therefore with the desires of their hearts God delivered them to impurity [consisting] of their bodies being dishonored through themselves,
> 25 the very ones who exchanged the truth about God for the lie, and venerated and worshiped the creature rather than the creator, who is blessed for infinite ages! Amen.
> 26 For this reason God delivered them to dishonorable passions, for their females exchanged the natural function for the unnatural,
> 27 and likewise also the males, in abandoning the natural function with females, were inflamed with their lust for one another, males committing unseemly acts with males, and receiving back within themselves the recompense which their deception was necessitating.

Verse 24 insists that God is directly[1] involved in a process of moral retribution, whereby the distorting and darkening of the heart (Rom. 1:21) results in God confining the heart within the twisted circle of its desires (1:24). Those who choose a dishonest heart are required to live out the life imposed by its twisted desires. The choice of the plural form of "desires" makes clear that Paul does not share the Stoic assessment that desire is in and of itself a root cause of the human predicament as an expression of the lower nature.[2] Paul has in mind the biblical understanding of "the devices and desires of the

1. C. H. Dodd discounts the subject of this active verb when he argues in *The Epistle of Paul to the Romans,* Moffat New Testament Commentary, rev. ed. (London: Collins, 1959), p. 29, that evil in this passage "is presented as a natural process of cause and effect, and not as the direct act of God. . . . The act of God is no more than an abstention from interference with their free choice and its consequences."

2. See Friedrich Büchsel, "θυμός κτλ," *TDNT* 3 (1965), pp. 168f.

heart," the complex and devious crosscurrents of human motivation that involve the entire person, not just one's bodily nature. The ultimate goal of the scheming heart encompasses the entire self, according to the earlier portion of this pericope, aiming to suppress and distort the truth about the relative status of God and humans. When humans live within the twisted prison of their desires, their inevitable direction according to this passage is "toward impurity." This word is used in the LXX to depict that which is ritually impure and thus fundamentally separated from the holy,[3] but it comes to be used in Hellenistic Judaism and the New Testament in a moral sense to denote behavior "which excludes man from fellowship with God."[4] Paul uses this term both in a moral[5] and a cultic sense, with regard to food not being impure,[6] revealing that instruction about purity/impurity constituted a fundamental part of instruction of converts (Rom. 6:19; 2 Cor. 12:21; Gal. 5:19; 1 Thess. 2:3 and 4:7). As we have come to learn from modern anthropologists, pollution is a state or action that is out of place, so inappropriate that it causes systems to become dysfunctional.[7] Although the ritual aspects of impurity were largely abandoned in the New Testament, the deep sense of revulsion about polluting behavior remains.

The clause defining "uncleanness" is connected with a genitive that has been interpreted in a variety of ways. If it is understood as a genitive of purpose in a final or consecutive sense "so that they might be dishonored,"[8] the idea would be that the ultimate goal of divine deliverance is to a state of bodily perversion. The more likely option is to understand the genitive of the articular infinitive as epexegetic, "consisting in becoming dishonored," because as Meyer

3. See Friedrich Hauck, "ἀκάθαρτος, ἀκαθαρσία," *TDNT* 3 (1965), p. 427; cf. also Helmer Ringgren, "טָהַד," *ThWAT* 3 (1978), pp. 306-15.

4. Hauck, p. 428.

5. Hauck, p. 428.

6. See Wilfried Paschen, *Rein und Unrein: Untersuchung zur biblischen Wortgeschichte,* SANT 24 (Munich: Kösel, 1970), pp. 170-72.

7. See the pioneering work of Mary Douglas, *Purity and Danger: An Analysis of Concepts of Pollution and Taboo* (London: Routledge & Kegan Paul, 1966), p. 35, which defines "dirt" "as matter out of place. . . . dirt is the byproduct of a systematic ordering and classification of matter insofar as ordering involves rejecting inappropriate elements." P. 30: ". . . if uncleanness is matter out of place, we must approach it through order. Uncleanness or dirt is that which must not be included if a pattern is to be maintained. To recognize this is the first step towards insight into pollution."

8. Theodor Zahn, *Der Brief des Paulus an die Römer,* Kommentar zum Neuen Testament 6, 3rd ed. (Leipzig: Deichert, 1925), p. 98; C. E. B. Cranfield, *The Epistle to the Romans,* International Critical Commentary, 2 vols. (Edinburgh, 1975, 1979), p. 122, prefers the "consecutive" to the "final" sense, as does H. Schlier, *Der Römerbrief,* Herders Theologischer Kommentar zum Neuen Testament (Freiburg, 1977), p. 60.

shrewdly observes, the term "dishonoring" "already constitutes the impurity itself, and does not merely attend it as a result."[9] The verb is clearly a passive, since the middle form has not been found in Greek literature,[10] probably reflecting the social dimension of honor. In reference to "their bodies," such dishonor could be achieved through inappropriate sexual intercourse,[11] but the body is also involved in most of the other forms of antisocial behavior listed in this pericope (1:29-30). And although such dishonor was alleged to be particularly characteristic of polytheism, seen from the perspective of Judaism,[12] Paul does not limit the range of his argument to those parameters here.[13]

Verse 25 reinforces and elaborates the theme of an aggressive campaign against God as stated in 1:23, with sin as the suppression of the truth, which is the leitmotif from 1:18 forward. The bodily dishonor for which persons are directly responsible, according to the final phrase of verse 24, is here connected with a reversal of the proper relationship between the creation and the Creator. It is unfortunate that the English term standing closest to the verb Paul employs at this point is the neutral-sounding "they exchanged," because the intensification of the word "change" used in 1:23 implies something like "travestied," implying an even more "odious" form of sin.[14] The aorist tense

9. Heinrich August Wilhelm Meyer, *Critical and Exegetical Handbook to the Epistle to the Romans* (New York: Funk & Wagnalls, 1884), p. 88. See also C. K. Barrett, *The Epistle to the Romans,* Black's New Testament Commentaries (London, 1957), p. 38.

10. Although Frédric Godet, *Commentary on St. Paul's Epistle to the Romans,* trans. A. Cusin, ed. T. W. Chambers (New York: Funk & Wagnalls, 1883), pp. 107f., recognizes this grammatical fact, he insists on the middle meaning with an active sense, "to dishonor their bodies in themselves," to convey the sense that self-imposed dishonor is "inherent in their very personality." This appears to impose modern conceptions of the self and honor onto the ancient text.

11. Most commentaries (e.g., Ulrich Wilckens, *Der Brief an die Römer,* EKK 6 [Zürich: Benziger; Neukirchen-Vluyn: Neukirchener Verlag, 1978-82], 1:108-9; J. D. G. Dunn, *Romans 1–8,* Word Biblical Commentary 38a [Dallas: Word, 1988], p. 62) assume the primary reference is sexual, since Paul takes up the sexual perversions first, and since there are Judaic parallels to connecting idolatry with sexual irregularities. See Sibylline Oracles 3:8-44 and Testament of Joseph 4:5f. and Wis. 14:24-27. Note, however, that the Wisdom reference includes other forms of antisocial behavior and criminality along with sexual promiscuity, just as Paul does later in this chapter.

12. O. Michel, *Der Brief an die Römer,* Meyer Kommentar, 4th ed. (Göttingen, 1966), p. 104.

13. Rolf Dabelstein, *Die Beurteilung der "Heiden" bei Paulus,* BET 14 (Bern and Frankfurt: Lang, 1981), p. 83, cites 3 Esdras 8:66 as evidence that Jews as well as Gentiles receive the accusation of impurity.

14. Godet, p. 108; also Meyer, p. 89; *LSJ,* p. 1113, lists "alter" and "substitute" as possible translations.

refers, as elsewhere in this pericope, to "the primal sin of rebellion against the Creator, which finds repeated and universal expression."[15]

The expression "truth of God"[16] picks up the theme of 1:18, making unequivocally clear that it is not truth in general or some limited truth that humans wish to suppress but the truth of God as the ultimate One who is disclosed by the creation. The choice of the term "the lie" as the antithesis to the truth of God emphasizes the intentionality of humans to distort and suppress the truth. As Conzelmann points out, "lying cannot be viewed merely as the opposite of truth,"[17] because it contains an element of deception which differentiates it from mere falsehood. And this is not simply "a lie" but "*the* lie,"[18] involving the fundamental ploy of humans to replace God with themselves, visible from the fall to the crucifixion of Christ. The prophets had referred to idolaters as speaking and trusting in "lies" about God (Hos. 7:13; Jer. 14:14; cf. Isa. 59:13),[19] but the singular use of "the lie" in Romans implies an antecedent act, from which all later lies about God derive, namely, the primordial desire of humans to "be like God," defining evil and good for themselves (Gen. 3:5). In the light of the gospel concerning the crucified Savior, Paul has radicalized the story of the fall by lifting up the element of willful distortion.

The description of the means by which humans express their commitment to "the lie" is drawn from Greco-Roman and Jewish religion. "To venerate" is used here for the first and only time in the New Testament, perhaps because the term was so intimately associated with polytheistic religion and the Roman civic cult.[20] The nominal form of this term was the exact equivalent of the Latin word "Augustus," used in the calendar, the coins, the state propaganda, and the cultic honors paid to the emperor Octavian and his successors.[21] Although commentators have not elaborated the political and ideo-

15. Ernst Käsemann, *Commentary on Romans* (Grand Rapids: Eerdmans, 1980), p. 47.

16. For a parallel to this expression in contrast to false worship, see Assumption of Moses 5:4.

17. Hans Conzelmann, "ψευδός κτλ," *TDNT* 9 (1974), p. 595.

18. Joseph Fitzmyer, *Romans: A New Translation with Introduction and Commentary* (New York: Doubleday, 1993), pp. 284f., refers to the "big lie . . . the deception that smothers the truth."

19. See Conzelmann, pp. 598f.

20. See BAGD, pp. 745f., and Werner Foerster, "σέβομαι κτλ," *TDNT* 7 (1971), pp. 173-75; the latter argues that the associated term σέβομαι (to worship, venerate) is used only for non-Christian worship. Fitzmyer, p. 285, cites an exception in Epistle of Aristeas 139, where Israel is spoken of as "venerating the only powerful God instead of all creation" (τὸν μόνον θεὸν καὶ δυνατὸν σεβόμενοι παρ' ὅλην τὴν πᾶσαν κτίσιν).

21. Foerster, pp. 174f. See Torben Christensen, *Christus oder Jupiter. Der Kampf um die geistigen Grundlagen des Römischen Reiches,* trans. D. Harbsmeier from Danish edition,

logical significance of this term, its use obliquely suggests the false character of the veneration of the emperor which was becoming so prominent a feature of Roman religion. The countercultural quality of Paul's argument, detected already earlier in the letter, expresses itself here in a subtle manner, because Paul's audience could scarcely have missed this allusion to the most prominent form of "venerating the creature" in Rome.

The second verb Paul employs, "to worship," is used broadly and positively in the LXX and the rest of the New Testament.[22] The same term is employed for his own activity in Romans 1:9. The selection of this term in coordination with "veneration" indicates that Paul does not wish to isolate Roman polytheism as the only prominent expression of false worship; the universal scope of his argument includes all forms of worship, which logically places Judaism on the same level as polytheism in Paul's argument.[23] Every religion infected by the universal urge to suppress the truth can be involved in worshiping "the creature rather than the creator."

The failure to worship God as creator violates the foundational belief in the Old Testament and in all later forms of Judaism, a belief shared by early Christianity. Paul had reiterated the basis for such a belief in 1:19-21. Now he provides the most memorable wordplay in the wide arena of discussion up to Paul's time, articulating the distinction between the creature and the Creator. The rhetorical eloquence rests on a profound emotional and theological foundation,[24] which evokes an ejaculation in the form of a traditional Jewish blessing.[25] Such blessings were used with meals and other family occasions as well as in religious services, and were taken over and developed in early Christianity. Paul "blesses"[26] God for "infinite ages," to use the wording of the

---

1970 (Göttingen: Vandenhoeck & Ruprecht, 1981), pp. 22-39; Bischoff discusses the calendric use of this term as an equivalent of the Latin *Augustus,* in "Sebastos," *PW,* 2, no. 2 (1923): 956f.

22. See H. Strathmann, "λατρεύω, λατρεία," *TDNT* 4 (1967), pp. 59-63.

23. For a less sweeping assessment, see Dunn, p. 63.

24. See Adolf Schlatter, *Romans: The Righteousness of God,* trans. S. S. Schatzmann (Peabody: Hendrickson, 1995), p. 43.

25. See Wolfgang Schenk, *Der Segen im Neuen Testament. Eine begriffsanalytische Studie,* Theologische Arbeiten 25 (Berlin: Evangelische Verlagsanstalt, 1967), p. 97; Claus Westermann, *Blessing in the Bible and the Life of the Church* (Philadelphia: Fortress, 1978), pp. 24-26, and Christopher Wright Mitchell, *The Meaning of BRK "To Bless" in the Old Testament* (Atlanta: Scholars Press, 1987).

26. To "bless" God in the Judaic sense implied here is to acknowledge God as the source of all blessings, according to Hermann W. Beyer, "εὐλογέω," *TDNT* 2 (1964), p. 756: "The One who possesses and dispenses all blessings is God the Lord. This is the sacred knowledge underlying all OT statements concerning blessing."

typical biblical formula.[27] A profound antithesis is expressed in this phrase, between the eternal Creator and the finite creatures who yearn for infinite status. As Michel says, "Paul praises the One Whom the pagans blaspheme."[28]

In a second refrain-like[29] statement of divine response to the great lie, verse 26 declares that "God delivered them . . . ," meaning that she confirmed and sustained the twisted bondage to a chaotic world.[30] The introductory phrase "for this reason" explains the deliverance to dishonest relationships as the fitting response to the deceptive assault of humankind on the status of God. The expression "to dishonorable passions" resonates with the wording of 1:24 except that "passion" is a more distinctive term in Greco-Roman ethics than "desires."[31] Paul had combined both expressions in an unusual expression found in 1 Thessalonians 4:5, "in passions of desires."[32] Paul's wording conveys the sense of an involuntary state that simply comes over a person.[33] Socrates, for instance, spoke of "the erotic passion" as a kind of "madness," a "being led away."[34] A tyrannical person, said Plato, is ruled by an even more tyrannical force within called "passion."[35] Aristotle defined passion as an emotional state marked by pleasure or pain.[36] The Stoics developed an entire philosophy on the premise of passion, teaching that the expectation of pleasure therefrom is irra-

27. Hermann Sasse, "αἰών, αἰώνιος," *TDNT* 1 (1964), p. 199, shows that the plural formula used here, εἰς τοὺς αἰῶνας, is typical for religious doxologies with roughly identical meaning with the singular formula except that the former "presupposes knowledge of a plurality of αἰῶνες, of ages and periods of time whose infinite series constitutes eternity." For an assessment of the semantic issues, see James Barr, *Biblical Words for Time,* SBT 33 (Naperville, Ill.: Allenson, 1962), pp. 119-21; for a theological appraisal, see Gerhard Delling, *Zeit und Endzeit. Zwei Vorlesungen zur Theologie des Neuen Testaments,* BibS(N) 58 (Neukirchen: Neukirchener, 1970), pp. 49-56, 98-101.

28. Michel, p. 105.

29. Marie-Joseph Lagrange, *Saint Paul. Epître aux Romains* (Paris: Gabalda, 1931; repr. 1950), p. 28.

30. Käsemann, p. 47.

31. See J. Hengelbrock, "Affect (πάθος, passio, Leidenschaft)," *HWP,* 1:89-91; BAGD, pp. 602f., shows the term is not used in the LXX with the connotation of passionate desire, whereas *LSJ,* pp. 1285f., lists a wide variety of classical and Hellenistic Greek usage, including the title of Zeno the Stoic's work, *περὶ παθῶν ("Concerning the Passions").*

32. See I. Howard Marshall, *1 and 2 Thessalonians* (Grand Rapids: Eerdmans, 1983), p. 110, who translates 4:5 as "*the passion of lust.* The former word expresses an overpowering feeling . . . and the latter word reinforces the thought of sinful desire."

33. *LSJ,* p. 1285: "that which happens to a person"; Wilhelm Michaelis, "πάθος," *TDNT* 5 (1967), p. 926: "The meaning 'mood,' 'feeling,' 'emotion' etc. is very common in both a good sense and a bad. . . ."

34. Plato, *Phaedrus* 265b.

35. Plato, *Republic* 575a-c.

36. Aristotle, *Nicomachean Ethics* 2.5.1-2.

tional, so that passion must be diagnosed as a sickness of soul to be rooted out.[37] Hellenistic Judaism shared this view, urging the taming of the passions.[38] To be without unreasonable passion was true wisdom for the Stoics, while the Peripatetics and Skeptics taught the ideal of "moderate passion."[39] The adjective "dishonorable"[40] and the context of 1:26b indicate that the plural term "passions" implies perverse, erotic passions for Paul,[41] not the broader philosophical sense of emotions in general.[42] To be confined within this realm of perverse passions would have had a horrific connotation for Paul and his audience, given this cultural background.

To substantiate the claim in 26a concerning dishonorable passions, Paul introduces with "for" the example of homoerotic intercourse. The example is a widely used means of proof in Greco-Roman rhetoric,[43] particularly suited for the demonstrative genre of a letter like Romans that concerns itself primarily with praise and blame of various types of behavior.[44] The most effective examples are drawn from everyday experience and derive their argumentative force from shared opinion or prejudice. In this instance, we have the most egregious instance Paul can find to demonstrate his thesis about human distortion, the arena of sexual perversity that created wide revulsion in the Jewish and early Christian communities of his time.[45] The depiction of a par-

37. Hengelbrock, p. 90, citing Chrysippus, in J. von Arnim, *Stoicorum Veterum Fragmenta* (Leipzig: Teubner, 1903), 1:121 and 3:443-55.

38. Michaelis, p. 927.

39. Hengelbrock, p. 91.

40. Cranfield, p. 125, defines ἀτιμίας as a "genitive of quality, the meaning of the phrase being 'passions which bring dishonour. . . .'" Ernst Kühl, *Der Brief des Paulus an die Römer* (Leipzig: Quell and Meyer, 1913), p. 57, suggests that dishonor in this context relates to the "perversion of the created order of the nature of humans, upon which their honor rests."

41. Michaelis, p. 928, acknowledges the plural form but translates in the singular, "erotic passion." He properly repudiates Schlatter's translation, "sufferings which are a disgrace," in *Römerbrief*, p. 68.

42. See M. Pohlenz, "Paulus und die Stoa," *ZNW* 42 (1949): 82.

43. For definition, see Aristotle, *Rhetorica* 1.2.13; Quintilian, 5.11.1; for general orientation, see Hildegard Kornhardt, *Exemplum. Eine bedeutungsgeschichtliche Studie* (Göttingen: Noske, 1936), and Heinrich Lausberg, *Handbuch der literarischen Rhetorik*, 2nd ed. (Munich: Hueber, 1973), par. 412-26.

44. Lausberg, par. 245.

45. Typical denunciations of pagan homosexuality may be found in Philo, *On Abraham* 135; *Special Laws* 1.50; 3.37-42; see also Jean-Claude Vilbert, "Aux origines d'une condamnation: L'homosexualité dans la Rome antique et l'église des premiers siècles," *Lumière et Vie* (Lyon) 29 (1980): 15-28, and Wolfgang Stegemann, "Paul and the Sexual Mentality of His World," *Biblical Theology Bulletin* 23 (1993): 161-66.

ticularly unpopular example for the sake of an effective argument leads him to highly prejudicial language, particularly to the modern ear. But it should be clear from the outset that his aim is not to prove the evils of perverse sexual behavior; that is simply assumed from the outset, both by Paul and in his view by his audience. The aim is to develop a thesis about the manifestation of divine wrath in the human experience of Paul's time. In contrast to traditional moralizing based on this passage, sexual perversion is in Paul's view "the result of God's wrath, not the reason for it."[46]

The same verb, "exchange," is used for homoerotic relations as had been used in verse 25 for religious perversion, suggesting a direct correspondence between the two.[47] In contrast to other discussions in the ancient world, however, intercourse between females[48] is mentioned first by Paul,[49] probably for rhetorical reasons. The silence about lesbianism in the Old Testament, the references to it in Greco-Roman literature,[50] and the conservative, chauvinistic sexual climate of the post-Augustan age suggest that this was a topic of vehement contempt for Paul and his audience.[51] Despite the appearance of lesbian scenes on the walls of Pompeii reported by

46. Käsemann, p. 47.

47. O. Kuss, *Der Römerbrief,* 3 pts. (Regensburg, 1957-58), 1:50: "The 'exchange' as punishment follows the 'exchange' as guilt." See also Richard B. Hays, "Relations Natural and Unnatural: A Response to John Boswell's Exegesis of Romans 1," *JRE* 14 (1986): 192: "The deliberate repetition of the verb *metêllaxan* forges a powerful rhetorical link between the rebellion against God and the 'shameless acts' (1:27, RSV) which are themselves both evidence and consequences of that rebellion."

48. Peter J. Tomson, *Paul and the Jewish Law: Halakha in the Letters of the Apostle to the Gentiles,* CRINT III.1 (Assen and Maastricht: Van Gorcum; Minneapolis: Fortress, 1990), p. 94, argues for unnatural intercourse between men and women, but this would make v. 26 a doublet of v. 27.

49. In "The Practices of Romans 1:26: Homosexual or Heterosexual?" *NovT* 37 (1995): 7, James E. Miller notes that in the few ancient references to male as well as female same-sex relations, including the important discussion in the Hellenistic Jewish *Pseudo-Phocylides* 190-92, "female homosexuality is never introduced first."

50. For general orientation, including the use of abusive epithets, see W. Kroll, "Kinaidos," *PW* 11. 1 (1921), pp. 459-62. See also K. J. Dover, *Greek Homosexuality,* 2nd ed. (Cambridge: Harvard University Press, 1989), pp. 171-73, and Mark D. Smith, "Ancient Bisexuality and the Interpretation of Romans 1:26-27," *JAAR* 64 (1996): 238-43.

51. In "Roman Attitudes toward Sex," Judith P. Hallett notes the tension between a puritanical view in older Roman thought and the permissive attitudes in the period from 220 B.C.E. to 150 C.E. Pp. 1265-78 in vol. 2 of M. Grant and R. Kitzinger, eds., *Civilization of the Ancient Mediterranean: Greece and Rome* (New York: Scribner, 1988). She observes that "homosexual liaisons of women never received as much attention as those of men. This disregard seems related to the Romans' much more negative assessment of female homosexual activity than of male homoeroticism . . ." (p. 1266).

Luciana Jacobelli,[52] Dover seems justified in referring to the "striking" element of male hostility with regard to female homoeroticism.[53] Bernadette J. Brooten has traced a broad pattern of such hostility in classical literature of the Greek and Roman periods, including magical papyri; astrological, medical texts; and guidebooks for interpreting erotic dreams.[54] She concludes that "the ancient sources nearly uniformly condemn sexual love between women," mainly because it involved women usurping the dominant place of men.[55]

Paul's description of lesbian behavior as exchanging "a natural use for an unnatural" employs philosophical language that originated with Plato[56] and gained particular prevalence among the Stoics.[57] They taught that proper use of objects is natural and that the failure to follow common sense and the inner law of one's being was unnatural. It is clear from various ancient references that "'natural' intercourse means penetration of a subordinate person by a dominant one," a female by a male.[58] One motif that Paul does not adopt from this philosophical tradition is "pleasure," referred to by a Hellenistic Jewish writer, Pseudo-Phocylides, as "Cyprian lawlessness."[59]

52. Roy Ward refers to her study, *Pitture erotische delle Terme Suburbane di Pompei*, Sopritendenza archaeologica di Pompei, Monographie 10 (Rome: Bretschneider, 1995).

53. Dover, p. 172; Eva Cantarella concludes in *Bisexuality in the Ancient World*, trans. C. Ó. Cuilleanáin (New Haven: Yale University Press, 1992), p. 166, that for Romans, "homosexuality was the worst form of female depravity." Miller also points out in "Practices of Romans 1:26," p. 6, that Pseudo-Lucian in *Amores* 28 "broaches the double standard of accepting male homosexuality but despising female homosexuality." Lucian satirizes this double standard, and the humor would not have been effective without the hostility of his male readers toward same-sex relations among women.

54. Bernadette J. Brooten, *Love between Women: Early Christian Responses to Female Homoeroticism* (Chicago: University of Chicago Press, 1996), pp. 31-186. Roman writers after Augustus satirize women who do not conform to the passive role expected of women while Greek writers in the same period "represent sexual love between women as masculine, unnatural, lawless, licentious, and monstrous" (p. 50).

55. Brooten, p. 359.

56. Roy Bowen Ward investigates this tradition, which has been largely overlooked by previous researchers, in "Unnatural or Unprocreative? The Tradition behind Romans 1:26-27," *HTR* 90 (1997): 263-84. See the authoritative discussions in John J. Winkler, *The Constraints of Desire: Essays in the Anthropology of Sex and Gender in Ancient Greece* (New York: Routledge, 1989), pp. 20-23, and in Brooten, pp. 41, 271-80.

57. See Helmut Koester, "φύσις κτλ," *TDNT* 9 (1974), pp. 262-65, 273.

58. Brooten, p. 241; see also Winkler, pp. 36-43.

59. The reference to "Cyprian lawlessness" implies behavior influenced by Aphrodite, whom tradition associated with Cyprus. On the importance of Pseudo-Phocylides, see Ward, p. 23. He points out the flaw in Furnish's comment that "a Hellenistic Jew like Philo could just as well have written it" (*The Moral Teaching of Paul* [Nashville: Abingdon,

Plato considered pleasure to be "natural" only when it resulted in legitimate childbearing.[60] There is no reference to parentage in Paul's discussion, either here or in other Pauline references to marriage, and there is a positive allusion to sexual attraction and pleasure between married partners in 1 Corinthians 7:4, 7.

In the light of various ancient parallels, it seems likely that Paul has in mind female homoeroticism in this verse, rather than women engaging in oral or anal intercourse with males[61] or heterosexual women committing homoerotic acts.[62] There is a strikingly egalitarian note in Paul's treating same-sex intercourse among females as an issue in its own right, holding women to the same level of accountability as men.[63] It is nevertheless clear that Paul's

---

1979], p. 77), showing that "erotic acts between spouses without a procreative intent were forbidden by Plato, Philo and Pseudo-Phocylides, but not by Paul" (p. 25).

60. See the discussion of *Phaedrus* 835c-e; 839a; 841d by Ward, pp. 4-10.

61. See Miller, "Practices of Romans 1:26," p. 10: "Thus the similarity in function described in Romans 1:26 refers to non-coital sexual activities which are engaged in by heterosexual women similar to the sexual activities of homosexual males. So females, described first, exchange natural function for unnatural, but an exchange of partners is not indicated."

62. See Klaus Wengst, "Paulus und die Homosexualität. Überlegungen zu Röm 1,26f," *ZEE* 31 (1987): 77-78; John J. McNeill, *The Church and the Homosexual* (Kansas City: Sheed Andrews & McMeel, 1976; Boston: Beacon Press, 1988, 3rd ed.), pp. 53-56; John Boswell, *Christianity, Social Tolerance, and Homosexuality: Gay People in Western Europe from the Beginning of the Christian Era to the Fourteenth Century* (Chicago: University of Chicago Press, 1980), pp. 109, 112-13; Else Kähler, "Exegese zweier neutestamentlicher Stellen (Römer 1,18-32; 1. Korinther 6,9-11)," in *Probleme der Homophilie in médizinischer, theologischer und juristische Sicht,* ed. T. Bovet (Berne: Haupt; Tübingen: Katzman, 1965), p. 31; A. M. J. M. Herman van de Spijker, *Die gleichgeschlechtliche Zuneigung. Homotropie: Homosexualität, Homoerotik, Homophilie — und die katholische Moraltheologie* (Freiburg and Olten: Walter, 1968), pp. 82-83; Arthur Frederick Ide, *Loving Women: A Study of Lesbianism to 500 CE*, Woman in History 3 (Arlington, Tex.: Liberal Arts, 1985), p. 65; Ide, *Zoar and Her Sisters: Homosexuality, the Bible, and Jesus Christ* (Oak Cliff, Tex.: Minuteman, 1991), pp. 189-92; Ide, *Battling with Beasts: Sex in the Life and Letters of St. Paul: The Issue of Homosexuality, Heterosexuality, and Bisexuality* (Garland, Tex.: Tangelwüld, 1991), p. 50. The refutation of this option by Brooten, p. 242, is compelling.

63. See Brooten, p. 246: "the active verb *(metellaxan)* with a feminine subject . . . is striking." While Ward affirms this egalitarian element in contrast to Stanley K. Stowers, he nevertheless suggests that 1:18-32 is placed in the mouth of the imaginary Jew of Rom. 2:1, 17, criticizing "the unnatural *pathos* of the Gentiles" with their "unprocreative acts, most obviously exemplified by same-sex acts by both women and men" (Ward, p. 27). This is most unlikely because the traditional Jew would not have argued as Paul does in this passage, dealing with female behavior as nonsubordinate to male behavior, and overlooking as he does the issue of procreation. The argument of Stowers also seems contrary to this

choice and description of the lesbian example reflect confidence that the audience, shaped by a similar philosophical and religious heritage, "will share his negative judgment."[64]

In view of the complex variations of sexual inclination discussed in ancient astrological and medical sources,[65] the popular application of the modern concept of individual sexual "orientation" based on alleged biological differences is anachronistic.[66] Such exegesis misreads Paul's argument as dealing with individual sins rather than the corporate distortion of the human race since the fall.[67] But this is not to claim that Paul's argument is unproblematic. In Paul's usage there is no awareness of the weaknesses in the Greco-Roman concept of nature: its cultural subjectivity and its threat to genuine human freedom in that one allegedly must conform to whatever "nature" as defined by that cultural group demands.[68] Paul is actually raising a cultural norm to the level of a "natural" and thus biological principle, which would probably have to be formulated differently today.[69] Finally, there is a residual element of chauvinism in the expression "their females,"[70] the only element in 1:26b that is not replicated in 1:27a.

There is no mistaking the direction of Paul's argument,[71] or its consis-

---

and other passages in the Pauline letters; in *A Rereading of Romans: Justice, Jews and Gentiles* (New Haven: Yale University Press, 1994), pp. 94-95, Stowers contends that Paul's argument in 1:26 was motivated by Paul's concern to retain "woman's status as inferior" by restricting sexual relations to the male dominance of penetrating females. This is implausible in view of the egalitarian sexual ethic of 1 Cor. 7:4.

64. Hays, p. 194.

65. See Brooten, pp. 242-43. See also William Schoedel, "Same Sex Eros: Paul and the Greco-Roman Tradition," chap. 2 above.

66. Boswell, p. 109; Furnish, p. 66; see the critique in Hays, p. 200.

67. See Hays, p. 200: "The charge is a corporate indictment of pagan society, not a narrative about the 'rake's progress' of particular individuals." See also the critique of Boswell in Fitzmyer, pp. 286-88.

68. For a brief discussion of these dilemmas, without dealing directly with the issue of cultural relativity, see Koester, p. 266.

69. See Margaret Davies, "New Testament Ethics and Ours: Homosexuality and Sexuality in Romans 1:26-27," *Biblical Interpretation* 3 (1995): 323-30.

70. The inclusion of αὐτῶν (their) is unexplained in the commentaries, but clearly implies the chauvinistic view that females stand under the responsibility and jurisdiction of males, a typical feature of Greco-Roman and Jewish sexual ethics. In *Love between Women*, p. 241, Brooten observes that the reference to "their females" "is a logical term in male-dominated societies, in which women belong to men and are seen in relation to them."

71. For a critique of Boswell's specious argument that there was "no general prejudice against gay people among early Christians" (p. 135), see Hays, pp. 202-4.

tency with all other known branches of ancient Judaism and early Christianity.[72] Convinced that heterosexuality was part of the divinely created order for humankind,[73] and that sexual identity is essential to humans as bodily creatures,[74] he presents deviations from traditionally Judaic role definitions as indicative of an arrogant assault on the Creator and as a sign of current and forthcoming wrath. The evidence in this verse is particularly damaging to the hypothesis by Robin Scroggs that the critique of homosexuality in this pericope aims solely to attack pederasty and thus has no bearing on homoerotic relationships between consenting adults.[75]

In verse 27 Paul turns to the example of male homoeroticism, the weaker case in his cultural setting because of its positive evaluation by some Greco-Roman writers[76] and its popularization in the Roman ruling class, in-

72. See Samuel H. Dresner, "Homosexuality and the Order of Creation," *Judaism* 40 (1991): 309-21.

73. See 1 Cor. 7 and 11; K. Holter, "A Note on the Old Testament Background of Rom 1,23-27," *Biblische Notizen* 69 (1993): 21-23.

74. See Robert Jewett, *Paul's Anthropological Terms: A Study of Their Use in Conflict Settings* (Leiden: Brill, 1971), pp. 268-71, 456; also Thomas Deidun, "Beyond Dualisms: Paul on Sex, Sarx and Soma," *Way* 28 (1988): 201-4.

75. Robin Scroggs, *The New Testament and Homosexuality: Contextual Background for Contemporary Debate* (Philadelphia: Fortress, 1983), p. 116; see particularly the critiques by Peter von der Osten-Sacken, "Paulinisches Evangelium und Homosexualität," *BThZ* 3 (1986): 34, and Smith, pp. 225-38, 43-44. The attempt by James E. Miller to answer these critiques is unconvincing: "Response: Pederasty and Romans 1:27: A Response to Mark Smith," *JAAR* 65 (1997): 861-66.

76. In "Greek Attitudes toward Sex," Jeffrey Henderson notes that "homosexual sentiment [was] pervasive in Greek culture" and that it played a key role in the transition from childhood to adulthood, both for men and women, and that it does "not interfere with heterosexual enjoyment or with a happy marriage"; see vol. 2 of *Civilization*, p. 1255. For similar assessments of Roman culture, see Vilbert, "Aux origines d'une condamnation"; Hallett, "Roman Attitudes toward Sex." Saara Lilja traces Roman celebrations of pederastic love in *The Roman Elegists' Attitude to Women*, Suomalaisen tiedeakatemian toimikuksia. Annales academiae scientiarum Fennicae, Ser. B, 135 (Helsinki: Suomalainen Tiedeakatemia, 1965; reprint, New York: Garland, 1978), pp. 217-25. Acknowledging that it is not always appropriate to use the modern term "homosexual" to describe Greco-Roman roles, Amy Richlin has shown that the social acceptance of males who penetrated other males was greatly in contrast to the prejudice against free adult males allowing themselves to be penetrated; such adult *cinaedi* (queers) were viewed as abnormal or diseased and could be prosecuted under Roman law. See "Not before Homosexuality: The Materiality of the *Cinaedus* and the Roman Law against Love between Men," *Journal of the History of Sexuality* 3 (1993): 523-73. Catherine Edwards discusses Roman hostility against the effeminacy of male citizens in *The Politics of Immorality in Ancient Rome* (Cambridge: Cambridge University Press, 1993), pp. 68-75.

cluding the emperor Nero.[77] This weakness is dealt with rhetorically by presenting homoerotic relations among males as similar to the more disreputable form among females: "and likewise also."[78] The language of "natural use" is consistent with the description of lesbianism in the preceding verse. The link between the two sentences clarifies that both male and female homoeroticism are seen as evidence of the same "dishonorable passions."[79] In the context of natural versus unnatural intercourse, the aorist participle "leaving, giving up" is the rough equivalent of the term "exchange" in 26b. It implies a departure from a divinely intended, originally heterosexual relationship between males and females. Except for the missing "their" in 27a, this first clause is a characteristic example of the effort in Paul's later letters to equalize the roles and responsibilities of males and females.[80]

The rest of verse 27 continues the rhetorical effort to evoke the despicable quality of male homoeroticism. "Inflamed with their appetite for one another" is rare and derogatory language for the New Testament,[81] implying an irrational bondage to an egoistic, empty, and unsatisfying expression of animalistic sexuality.[82] The next clause is equally derogatory, "males committing shameful acts with males," alluding to the language of Leviticus 18:22 and 20:13 that prohibits "same-sex relations between males of all ages, not only pederasty."[83] The term "shame" was used both for "shameless deed" and for

77. See Boswell, pp. 82, 130; Richlin, p. 532, describes Nero as "a no-holds-barred omnisexual Sadeian libertine."

78. See Zahn, p. 100, and Michel, p. 105; for ὁμοίως as a commonly used term to indicate similarity or commonality, see Johannes Schneider, "ὅμοιος κτλ," *TDNT* 5 (1967), pp. 186-88.

79. See Brooten, pp. 253-55, for a compelling argument concerning the "parallel" between male and female actions in 1:26-27.

80. See Jewett, "The Sexual Liberation of the Apostle Paul," *JAAR* Supplement (March, B) 47.1 (1979): 68-77; see also Scroggs, pp. 114f., who comments that the complementarity of the female and male examples indicates "that the false world is lived in equally by women as well as men. . . ."

81. Both ἐκκαίω (be inflamed) and ὄρεξις (sexual desire, lust) are *hapax legomena* in the New Testament; see BAGD, pp. 240, 580.

82. See Wilckens, 1:110. See the similar expressions in Wis. 14:2; 15:5; Sir. 18:30; 23:6, pointed out by Brooten, p. 255.

83. Brooten, p. 256; she builds her case on the work of Saul M. Olyan, "'And with a Male You Shall Not Lie the Lying Down of a Woman': On the Meaning and Significance of Leviticus 18:22 and 20:13," *Journal of the History of Sexuality* 5 (1994): 179-206, and Daniel Boyarin, "Are There Any Jews in 'The History of Sexuality'?" *Journal of the History of Sexuality* 5 (1995): 333-55. For a discussion of other Old Testament passages that condemn homoerotic relations between males, see Maurice Gilbert, "La Bible et l'homosexualité," *NRTh* 109 (1987): 80-84, and James B. De Young, "The Contributions of the Septuagint to

sexual organs,[84] whose privacy remained a matter of substantial taboo in first-century Judaism (e.g., Exod. 20:26; Lev. 18:6-18).[85] The term is clearly a euphemism for sexual intercourse of a shameful type.[86] For Jewish hearers reared in an atmosphere of sexual modesty and for Greco-Romans who had been taught moderation, honor, and dutifulness, Paul's language served to remove any vestige of decency, honor, or friendship from same-sex relations. Making no distinctions between pederasty and relationships between adult, consenting males,[87] or between active and passive partners as Roman culture was inclined to do,[88] Paul is acting consistently with his Jewish cultural tradition by construing the entire realm of same-sex relations as a proof of divine wrath.[89]

The final clause returns to the leitmotif of suppressing the truth which produces its twisted consequences, referring to an active "deception" about the created order.[90] Rather than the bland translation of "error,"[91] perhaps even the sexually related term "seduction" might be appropriate here.[92] Such suppression of the truth "necessitates" a retribution, whose divine origin is emphasized by the use of the term translated "it is necessary,"[93] a term used

---

Biblical Sanctions against Homosexuality," *Journal of the Evangelical Theological Society* 34 (1991): 157-77. Michael L. Satlow concludes that "the Hebrew Bible forbids anal intercourse between men . . . ," a stance echoed in later Jewish writings; see "'They Abused Him Like a Woman': Homoeroticism, Gender Blurring, and the Rabbis in Late Antiquity," *Journal of the History of Sexuality* 5 (1994): 6.

84. BAGD, p. 119.

85. S. Safrai, "Home and Family," in *The Jewish People in the First Century,* ed. S. Safrai and M. Stern (Philadelphia: Fortress, 1976), 2:762, reports that a married partner had to be divorced after appearing in public in torn clothing or participating in public baths, following the Greco-Roman custom, because of the violation of the privacy laws.

86. See Hans Lietzmann, *An die Römer,* 5th ed., HNT 8 (Tübingen: Mohr [Siebeck], 1971), p. 34.

87. For this distinction, see Scroggs, pp. 115-17.

88. See Richlin, pp. 532-40.

89. See particularly James B. De Young's discussion of the longer recensions of 2 (Slavonic) Enoch 10:4-5 and 34:1-3, Jub. 16:5-9, Epistle of Aristeas 151-52 in "A Critique of Prohomosexual Interpretations of the Old Testament Apocrypha and Pseudepigrapha," *Bibliotheca Sacra* 147 (1990): 446-52.

90. Herbert Braun, "πλανάω κτλ," *TDNT* 6 (1968), p. 243; the other uses of πλάγνη by Paul in 1 Thess. 2:3 and 2 Thess. 2:11 imply demonic deception rather than simple, human error.

91. Dunn, p. 65; Leon Morris, *The Epistle to the Romans,* Pillar New Testament Commentary (Grand Rapids: Eerdmans, 1988), p. 93.

92. See Zahn, p. 101.

93. BAGD, p. 172.

elsewhere by Paul and other biblical writings to denote divinely imposed exigency.[94] The term "recompense" is only found in Christian sources, reflecting the "reciprocal nature" of the punishment.[95] In this instance, it appears clear that the perverted relationships are themselves the punishment "received back"[96] in return for the perverted mind which is captured by its deception about God and the created order.[97] These indications of divine involvement in the wrath are consistent with the thrice-repeated "he delivered them."[98] The repetition of the pronouns "their" and "themselves" serves to underscore the human responsibility for this primal deception and its social consequences. The broad scope of this responsibility is eroded somewhat in most translations, since the antecedents for the two pronouns in 27d are usually construed as the males mentioned in 27a-c.[99] But if 1:26-27 is a single example, and if one accepts Paul's argument about the correspondence between male and female perversion noted above, there is no reason to limit the responsibility to the males. The final clause of 1:27 should be seen as a theological comment on same-sex relations, both among women and men. Taken as a whole, this effort in 1:26-27 to provide a theological approach to the issue of perceived homoeroticism is unique in the ancient world.[100]

While the Jewish background of the social context for Paul's argument has been frequently lifted up as decisive by previous researchers, little attention has been given to the correlation between homosexuality and slavery.[101] This is potentially very significant in grasping the impact of Paul's rhetoric, because slavery was so prominent a feature of the social background of most

94. See 1 Cor. 15:25, 53; 2 Cor. 5:10; 1 Thess. 4:1; and 2 Thess. 3:7, some of which are noted by Schlier, p. 62; for the shift from the Greek concept of fate to the biblical concept of the divine will, see Walter Grundmann, "δεῖ," *TDNT* 2 (1964), pp. 22f., and Erich Fascher, "Theologische Beobachtungen zu δεῖ," in *Neutestamentliche Studien für Rudolf Bultmann zu seinem siebzigsten Geburtstag am 20. August 1954, ZNW,* ed. Walter Eltester, Beiheft 21 (Berlin: Töpelmann, 1957), pp. 247f.

95. See BAGD, p. 75, and H. Preisker, "μισθός κτλ," *TDNT* 4 (1967), p. 702.

96. See Dunn, p. 65.

97. See Kühl, p. 58, who refutes the view of Zahn, p. 101, who thinks instead that the recompense is the "bodily deterioration" that comes upon those involved with sexual perversity.

98. Kühl, p. 58.

99. The issue of the antecedents is not explicitly discussed in any of the commentaries I have consulted.

100. Schlier, p. 62; Richard M. Price, "The Distinctiveness of Early Christian Sexual Ethics," *Heythrop Journal* 31 (1990): 261-73.

101. Jean-Claude Vilbert points out this correlation, without connecting it with Paul's letter to the Christians in Rome, in "Aux origines d'une condamnation," p. 19. As evidence he cites Plutarch, *Moralia, Roman Questions* 288A, and Plautus, *Curculo* 23.

of Paul's audience in Rome.[102] Werner Krenkel writes that "Intercourse between masters and their male slaves was normal and in accordance with the standards of a male-dominated society,"[103] citing Seneca the Elder: "Sexual servicing is a crime for the freeborn, a necessity for a slave, and a duty for the freeman."[104] Paul Veyne reports that a "much repeated way of teasing a slave is to remind him of what his master expects of him, i.e., to get down on all fours."[105] Krenkel notes that in fourth-century Athens the minimum fee for a male prostitute was higher than that for females, and that "to meet the demand for male prostitutes, beautiful boys were captured, imported . . . sold . . . and prostituted."[106] Krenkel describes the double standard in Greek culture, in that it was acceptable for one male to dominate another, but to be "'the beloved boy' after reaching adulthood, was frowned upon."[107] The Romans, in contrast, forbade the passive sexual role for free males and enforced laws against pederasty when it involved the sons of citizens.[108] In general, sexual freedom was granted to freeborn males in relation to all slaves, clients, and persons of lower standing, so that sexual relations were clearly an expression of domination.[109] Observing that there are no firsthand accounts of the feelings of those being exploited, Krenkel cites the elder Seneca's words describing prostitution as "unhappy and sterile submission."[110] I wonder if

102. See the introduction above, and especially the work of Peter Lampe, *From Paul to Valentinus: Christians at Rome in the First Two Centuries,* trans. J. L. Holland and M. Steinhauser (Minneapolis: Fortress, 1999), pp. 170-83.

103. Werner A. Krenkel, "Prostitution," in *Civilization,* p. 1296.

104. Seneca, *Controversiae* 4 preface 10; this view is similar to *Satyricon* 75.11.

105. Paul Veyne, "Homosexuality in Ancient Rome," in *Western Sexuality,* ed. P. Ariès and A. Béjin, trans. A. Forster (Oxford: Oxford University Press, 1985), p. 29, cited by Cantarella, p. 99. Winkler, p. 211, cites Artemidoros, *Dream Analysis* 78: "To have sex with one's own female slave or male slave is good, for slaves are the dreamer's possessions. . . . To be penetrated by one's house slave is not good. This signifies being despised or injured by the slave."

106. Krenkel, p. 1296; Macrobius, in *Saturnalia* 3.17.4, reports that in 161 B.C.E. "Most of the freeborn youths sold their modesty and freedom." David M. Halperin discusses the high price of young male prostitutes in *One Hundred Years of Homosexuality and Other Essays on Greek Love* (New York: Routledge, 1990), pp. 108-9. Cantarella, p. 102, notes that in Rome male prostitution became "a luxury item."

107. Krenkel, p. 1297.

108. Cantarella, pp. 97-186, 217-18; see also Hallett, pp. 1268, 1272-78.

109. Cantarella, p. 217, concludes that the Roman male was socialized to be "an aggressive dominator," so that under a bas-relief of an erect phallus one reads the inscription *hic habitat felicitas* ("here dwells happiness"). See also Halperin, p. 33.

110. Krenkel, p. 1297; Halperin, p. 96, observes that "Prostitution can be spoken of, especially in the case of males, as hiring oneself out 'for *hybris*' *(eph' hybrei)* — meaning,

Paul's rhetoric may not provide entree into the similarly unhappy experience of slaves and former slaves who had experienced and bitterly resented sexual exploitation, both for themselves and for their children, in a culture marked by aggressive bisexuality.[111] Their countercultural stance as members of the new community of faith entailed a repudiation of such relationships and, from all the evidence available to us, a welcome restriction of sexual relations to married, heterosexual partners. For those members of the Roman congregation still subject to sexual exploitation by slave owners or former slave owners who were now functioning as patrons, the moral condemnation of same-sex and extramarital relations of all kinds would confirm the damnation of their exploiters and thus raise the status of the exploited above that of mere victims.

The difficulty in applying Paul's argument to current circumstances derives partly from the vast disparity in the social situation of modern readers as compared with Paul's original audience. Paul and his audience were resisting an aggressively bisexual society whereas the current debate takes place in a predominantly heterosexual society. The patterns of abuse and exploitation are therefore very different, with discrimination in the current setting largely directed against those who dissent from a heterosexual norm. A text that functioned as liberating in a bisexual environment thus appears discriminatory in a heterosexual context. But it is not adequate simply to dismiss Paul's stance because he does not share the premises of sexual "orientation" that emerged in recent Western societies. He and his congregations were attempting to cope with a social situation that the liberating impulses in the United States in particular may inadvertently be re-creating. With the abandonment of normativity in sexual identity and behavior, the door is currently open for increasingly exploitative bisexual behavior, which by its essential nature will not restrict itself to a single partner. Although it will not be exercised in an environment in which two-thirds of the population consisted of slaves or former slaves, which greatly enhanced the possibility of exploitation, it could well be that the protection of the weak can still be best achieved by something like the standard accepted so broadly in early Christianity. While there was no possibility of enforcing this standard on the society as a whole, the heterosexual preference seems quite appropriate for the countercultural community of the early church, given the likely exploitation of many of its members in an

'for other people to treat as they please.' . . . It was understood, for example, that a man went to prostitutes partly in order to enjoy sexual pleasures that were thought degrading to the person who provided them. . . ."

111. See especially Cantarella, pp. 156-64.

aggressively bisexual society. When the social context and ethical implications of Paul's argument are understood, this text could provide significant guidance for thinking through the issues of sexual identity and formation in the modern world.

CHAPTER 9

The Logic of the Interpretation of Scripture and the Church's Debate over Sexual Ethics

KATHRYN GREENE-MCCREIGHT

In 1973, after several years of bitter dispute, the Board of Trustees of the American Psychiatric Association decided to remove homosexuality from the *Diagnostic and Statistical Manual of Psychiatric Disorders,* its official list of mental diseases. Infuriated by that action, dissident psychiatrists charged the leadership of their association with an unseemly capitulation to the threats and pressures of Gay Liberation groups, and forced the board to submit its decision to a referendum of the full APA membership. And so America's psychiatrists were called to vote upon the question of whether homosexuality ought to be considered a mental disease. The entire process, from the first confrontations organized by gay demonstrators at psychiatric conventions to the referendum demanded by orthodox psychiatrists, seemed to violate the most basic expectations about how questions of science should be resolved. Instead of being engaged in a sober consideration of data, psychiatrists were swept up in a political controversy. The American Psychiatric Association had fallen victim to the disorder of a tumultuous era, when disruptive conflicts threatened to politicize every aspect of American social life. A furious egalitarianism that challenged every instance of authority had compelled psychiatric experts to negotiate the pathological status of homosexuality with homosexuals themselves. The result was not a conclusion based on an approximation of the scientific truth as dictated by reason, but was instead an action demanded by the ideological temper of the times. . . . To assume that there is an answer to this question that is not ultimately political is to assume that it is possible to determine, with the appropriate scientific methodology, whether homosexuality is a disease given in nature. I do not accept that assumption, seeing in it a mistaken view of the problem. The status of homosexuality is a political question, representing a historically rooted, socially determined choice regarding the ends of human sexuality. It requires a political analysis.[1]

In some respects the church in the West, particularly in its American Protestant denominational instances, is in much the same situation as was the American Psychiatric Association (APA) in the early 1970s when it struggled with whether or not to remove homosexuality from its diagnostic list of mental disorders. Now we, in our turn, struggle over how to assess the theological status of homosexuality as opposed to its psychological status. Specifically, we are being called to reevaluate, in light of the conflicting evidence from the world of science and the reports of our homosexual brothers and sisters in Christ, the church's position on homoerotic activity.[2] The "historical roots" and "social determinants," of course, which guided the work of the APA will differ from those which govern the work of the church, and therefore the very term "political decision" will carry different connotations for us and shape our debate in a distinct way. I therefore offer for the purposes of this essay the following definition of the term "political": the dialogical-dialectical charac-

1. Ronald Bayer, *Homosexuality and American Psychiatry: The Politics of Diagnosis* (New York: Basic Books, 1981), pp. 3-5.

2. Our gay and lesbian friends and colleagues remind us that they understand homosexual desire to be their natural God-given "orientation." Gays and lesbians therefore often object to the heterosexual majority asking them to deny or control their desire for homoerotic pleasure, since they feel that desire to be something they do not choose and, so it is often said, would not choose in the best of all possible worlds. This understanding, however, tends to dull the distinction between desire and action, a distinction which is consistent with the tradition of Christian moral reflection. That is, regardless of the desires and activities being discussed, it has generally been assumed throughout the centuries of Christian moral theology that the human will plays a role in how we shape our response to our desires as we live in obedience to the Word of God. I will therefore assume in the course of this chapter the validity of the distinction between homoerotic desire and activity. This distinction will, among other things, help us to speak productively again about what we used to call "friendship." For the purposes of this chapter, the term "homosexual relationship" will be reserved for the general category of relationships between people of the same sex, whereas the term "homoerotic relationship" will refer to relationships between people of the same sex which seek out and/or result in genital gratification between the partners. Homoerotic relationships may be based on homosexual love, or may not be, and homosexual love need not result in homoerotic relationships. The gay and lesbian communities with which I am familiar will not be happy with such distinctions, needless to say, but it seems to me that the distinctions are consistent with those made in other areas of Christian moral theology.

ter of the attempt, via the power of theological rhetoric and argument within the constraints of Christian theological discourse and within the body of Christ, to persuade. In this sense alone can the debate be "political" in the church. We might do well therefore to understand the notion of *sensus fidelium* as the analogue within the body of Christ to the ideological struggle of the APA's decision. In the process of this attempt at mutual persuasion, we will at best come to some agreements: if not on the content of the issue at hand, at the very least on how different arguments can be mounted and defended within the logic of the types of Christian theological discourse represented by the participants here. Since the constraints of theological discourse will govern our mutual attempt at persuasion, one of the most important tasks will be to come to some understanding among ourselves regarding these constraints.

In attempting to frame an appropriately Christian response to the last quarter-century of research and political positioning on homosexuality, our respective denominations are struggling with a potentially communion-splitting issue.[3] This is, of course, no reason to avoid the task of framing such a response. The turmoil in our denominations will not subside by our ignoring the issue, nor will it disappear once such responses have been articulated. This is because, for both sides of the debate within the church, the integrity of the gospel itself is at stake.[4] It has come to the point where each "side" of the debate is drawing its line in the sand, arguing that those who disagree simply do not understand the heart of the gospel message. Yet we cannot resolve the problem by easy appeal to either science or experience, because the data from these arenas are contradictory and inconclusive. Nor can we make a simple appeal to isolated biblical texts, for the Bible is used to support the arguments of both sides of the debate. We try to discern in the midst of this cacophony the will of God, and find ourselves coming to very different conclusions. Some chalk this situation up to each side trying to shore up its own power base. Since we are all "fallen," this must be true to some extent. However, we would profit from exploring what is at work beyond mere power struggles: How is it that Christians committed to following their Lord and Savior could come to such absolutely opposed conclusions on this issue? I would suggest that what fundamentally divides us here is not our attitudes toward sexuality, embodied-

3. I shall assume here general agreement on the importance of unity, that broken communion is to be avoided at all possible costs short of full apostasy.

4. See, for example, the introductory essay by Choon-Leong Seow in *Homosexuality and Christian Community* (Louisville: Westminster/John Knox, 1996).

ness, difference, ethics, or even our most cherished understandings of the nature of the gospel, but more centrally and decisively our attitudes and postures toward Scripture. The argument we see raging in the church, fought passionately from each side, is really about hermeneutics, about the interpretation and use of Scripture.

Let me say for the record that I am among those who wish they could be convinced that Scripture and tradition could be read to support the revisionist position, which would argue for the theological and religious appropriateness of homoerotic relationships for Christians who feel drawn to them. It seems clear to me, however, that the Bible rejects homoerotic activity whenever the topic is dealt with, which is indeed quite infrequently, and that Scripture read holistically upholds the norm of fidelity in marriage between one man and one woman, and of chastity in singleness. This seems so obvious to me that, since space is limited here, I will leave to the biblical scholars to debate the issues of translation of *arsenokoitai* and what forms of homosexuality Paul would have been talking about in Romans 1, etc.[5] While I have not yet been convinced by the revisionist position, I keep listening in hopes that someone will come up with something new.[6]

This is the aspect of our present debate in the church which mirrors

5. I will say, however, that for me the decisive biblical texts when it comes to sexuality are Gen. 1–3 and Eph. 5. This is not to discount Romans, Leviticus, etc., etc., but even if I retranslate Rom. 1 and bracket the purity laws, I still cannot get past the compelling vision of the creation of humankind male and female as a unit in the image of God, and the morphological fit between this and the "mystery" of the new creation in which the church is portrayed as Christ's bride.

6. There was much discussion among the authors of the essays collected here over how to describe the different positions and opinions represented. I objected to Mark Toulouse's typology of opinions adapted from James Nelson because its descriptive capacity seemed very shallow. Nancy Duff objected to the dichotomy of "traditionalist" and "revisionist" insofar as she embraces a position which I would attribute to the revisionist hermeneutic, whereas she sees herself as a "traditionalist" and in no way understands herself to be "revising" the gospel. I recognize the weakness of the terms "traditionalist" and "revisionist," but nevertheless find them useful to indicate the hermeneutical substructure which grounds the opinions. That is, to say someone is a revisionist is not necessarily to say he or she is "revising the gospel," but that the interpretive assumptions and moves of that person are revised from that indicated in the wide corpus of the tradition. "Traditionalists" may indeed have a range of different opinions as to how the matters at hand will be adjudicated, as also will "revisionists," but each group will nevertheless share some very basic assumptions about how Scripture is to be read normatively. In other words, my use of the terms "traditionalist" and "revisionist" points not so much to the outcomes of interpretation or to "opinions" as per Toulouse's typology, but to the logic of interpretation which undergirds these outcomes and opinions.

that in the APA in the early seventies, and yet simultaneously the one in which it must differ. Like in the APA debate, there is room for each side to attempt to persuade the other. Unlike the APA, however, we in the body of Christ are held accountable to a different authority, and therefore different rules for discussion and behavior among ourselves will obtain. We must speak to each other, even to those whose view contradicts our own, as brothers and sisters in Christ. We have a deeper unity at stake than merely membership in a professional society with its own unique bases for authoritative decision making. For the sake of the unity of the body of Christ, therefore, it will be even more important than in the APA that crowding out or shouting down the opposition be avoided at all costs. This must be emphasized. If we cannot manage to display the fruits of the Spirit, if we cannot manage to love each other despite our differences of conviction, we will seriously compromise our witness to Christ's redeeming love for the world.

When a new convention or interpretation is offered within the community of Christian theological discourse which contradicts an interpretation or set of interpretations traditionally held, its warrants need to be presented in order for the proponents to argue for its validity. Furthermore, its warrants must be coherent within the structure of Christian theological discourse.[7] That is, we cannot just unilaterally demand change for the sake of change, or even change for the sake of a noble goal, without coherent reasons, or without reasons that cohere with the way we give reasons for anything else. On this basis, I would reject the assertion that the burden of proof (regarding the failing of homoerotic activity to attain covenant righteousness) rests on the church, even while I affirm the clear obligation of the church to repent for any and all participation in hostility and cruelty toward homosexuals throughout the ages.[8] My point here is that the "burden of proof" always rests on those who propose something novel. In order for traditional readers to be convinced of the righteousness before God of homoerotic relationships, they

7. "Anyone wishing to introduce a new convention owes us first an account of how it squares with such existing conventions, and secondly, what motivates the introduction of the convention." John Searle, *Speech Acts: An Essay in the Philosophy of Language* (Cambridge: Cambridge University Press, 1969), p. 76.

8. See, e.g., Dale Martin, "*Arsenokoites* and *Malakos:* Meanings and Consequences," in *Biblical Ethics and Homosexuality: Listening to Scripture,* ed. Robert L. Brawley (Louisville: Westminster/John Knox, 1996), p. 131: "The burden of proof in the last twenty years has shifted. There are too many of us who are not sick, or inverted, or perverted, or even 'effeminate,' but who just have a knack for falling in love with people of our own sex. When we have been damaged, it has not been due to our homosexuality but to your and our denial of it. The burden of proof now is not on us, to show that we are not sick, but rather on those who insist that we would be better off going back into the closet."

would need to be convinced on "traditionalist" grounds.[9] This will mean that if we are to offer a revisionist interpretation of Scripture, either the revisionist interpretation must follow the same "rules" as the traditional interpretation or the revisionist side must convincingly show how and why the rules must be changed. Otherwise, both sides will continue to talk past each other.

If indeed reading Scripture and doing Christian theology and ethics is like a language game, as those influenced by Wittgenstein will say, we need to acknowledge the rules by which we "play." To illustrate, when we play chess, we know that the king may move in any direction but only one space at a time, that pawns may move only straight ahead unless capturing an opponent's piece, that knights move in an L-shaped pattern, etc. One move may be more strategic than another, to be sure, but the rules of the game apply no matter the myriad constellations of possible moves and countermoves. If one of the players refuses to follow the fundamental rules, however, the game ends abruptly because all coherence which is the basis for the give-and-take of play disappears. So with the logic of interpreting Scripture. Since it is almost universally true that both "sides" of the debate agree on the fundamental importance of Scripture, maybe we could begin there and push further to see if we can agree also on the constellations of moves and countermoves which one can make with Scripture in this debate.

Before we can do that, we must first set out some of the characteristics of traditional biblical hermeneutics. Probably even more important than any "methodology" for traditional biblical hermeneutics are the postures and attitudes with which the interpreter approaches the text. One of the "rules" of this game, then, is that one approaches Scripture expecting to be taught.[10] Therefore, one assumes that the writers of Scripture were at least as intelligent as the present-day readers and that God works through the text to address us. Even if the biblical authors expressed themselves differently and viewed the world differently from the present-day reader, traditional interpreters assume that the biblical authors correctly perceived and depicted God's relationship

9. This is why most "revisionists" tend to base their arguments on biblical texts and concepts. In spite of this, the traditionalists tend to accuse the revisionists of not "starting with the Bible." This accusation is completely unhelpful. First, the act of interpretation is epistemologically too complicated to find the Archimedean point where one "starts." Second, it is not a matter of simply "starting" with a text, but how the text is read. I hope to shed more light than heat here by exploring the constellation of fundamental beliefs, postures, and attitudes which the traditional side in particular brings to the act of biblical interpretation.

10. Almost all of these postures and attitudes are mentioned in book 4 of Augustine's famous treatise *On Christian Doctrine.*

to the world: the world hangs on God's creating breath and will return to chaos without it. Therefore, one approaches the witness to that God with the same reverence and humility with which one would approach the Holy One. One approaches the text waiting to be transformed, to be built up in the love of God and neighbor and in trusting devotion to God.

In addition to these basic assumptions, traditional hermeneutics sought to "do" specific work with the biblical text. Again, it is not so much methodology which preoccupies the attention of the traditional interpreter as it is a certain degree of "function." Any interpretation offered had to fit certain functional criteria, as is hinted above: it was deemed valid if it built up love of God and neighbor, and if it at the least did not contradict the faith of the church. Basing a theological or ethical argument successfully on Scripture almost universally until the Enlightenment meant therefore the convincing demonstration of the argument's resting on the publicly accessible verbal sense of a passage or passages interpreted according to the rules of faith and charity, which resulted in what we might call the "plain sense" of Scripture.[11] The rule of faith disallowed any interpretation that contradicted the basic tenets of the *regula fidei,* the precreedal "creed," or the overarching Christian canonical plot with its beginning, climax, and denouement. The rule of love disallowed any interpretation that was nonconducive to love of God and love of neighbor, and this as defined within that web of belief indicated by the *regula fidei.* Indeed, this kind of reading is what the Reformers meant with their cry for *sola Scriptura:* neither random proof texting nor the physical book of Scripture itself, but rather the practice of reading parts of Scripture

11. The term "plain sense" has received attention in recent times as referring to a discrete area of theological discussion which is also investigated under the rubric of *sensus literalis* in Christian interpretation and *peshat* in Jewish interpretation. Recent discussion of "plain sense" readings of Scripture tends to include consideration of communal norms and decisions, such as the fact of canonicity, which tended not to be accounted for in former discussions of *sensus literalis.* See Kathryn E. Tanner, "Theology and the Plain Sense," in *Scriptural Authority and Narrative Interpretation,* ed. Garrett Green (Philadelphia: Fortress, 1987), pp. 59-78; Raphael Loewe, "The Plain Meaning of Scripture in Early Jewish Exegesis," in *Papers of the Institute of Jewish Studies, London,* ed. J. G. Weiss (Jerusalem: Magnes Press, 1989), pp. 140-85; Brevard Childs, "The Sensus Literalis of Scripture: An Ancient and Modern Problem," in *Beiträge zur alttestamentlichen Theologie: Festschrift für Walther Zimmerli,* ed. Herbert Donner et al. (Göttingen: Vandenhoeck & Ruprecht, 1977), pp. 80-93; James Barr, "The Literal, the Allegorical and Modern Biblical Scholarship," *JSOT* 44 (1989): 3-17; Rowan Williams, "The Literal Sense of Scripture," *Modern Theology* 7 (1991): 121-34; and Kathryn Greene-McCreight, "Restless until We Rest in God: The Fourth Commandment as Test Case in Christian 'Plain Sense' Interpretation," *Ex Auditu* 11 (1995): 29-41.

according to the whole. This was, after all, one of Augustine's cardinal hermeneutical guidelines. When the Reformers claimed that Scripture is its own interpreter, they did not mean that one need not think in order to read the Bible, but rather that Scripture is to be read according to its own logic, a logic that was stated and summed up in the rules of faith and love. Since these rules are drawn from Scripture itself, they are not considered extratextual interpretive devices (such as would be Augustine's dearly held Neoplatonic philosophy, Lombard's *Sentences,* Thomas Aquinas's *Summa,* or in our day, existentialist philosophy, evidentialist epistemology, or the Constitution of the United States of America). To be sure, the Reformers did not usually use the words "rules of faith and love," but more often spoke of this by insisting that Jesus Christ is the center of Scripture.

The following five observations about the overall structure of the constraints on traditional biblical interpretation may seem not to be directly related to the matter of homosexuality per se, but they in fact are. They point to fundamental constraints on biblical interpretation for those who seek to follow the hermeneutics of the "Great Tradition" (itself a complex matter), and are therefore quite pertinent to our discussion if we are going to find a way to speak to each other on this topic.[12] It will be shown when we turn our discussion to one of the dominant revisionist arguments from Scripture how these points can be disregarded in some very basic ways.

1. Traditional hermeneutics offered a coherent theological relating of the two covenants of our Bible. If we are to argue for a novel interpretation, we in our own day need to account for the relationship between the two Testaments. What do we do with testimony from different cultures and historical periods? How do we affirm that both are equally God's word without the New Testament stifling the witness of the Old, or vice versa? More importantly, how do we affirm that Jesus Christ is the goal of the Law, *telos nomou,* while affirming the impossibility of a "newer" revelation claiming priority over the New Testament's witness? This was the case with Montanism, and is the case with Mormonism. It will not be sufficient to argue that God is doing a new thing in shedding his grace on homoerotic relationships without, first, ac-

12. Several readers have asked me where in the corpus of Christian theology I find these five points. It seems that the posing of the question itself points to our hermeneutical problem: these "points" are present virtually throughout classical Christian theology, but are never explicitly stated in this way as far as I am aware. The most obvious and earliest place they "appear" in Christian writings is in the sustained argument which Paul weaves throughout Rom. 9–11, but again, they are not explicitly spelled out. Instead, they implicitly ground and guide Paul's exegesis of the Old Testament as he grapples with the faithfulness of the God of Israel in Jesus Christ.

counting for how this revelation is to be judged vis-à-vis the unsurpassability of the revelation in Christ, and second, assuring the rest of us that those who offer the revisionist view are reliable prophets of God's will.

2. Without the adequate relating of the two Testaments, Christian appropriation of Old Testament Law becomes problematic, as was the case with Marcion in the ancient church, and with so-called "German Christian" theologians of the Third Reich. Traditional hermeneutics at its best holds a place for Old Testament Law, interpreting it through the lens of the narratives of Jesus. If we are to argue for an interpretation which contradicts that of the tradition, we must make a move analogous to that of the tradition. It will therefore not be adequate to sweep aside an item within the "Holiness Code" on the basis that Christ has set us free from the burdensome old yoke of Torah.[13] This is the antinomian danger of a flat-footed relating of the covenants. Far more pernicious and pervasive, however, is a modernist version of this: Israel's law is ancient; we are moderns; and no self-respecting person in his or her right mind would follow those ridiculous laws.[14] This is ethnocentric, theologically suspect, and borders on anti-Semitism. If one finds the traditional venue for reinterpreting Old Testament Law unacceptable, one must

13. For example, see Jeffrey Siker, "How to Decide: Homosexual Christians, the Bible, and Gentile Inclusion," *Theology Today* 51 (1994): 227: "So, if one chooses to take the prohibitions about a man lying with another man out of context and apply them to today, what is the rationale for not abiding by the other levitical prohibitions? To read and apply the biblical texts out of context leads inevitably to misreadings and misapplications." The context within which the Levitical prohibitions are traditionally read in Christian circles is the law of Christ, which may overthrow some of the Levitical laws but not others, depending on their witness in other parts of the canon. For example, unclean foods are made clean in Christ, but we do not also thereby assume that witchcraft (Lev. 19:26b; etc.) has been made clean, for the New Testament itself witnesses to its impurity.

14. An example of this is the argument that since Jews no longer kill homosexuals, clearly they realize that this command is outdated and barbaric ("If a man lies with a male as with a woman, both of them have committed an abomination; they shall be put to death . . ." [Lev. 20:13 NRSV]). However, the Orthodox Jewish community's failure to act literally on this command regarding the death penalty has nothing to do with the command's being cruel or outdated. Rather, it is because of the Diaspora: when the temple is rebuilt and the ruling structures of Orthodox Judaism "re"established, so goes the argument, those *Jews* who engage in homosexual genital gratification will indeed be subject to the death penalty. Of course, the process by which the death penalty is finally declared and enacted is itself quite complex. The careful reader will note that this example is *not* used in the present essay as a warrant for punishment of homosexual behavior, but rather simply to point out that lack of literal action on a specific law does not indicate its "outdatedness" but has to do with the present location of the religious community on the eschatological time line. This is, of course, one of the key factors in Christian relating of the two Testaments.

find another venue which at least allows for the integrity of the theological witness of the Old Testament.

3. In addition, traditional hermeneutics gave a coherent account of God's unity, integrity, and faithfulness in his dealings with Israel and with those of us of the New Covenant. This is, after all, what Paul is trying to do in Romans 9–11: Given that the death and resurrection of the crucified Jesus has ushered in the dawning of the eschatological age, does this mean that God has changed his mind? What of the promises to the patriarchs, indeed of the very righteousness of God? If we are to offer an interpretation which contradicts traditional interpretation, we must at least give a coherent account of the unity of God's will for humanity. It will not be adequate to say that God has changed his mind and given up on the Jews with their vision of righteousness (as though they themselves invented it in the first place!) and turned to the more enlightened Gentiles of postmodern Western culture. How can God's will for our embodied lives be so radically different from that set forth for Israel? I am not saying that such radical difference is theologically impossible; indeed it is not impossible. I am simply saying that an adequate account of it needs to be given.

4. Traditional hermeneutics would tend to have us seek our "place" in the biblical narrative in order to interpret the text. That is, we resist adopting certain biblical practices but embrace others depending upon our location in the story in comparison with the location of the characters, incidents, or activities depicted. We do not chide Judah or Tamar for the episode in Genesis 38, or Abraham and Sarah for their activities in Genesis 16, nor do we emulate them. They come before the giving of the Law in the story line; we come after — indeed, in the *nova lex.* In the same way, we do not hold David's affair with Bathsheba up as an example of heterosexual sex to be emulated; David had read the Law and knew that what he was doing was wrong. We stand in the dawning of the eschatological age, where there is neither Jew nor Greek, slave nor free, male nor female, yet where we await with eager longing the redemption of our bodies. This means that we stand in a fundamentally different place than did the patriarchs and prophets of the Old Testament, but in the same place as those witnesses of Jesus' resurrection appearances and the early church. We are not fundamentally more eschatologically informed or hermeneutically privileged than Mary Magdalene, for example. But in order to contradict a traditional interpretation of Scripture, particularly on sexual ethics, it seems that we must rely heavily on a confidence in our eschatological privilege over all those who came before us. This tends to lead us into arrogance, an attitude ruled out logically by traditional interpretation.

5. To state the obvious, traditional hermeneutics knew nothing of his-

torical criticism, although very similar questions indeed to those asked by the methods of historical criticism were asked by the Fathers, Scholastics, and Reformers. Questions of consistency and contradiction in biblical accounts, questions of historicity and correspondence to the time-space continuum were asked, but they were always submitted to the overarching conviction that the Scriptures could be trusted to express the divine voice and will. Therefore, it will not be adequate to analyze Scripture's depictions of communities of faith, whether ancient Israel or the New Testament communities, according to, e.g., a caricature of form-critical methodology. Such might result in a conclusion similar to the following: since the texts were developed to deal with certain crises, power imbalances, or (less titillatingly) liturgical celebrations, we can discount any element which exhibits this tendency on the grounds that it is culturally conditioned. Traditional claims about the divine voice speaking through the text, whether articulated in terms of the doctrine of revelation, or inspiration, or *sola Scriptura,* or the mere fact of canon, cannot be honored by such moves. Traditional hermeneutics at its best, therefore, attempted what Clifford Geertz has dubbed a "thick description" when and insofar as it allowed the biblical story to unfold on its own terms and in its own categories. If we are to attempt such a "thick description" in our own biblical interpretation, we will need to avoid the ethnocentric use of historical judgments and categories when they are foreign to the unfolding of the biblical story.

While most revisionists and traditionalists alike will use the Bible and are dedicated to supporting their position via the interpretation of Scripture, the fault line between the two tectonic-hermeneutical plates runs underneath the line sketched out in the above discussion. Ironically, the revisionists more often than not rely on a hermeneutic which does not submit to the rules of faith and love, despite the appeal to the integrity of the gospel message ("faith") and to compassion and mercy toward gays and lesbians ("love"). Oftentimes, the "love" and "faith" of the revisionist position rely more on Enlightenment notions of equity and tolerance than on a biblically shaped understanding of the righteousness of God and the grace of God toward fallen humanity.[15] The revisionist hermeneutic therefore tends to be less holistic

15. E.g., Dale Martin argues that "any interpretation of scripture that hurts people, oppresses people, or destroys people cannot be the right interpretation, no matter how traditional, historical, or exegetically respectable. There can be no debate about the fact that the church's stand on homosexuality has caused oppression, loneliness, self-hatred, violence, sickness, and suicide for millions of people. If the church wishes to continue with its traditional interpretation it must *demonstrate,* not just claim, that it is more loving to condemn homosexuality than to affirm homosexuals. Can the church *show* that same-sex

than the traditional one, more reductionist despite its claim to openness in its including "experience" as an authority in interpretation. Those who argue in favor of the righteousness before God of homoerotic relationships often reject certain parts of Scripture and choose isolated texts to be used as a lever over against the whole to pry open a new venue on the matter. More often, but not always, the traditionalists who do not acknowledge the righteousness before God of homoerotic relationships tend to read Scripture according to the rules of faith and love, resulting in a more holistic, less reductionist use of Scripture.[16]

One of the most compelling revisionist arguments which uses Scripture to affirm the righteousness before God of gay and lesbian sexual activity is that of Jeffrey Siker and others. This view proposes that homoerotic union (my term; Siker uses the term "homosexual expression") is to be embraced within the Christian community just as Gentiles, who were once considered outsiders to Israel, were included in the people of God with the advent of Christ.[17] On the surface this seems a rather straightforward argument, but it in fact is quite complex and operates on the basis of several key but un-

---

loving relationships damage those involved in them? Can the church give compelling reasons to believe that it really would be better for all lesbian and gay Christians to live alone, without the joy of intimate touch, without hearing a lover's voice when they go to sleep or awake? Is it really better for lesbian and gay teenagers to despise themselves and endlessly pray that their very personalities be reconstructed so that they may experience romance like their straight friends? Is it really more loving for the church to continue its worship of 'heterosexual fulfillment' (a 'non-biblical' concept, by the way) while consigning thousands of its members to a life of either celibacy or endless psychological manipulations that masquerade as 'healing'? . . . What will 'build the double love of God and of our neighbor'? . . . We ask the question that must be asked: 'What is the loving thing to do?'" (pp. 130-31, italics Martin's). This is indeed a compelling and passionate statement, but if we define the concept "love" via its depiction in the biblical narrative, it is arguably more "loving" to condemn homoerotic acts while affirming the homosexual as brother or sister in Christ. Notice my reworking here of the phrase in Martin's first italicized sentence: the alternatives are not between condemning homosexuality and affirming homosexuals. This is an example of the usual but unhelpful oversimplification of the dilemma.

16. To be sure, this is not always the case. Sometimes, in fact, those who oppose homoerotic relationships on religious grounds use the Bible in very reductionistic and simplistic ways, citing only the phrases which can allow them to vent their hostility at the dawning cultural acceptance of gay and lesbian life. These people often do not follow a "traditionalist" hermeneutic, however, as I have defined it above. The above sketch of a "traditionalist" hermeneutic would appear too catholic for the brand of American Protestantism highly influenced by the individualistic piety of the Second Great Awakening out of which comes some of the most vocal religious opposition to homoerotic relationships.

17. See Siker, pp. 219-34; Luke Timothy Johnson, "Homosexuality: Debate and Discernment, Scripture and the Spirit," *Commonweal,* 28 January 1994, pp. 11-13.

articulated assumptions which must be examined before we can consider its use of Scripture. These assumptions are as follows:

a. Sexual "orientation," whether heterosexual or homosexual, is such a fundamental aspect of one's God-given identity that not to express it is to diminish one's humanity, and expressing one's sexual orientation will involve at least genital gratification. Other expressions may or may not be attendant. [Note that "homosexual expression" would not be negated by a traditional reading of the Bible if it referred to, for example, homosexual friendships or partnerships which did not engage genital gratification; hence my distinction in terms.]
b. The Old Testament in particular consists not so much of divine law, writings, prophecies, and stories, as of "social constructs" projected onto a religious screen. The ancient Israelites were Feuerbachians without knowing it. Since "that was then and this is now," we are not bound by Old Testament Law. No direct appeal is made to the work of Christ in arguing for the Christian's "freedom" from the law.[18]
c. Those who affirm homoerotic relationships within the Christian life have received a new revelation of the Spirit, and those who reject such union assume that homosexuals are bereft of the Spirit.[19]

In order for Siker's argument to convince, then, it would need first to persuade traditionalist readers of what the argument itself assumes, namely, that genital gratification is indeed such a fundamental part of our identity that to deny it would be to diminish our humanity. To convince the traditionalists, this assumption would need to be shown to be supported by the biblical witness. It seems, however, to add one codicil too many to the biblical depiction of our identity as made in the image of God, male and female. Our identity depiction in the Bible does not include what we do with our maleness and femaleness apart from our being fruitful and multiplying. In comparison with the other creatures who are created "according to their kind," the only distinction which obtains within the class of creatures known as *'adam* is that between male and female — neither species nor race nor orientation of any other sort. What does Siker's first assumption implicitly say of those who abstain from genital gratification with a partner of either sex for

18. E.g., "Do we blithely adopt first-century (or ancient Israelite) social constructions of human sexuality and sexual relations and apply them to today?" (Siker, p. 228).

19. Again, "I was like the hard-nosed doctrinaire circumcised Jewish Christians who denied that Gentiles could receive the Spirit of Christ as Gentiles" (Siker, p. 230).

religious or social reasons? What does it say about children, the celibate elderly or disabled? Does it make them less than human simply because they do not find genital gratification with a partner? Siker would need to be explicit here about how he arrives at such an understanding of human identity.

Secondly, Siker would need to show that he values Scripture other than for its collecting of ancient social conventions. How does Siker ground the authority of Scripture? I am *not* saying that Scripture is not authoritative for him; clearly, it is indeed a highly valued authority. If he is going to play by the rules of the "game," however, dismissing parts of Scripture as "social construct" will not do, as was apparent in observation 5 above, theological misappropriation of historical-critical methods. His argument would need to address such questions as what it is about Scripture, or what it is which one does with Scripture, which makes one able to hear the divine voice. He would need to have a more coherent theological understanding of both the integrity of the Old Testament and of its use within Christian discourse, as is apparent from observations 1 and 2 above, the hermeneutical relating of the two Testaments and Christian appropriation of Old Testament Law. Again, I am *not* saying that this would need to be explicit for the purposes of such an article as his, but that the arguments he makes would need to be supported by a more theologically coherent position than the one which seems to underlie that in the article cited.

Thirdly, Siker would need to document his depiction of those who take the traditional line. In other words, Siker's "solution" (of reading Acts 10 as an allegory of the inclusion of self-affirming practicing homosexuals into the life of the Spirit) needs to fit the problem it purports to solve. Where and when do traditionalists say that homosexuals are not recipients of the Spirit? I have not heard such an argument except from very angry fundamentalists, but maybe I have not listened carefully enough. Not only is this depiction not self-evidently accurate, it breaks the rules of this game. Christian theology generally says of the Spirit that it is the gracious gift of God to all who are baptized into Christ, despite the lack of any individual's own righteousness before God.[20] Reception of the Spirit according to a holistic reading of Scripture has nothing to do with one's bodily desires, but has to do with baptism, which itself is in the theological sphere of election.

Ultimately, the analogy between sexuality and election proves the undoing of any ties to the rules of our game. Siker quite clearly claims that "[t]he crux of the analogy, however, lies in the observation that early Jewish-

20. The episode in Acts 10 is the sole instance in the New Testament in which reception of the Spirit actually precedes baptism.

Christians saw Gentiles as being sinners because they were Gentiles, just as today most heterosexual Christians see active homosexuals as being sinners because they engage in homosexual activity."[21] According to a holistic reading of the Bible, however, Gentiles are not "sinners" per se. They are a category apart; they are those without the law, without God in the world. Without the law, there is no such thing as sin, since sin is transgression of the law, or so Paul argues in Romans. Gentiles are to be avoided, yes, but not because of what they do but who they are: the nonelect, and their nonelection expresses itself in their remaining bound in idolatry. In Christ they are grafted into the body of the elect, viewed as clean, not because of what they do or who they are, but in spite of it, and yet as a result of this new grace they are enabled and required to turn from their idolatry. The same, however, goes for Jews: in Christ they are righteous in the sight of God not because of what they do or who they are, but in spite of it. That is what we mean by the term "grace." The inclusion of the Gentiles has to do with God's election of Israel and nonelection of other nations, and with the grace of God in the face of Jesus Christ overcoming the alienation of both the elect and the nonelect alike. I am at this point familiar with no theological argument to the effect that heterosexuals are more "elect" than homosexuals. Indeed, the categories of sexuality (homosexuality, heterosexuality, practicing or nonpracticing, orientation or choice) are completely unbiblical and so cannot possibly have any bearing with regard to the notion of election, as Siker and others are quick to point out but slow to digest. The only sexual categories that are significant according to a holistic reading of the Bible are those of male and female, just as the only racial categories of significance in the Bible are Jew and Gentile, and that only after the "fall" of Genesis 3 to the final "splat" in Genesis 11 through to the resurrection of Jesus. To suggest that there is an analogy between Jew/Gentile and hetero/homosexual is a major category error; it is to compare apples and paper clips. The argument takes one biblical image, the inclusion of the Gentiles, and pulls it out of its canonical context to serve as the primary if not sole biblical touch point to support the weight of the revisionist position here. What can such an argument do with the pluriform witness of the Old Testament itself to the inclusion of the Gentiles?

Finally, Siker's argument assumes a fundamentally different eschatological "location" for the present Christian community vis-à-vis that of the writers of the New Testament. It would logically need to assume that present-day Christians can receive visions which contradict the revelation of the New Testament. This hinges on the implicit belief that the revisionists have received a

21. Siker, p. 231.

"revelation" or "gnosis" which supersedes the New Testament witness regarding sexuality. This is not the case with all arguments on behalf of the revisionist position, for some of them simply say that Scripture does not countermand lifelong loving homoerotic relationships. This argument would go as follows: The writers of the New Testament did not know homosexuality as we know it today, as instantiated in the covenantally committed love of two people of the same sex. They condemned not this genre of homosexuality, but that which was abusive, coercive, between adults and children, etc.[22] Such an argument does not necessarily imply that new "revelation" has been received to reinterpret the Scriptures so much as that the words of Scripture have been improperly translated. But Siker's argument must assume some such revelatory experience because it rests on the analogy to Acts 10, where it is Peter's vision which prompts his change of mind and heart regarding table fellowship and Gentile Christianity. However, we would not want to reject Siker's argument simply on the basis that it claims to be "prophetic," for it would seem wise to welcome study of how to discern the spirits. That is, even if we determine that it is false prophecy, or especially so, we should attend to it. At the same time, it must be acknowledged that the claim to a different eschatological "location" has never been easily met in the history of the church. It seems indeed to be one of the "rules" indicated in observations 1 and 4 above (the hermeneutical relating of the two Testaments and the hermeneutical discernment of our placement in the story line) that, barring the return of Jesus, our eschatological location is in no position of superiority to that of the New Testament writers. In fact, our location could only be argued to be that of inferiority, for they were closer to the Alpha and Omega himself, fished and talked with him, ate and drank with him, stuck their hands in his wounds.[23] Siker's argument would at the very least need to address these matters.

The implicit appeal to eschatology here is formally similar to that in the arguments from Scripture in favor of the abolitionist position and women's ordination. Indeed, it is often argued that as the church learned over time that slavery was inconsistent with the gospel, and as the church (or parts of it) learned over time that women called by the Holy Spirit and the body of the faithful could not be denied Holy Orders, so eventually the church will realize that homoerotic relationships are righteous in the sight of God. However, the similarity of appeal to eschatology in these three cases actually undercuts the

22. So John Boswell and Dale Martin.

23. E.g., Matt. 24:9-14; Rev. 1–3. Even Joachimite thought supports the view of deterioration within each epoch rather than amelioration. Many thanks to Ephraim Radner for pointing this out.

revisionist position with regard to homosexuality. This is because the appeal functions differently in the arguments regarding slavery and women's ordination than it does in those regarding homosexuality. The biblical witness regarding slavery, for example, never commends the holding of slaves as a witness to human redemption in Christ. The New Testament does indicate that slavery is a condition to be tolerated within the confines of fallen reality, but that eschatologically in fact there is no distinction between slave and free (Gal. 3:28). Thus, the church learned over time not a different hermeneutic to apply in these cases, but to see itself as the body of Christ in the light of the eschaton. "And so, when in the Christian tradition men and women rose up in later historical periods and questioned the social and political tolerance of slavery, they were *not changing* the church's mind from what the Bible teaches on this matter. Instead, they were *making present in society* what the New Testament writers anticipated would happen in *God's own* future reversal of human institutions."[24] Arguments in favor of the revisionist position regarding homosexuality want to claim that the eschatological gift of the Holy Spirit would have the almost two thousand years of the church's biblical interpretation on this matter proven wrong.[25] Can we say that the way of life held up for consideration in the revisionist position is consistent with the biblical depiction of God's intention for our eschatologically-present life in Christ?

This, then, is the question: Can an argument be framed according to the inner logic of traditional Christian discourse which can allow us to arrive at the revisionist position? One could easily choose to reject the logic of traditional Christian discourse itself, and indeed some are willing and eager to do this. But such a move would lead to sectarianism, further threatening the already-fragile unity of the body of Christ as we find it in North America. The "rules" which form the logical structure of traditional Christian discourse are not my rules; they are not our rules; they are not the rules of those who "won," or even of those who "lost." They are the rules we inherited from our brothers and sisters in Christ who, throughout the centuries, struggled together in the power of the Holy Spirit to understand the will of God. They are rules to the game we entered into at our baptism. Short of renouncing them,

24. Stephen Holmgren, "Human Sexuality from a Theological Perspective: Part of Our Walk in Holiness and Righteousness All Our Days," *Harvest* 6 (1996): 21.

25. John Boswell's "same-sex unions" only serve to strengthen the traditionalist argument on this account: the "fact" that such unions, if they did indeed involve genital gratification, were "kept a secret," if indeed this is an adequate description of why they were unheard of until recently, proves the point that the practice never convinced anyone apart from a tiny minority. John Boswell, *Same-Sex Unions in Premodern Europe* (New York: Vintage, 1994).

do we have the authority to pronounce homoerotic relationships to be righteous in the eyes of God?

Even if we come to the conclusion that such a pronouncement is impossible, we do indeed have something positive to add to our society's debate over matters of sexuality. First, the church could and should take the lead in publicly repenting for any and all times and instances in which its teaching has implicitly or explicitly allowed or promoted violence and hostility to gays and lesbians. This means that all Christians, exercising the priesthood of all believers, in the presence of those who from either "side" engage in hostile rhetoric, do everything in their power to denounce and defuse it. Secondly, the church could take the lead in publicly repenting for its hypocrisy manifest in its willingness to ignore the less culturally repugnant forms of sexual sin while focusing on the sexual activity of homosexuals. Thirdly, the church could take the lead in publicly proclaiming its own unique word on the goodness of God's gift of sexual pleasure shared between husband and wife, the normativity of fidelity within marriage, and the normativity of chastity in singleness. To declare the normativity of fidelity in marriage between one male and one female and of chastity in singleness would be a radical stand indeed in late twentieth-century North America. We would need to make clear that declaring the normativity of fidelity in marriage and chastity in singleness is *not* to open the door to spying on one another's sex lives and playing tattletale. We have all sinned and fall short of the glory of God, and this brings a unique perspective on any finger-pointing. Fourthly, the church could strengthen its proclamation of God's mercy and grace shed on all sinners who repent and turn to Jesus Christ for wholeness.

In addition, the church could indeed go so far as to acknowledge the "goods" which can come from homosexual relationships. The self-giving of two individuals in a committed relationship can, after all, reflect the sacrificial love of Christ. The contribution to the wider community which may come of homosexual relationships can also be acknowledged as a "good," such as the time and talents given in service to the church and the love and care rendered to the adopted children of gay and lesbian couples. The church can recognize as a "good" the pastoral, preaching, and teaching ministries of gays and lesbians which further the church's witness to Christ. To recognize these goods, however, is not to sanction the sexual activity which may (or may not) accompany such relationships. It does not follow from the church's freedom to recognize these goods which may issue from homosexual relationships that the church therefore has the freedom to bless such relationships. The church has neither such freedom nor such authority. To insist on this would be to insist on consequentialist ethics, that the "ends justify the means," so to speak.

Some denominations have called for a period of reflection on this issue, after which they will presumably vote to enact policy either pro or contra the traditional theological status of sexual union. These periods of reflection tend to be quite short — e.g., three years in the Presbyterian Church (USA). That a denomination would deem itself able to discern the spirits on this issue in the space of three years seems either a gross overestimation of its spiritual capacities or an underestimation of the magnitude of the issue at stake. Seeking God's will surely means more than gathering "evidence" from the world of science or commissioning studies in human sexuality from our denominational headquarters. We should first of all confess our individual and communal sins before God. If there is anything that we should learn from Romans on this issue, it is that we all have sinned and fall short, that if God were to exact judgment not one of us would be left standing. We should not only study together, we should also repent, pray, fast, worship. If there is anything we should learn from Leviticus on this issue, it is that God calls us to lives of holiness.

Ultimately, this issue has presented the church with a contemporary "Athanasian moment," a fork in the road so to speak, where there is little prospect for happy resolve or compromise. The matter of the theological and moral status of homoerotic activity has raised afresh questions which touch the very nerve center of the faith, and once again presents us, in an especially painful and poignant way, with the choice of life over death. We all want to choose life, not death, as we are enjoined in Deuteronomy. The question is this: Is the life of God something we can know on our own, with the guidance of our experience (in this case) over against the witness of Scripture and tradition? Or is the life of God something we cannot know on our own apart from God's unprompted and gracious depiction of it in the life of Israel, and in the life, death, and resurrection of Jesus? While we all hope to convince each other on the basis of Scripture, on the basis of "the gospel," however that may be understood, I fear that this debate may ultimately be "resolved" as it was in the APA, that is, with political lobbying and jockeying for power. If this is the case, whichever side "wins," the church will have lost an opportunity to witness to the love of Christ, that perfect love which casts out all fear and which demands our obedience and our deepest gratitude.

CHAPTER 10

Christian Vocation, Freedom of God, and Homosexuality

NANCY J. DUFF

In my eleven years of seminary teaching, three issues have proven to evoke the most controversy: homosexuality, abortion, and (oddly enough) vegetarianism. Of these three, debate over homosexuality has left me the weariest. Along with many allies and opponents I find my energies depleted by the persistent and heated nature of the argument. I remain in the conversation, in part, to look for mutually acceptable ways to live together as the body of Christ in light of this serious disagreement. I have addressed this concern in a previous essay.[1] In this present work, however, I argue my own position on homosexuality, seeking to persuade those who have not yet made up their minds and to explain to opponents why I stand where I do.

Drawing on the doctrine of vocation and the freedom of God, I contend that while most human beings are called by God into heterosexual relationships and some are called into the celibate life, still others are called into homosexual relationships. This affirmation of faithful, homosexual unions does not challenge the essential value of the male-female relationship (as some fear that it will) any more than the affirmation of celibacy does.

Although the doctrine of vocation is usually considered in light of the

1. "How to Discuss Moral Issues Surrounding Homosexuality When You Know You Are Right," in *Homosexuality and Christian Community,* ed. Choon-Leong Seow (Louisville: Westminster/John Knox, 1996), pp. 144-59. This is a book of essays written by members of the faculty at Princeton Seminary.

work we do, a broader understanding of it is intended here.[2] In its most fundamental form the doctrine of vocation affirms that each individual life with its unique combination of gifts and limitations has divinely appointed purpose. Each of us was brought into the world for a purpose, so that we can say to one another, "Your life matters." The doctrine of vocation also says that we are called to glorify God in all that we do. While this affirmation should not be misinterpreted as a command to give glory to God no matter how awful the circumstance or the task, it lends dignity to people and the tasks they perform even when others aim to take that dignity away.

The affirmation of the freedom of God is essential to the doctrine of vocation. In the claim that God calls each of us into the world for a purpose, the object of the claim is humanity but the subject is God. The doctrine of vocation initially focuses our attention on the activity of God and subsequently on the activity of human beings. The doctrine of vocation challenges arguments which deny the freedom of God to call people to different identities and tasks.

My position regarding Christian vocation, the freedom of God, and homosexuality relies on four presuppositions within the discipline of theological ethics which provide the framework for this essay. (1) The starting point for theological reflection on moral issues is not human freedom but divine freedom. (2) A theological ethic built on the freedom of God rejects casuistry as the application of absolutes to particular situations. (3) The doctrine of the incarnation assigns significance to particular situations and tangible consequences even though it does not promote a utilitarian ethic. (4) The doctrine of creation, which affirms both the goodness and sinfulness of creation, celebrates the goodness of human sexuality while acknowledging that, because of sin, human sexuality requires redemption.

Part I of this essay describes how these four presuppositions inform a Christian sexual ethic in general. Part II indicates how these presuppositions inform the moral issues surrounding homosexuality in particular.

2. See my article "Call/Vocation," in *Dictionary of Feminist Theologies* (1996), and "Vocation, Motherhood, and Marriage," in *Women, Gender, and Christian Community*, ed. Jane Dempsey Douglass and James F. Kay (Louisville: Westminster/John Knox, 1997), pp. 69-81. Finally, see my essay, "Reformed Theology and Medical Ethics: Death, Vocation, and the Suspension of Life-Support," in *Toward the Future of Reformed Theology*, ed. David Willis and Michael Welker (Grand Rapids: Eerdmans, 1999), pp. 302-20.

Part I: Christian Ethics and Human Sexuality

1. Theological Shift from Human Freedom to Divine Freedom

The church rightly resists the claim that the freedom to choose between options stands at the heart of a Christian approach to ethics. Centering our attention on free choice not only misses the point that not all free choices are moral ones, it also runs counter to the Reformed theological claim that human will is not free, but bound by sin. Theologically, true freedom occurs not when one chooses between options, but when human will is consistent with the will of God.[3] Cigarette smoking provides a case in point.

When a person addicted to nicotine seeks to quit smoking, choosing between options does not represent freedom, but bondage. The struggle which ensues over making the right choice indicates that the smoker is enslaved to a power that must be resisted. The apostle Paul knew that sin always involves this kind of bondage: "I can will what is right, but I cannot do it. For I do not do the good I want, but the evil I do not want is what I do. Now if I do what I do not want, it is no longer I that do it, but sin that dwells within me" (Rom. 7:18b-20 NRSV). Theologically, freedom occurs when one's will is consistent with the divine will and no struggle to make and carry out the right decision is necessary. Hence, for the ex-smoker true freedom occurs when a pack of cigarettes does not invoke the need to choose; smoking has, quite literally, ceased to be an option.

Rejecting freedom of choice as the heart of moral responsibility holds significant implications for a Christian sexual ethic. As Max Stackhouse points out, some ethicists (wrongly in his opinion and mine) put human freedom of choice at the center of ethics. According to *them:* "People inevitably exercise a substantial measure of freedom over how they will live their sexual lives, and that is how it should be. Is it not so that the highest value is freedom? that each person must be free to decide how to live his or her life as he or she wishes? and that no one has a right to impose any values on that freedom?"[4] In its most antinomian form, an ethic built on human freedom (when freedom is understood as choice) assumes a nonessentialist stance, claiming that human beings are not born into a predetermined definition of

3. In the political and social arena, of course, freedom to choose between options must be protected. Free choice is being evaluated here from the theological perspective of making moral decisions.

4. Max L. Stackhouse, "The Heterosexual Norm," in *Homosexuality and Christian Community,* p. 138. Although Stackhouse and I agree that freedom of choice does not stand at the heart of Christian ethics, our alternative proposals differ.

what it means to be human, but define who they are by what they do. "Existence precedes essence," claimed Jean-Paul Sartre, i.e., there is no given human essence to which human beings conform or against which they rebel.[5] Instead, human beings define their individual essence by making free choices. Even those who fall short of a nonessentialist or antinomian position often give moral priority to freedom of choice. Hence, some people identify any sexual behavior between consenting adults as not only legally but also morally acceptable, failing to recognize that not all choices freely made are morally good.

In opposition to this nonessentialist position, some ethicists give moral priority to absolute standards of behavior. Christian sexual ethicists, for instance, often invoke the norm of heterosexual marriage, stressing "faithfulness in marriage and celibacy in singleness" (a phrase coined by the United Methodists). Drawing from commandments in the Bible as well as from reason and tradition, the right pattern and rules for human sexual behavior are known in advance and then applied to each situation, thereby bringing order to moral chaos. This casuistical route, however, is not the only one available to those who wish to avoid the moral chaos that can arise from the nonessentialist position. The alternative to both nonessentialism *and* an ethic of absolutes acknowledges that divine freedom provides the starting point for Christian moral reflection.[6]

Early in his writing Karl Barth compared the movement of God in history to a bird in flight, thus identifying the central theme of theology as the freedom of God.[7] This emphasis on divine freedom indicates that God's reve-

5. Jean-Paul Sartre, "Existentialism and Humanism," in *Existentialism and Humanism* (London: Methuen, 1948), pp. 28-29. See my discussion of this essay in *Humanization and the Politics of God: The* Koinonia *Ethics of Paul Lehmann* (Grand Rapids: Eerdmans, 1992), pp. 40-45.

6. Some ethicists acknowledge this starting point while upholding a casuistical ethic. I agree with Karl Barth, however, that beginning with the freedom of God necessitates the rejection of casuistry (as well as "piecemeal" or "nonessentialist" ethics). See *Church Dogmatics,* III.4, *The Doctrine of Creation,* ed. Thomas F. Torrance, trans. Geoffrey W. Bromiley (Edinburgh: T. & T. Clark, 1961), pp. 6ff. Also see my discussion of Barth's theological ethic in *Humanization,* pp. 51-56.

7. Karl Barth, "The Christian's Place in Society," in *The Word of God and the Word of Man,* trans. D. Horton (Grand Rapids: Zondervan, 1935), p. 282. The "bird in flight," of course, represents the movement of God in history, a movement "whose power and import are revealed in the resurrection of Jesus Christ from the dead" (p. 283). The freedom of God provides the foundation for all of Barth's work; his entire dogmatics is built upon this affirmation. See also, Paul Lehmann, "The Dynamics of Reformation Ethics," *Princeton Seminary Bulletin* 14, no. 4 (spring 1950): 18.

lation is dynamic (never static or stationary) and cannot be captured by a snapshot or fixed in print through the formulation of an exact definition. The freedom of God also indicates that human beings have no power over the movement of God; they cannot define it or maneuver it to suit their liking. God cannot be manipulated or coerced by human will or human action.

Christian ethics, therefore, begins not with reflection on human action and freedom but on the action and freedom of God. God's activity creates the arena in which human beings are called and enabled to live as God would have us live. Theological ethics seeks to describe the dynamic movement of God and the ethos or arena of human life created by God's activity. As Paul Lehmann taught, God's action creates a world fit for being human in; human action seeks to become a parabolic expression of this divine action.[8]

2. Rejection of Casuistry as the Application of Absolutes to Particular Situations

Although the precise definition of casuistry stands in dispute, I use it here in its general meaning as "the application of principles or norms to specific cases."[9] Such a casuistical approach claims that there are set laws, principles, or norms which, once known, can be applied to specific situations. Such an approach seeks to avoid the nonessentialist or antinomian ethic in which the denial of laws, principles, or norms leads to moral chaos. It also seeks to avoid the pitfalls of legalism by taking exceptions into account when applying the moral law to particular cases. One can legitimately charge, however, that casuistry is inconsistent with divine revelation and cannot prevent the legalism it seeks to avoid. When one rejects casuistry as antithetical to divine freedom, one discovers the possibility of affirming homosexual orientation as a divinely appointed vocation for some individuals. Hence, not all homosexual behavior is deemed sinful.

That God's grace is "new every morning" (in Karl Barth's words) indicates that what God demands in one situation may be different from what God demands in another.[10] God's will can never be captured and tightly grasped in our hands or so firmly fixed in our hearts and minds that we are no longer able to hear God's word anew. When revelation is understood to be

8. See Paul Lehmann, *Ethics in a Christian Context* (New York: Harper & Row, 1963), p. 99.

9. Albert R. Jonsen and Stephen Toulmin offer a persuasive alternative to this definition in *The Abuse of Casuistry: A History of Moral Reasoning* (Berkeley: University of California Press, 1988).

10. Barth, *Church Dogmatics*, III.4, p. 16.

a movement of God's freedom and power, it cannot be reduced to an absolute law which we in turn apply to situations. Barth points out that such a casuistical reduction of divine revelation implies that we can control and manipulate the divine will.[11] Brunner (although he finally betrayed his own position) rightly claimed: "Therefore we can never know beforehand what God will require. God's command can only be perceived at the actual moment of hearing it. It would denote a breaking away from obedience if we were to think of the Divine Command as one which had been enacted once for all, to be interpreted by us in particular instances."[12] Against this view which claims to know the will of God as prescribed beforehand and subsequently applied by us to each situation, we can claim that the will of God is dynamically revealed in each situation.

Furthermore, casuistry cannot prevent the legalism it seeks to avoid. It is certainly true that an ethic built on absolute moral laws with no concept of casuistry (i.e., of how to apply those laws to various situations) would produce unbearable legalism, for one would be compelled to follow the law without *any* exceptions or adjustments. On the positive side, casuistry identifies situations where laws can be suspended, e.g., lying to save the life of a friend or allowing abortion in situations of rape or incest, even though one believes that lying and abortion are under most circumstances morally prohibited. Even the most responsible casuistry, however, cannot always avoid legalism. Sometimes casuistry leads to an intricate system of defining exceptions and subsequently becoming indifferent or even callous toward those people whose situations do not fall within the exception. More importantly, when no room is found for making an exception, a casuistical approach can justify overlooking the consequences of action, allowing one the moral justification of claiming, "At least my conscience is clear; I did what was right," even if the consequences of one's action caused great harm.

Within Christian moral tradition it makes a difference if one believes that commandments given in the Bible constitute prescriptive rules which are to be applied to each situation, making exceptions when necessary, or if one interprets divine commands as *descriptive* accounts of the world God has made fit for being human in. The latter position shifts attention from obeying the rules to obeying the living God. Far from embracing moral chaos, obedience to God never means assuming an attitude of "anything goes." Rather,

11. Karl Barth, *Church Dogmatics,* ed. G. W. Bromiley and T. F. Torrance (Edinburgh: T. & T. Clark, 1957), II.2, pp. 664ff.

12. Emil Brunner, *The Divine Imperative* (Philadelphia: Westminster, 1947), p. 117.

Christians seek to act in ways consistent with their vocation as believers in Jesus Christ and members of Christ's church.[13]

While the casuistical approach does not in every instance lead to legalism (which, of course, it seeks to avoid), its tendency to excerpt laws from Scripture and emphasize their absolute nature can lead to a rigidity which unintentionally denies the freedom of God. This is especially true when Christian sexual ethics combines absolute laws gleaned from Scripture with moral laws gleaned from biology.[14] For instance, when a Christian sexual ethic combines the command to be fruitful and multiply with women's physical ability to conceive, bear, and nurture children, women are deemed better suited to take care of children than men, and are often deemed better able to take care of children than to fulfill any other task. As a result, one denies the freedom of God to call women to tasks according to their unique combination of gifts and limitations, of circumstance and promise. Rather, God is bound to an order that universally defines the vocation of women.

Against this approach, the doctrine of vocation claims that identical roles cannot be assigned to all members of any one race, class, culture, or gender. Not all women are called to be mothers no matter what their biological potential. God is free to call some women to be pastors or physicians as well as mothers, just as God is free to call some men into full-time child care. When the church excludes all women from a particular vocation for which they are well suited, it has challenged the freedom of God to address particular individuals according to their calling. When the church claims that it is unacceptable for men or women to assume untraditional vocations (by society's standards), it has overlooked the particular circumstances, limitations, and gifts of each individual as well as the freedom of God to call people to different identities and tasks.

3. Incarnation Indicates that Consequences Matter

The doctrine of the incarnation affirms that God chose not to be aloof, but present in "this world of time and space and things."[15] While the incarnation does not affirm the world the way it is by justifying the status quo, it does in-

13. See Lehmann, *Ethics.*

14. See James Dobson, *Straight Talk: What Men Need to Know, What Women Should Understand* (Dallas: Word, 1991), p. 184. Dobson provides one of the leading voices in the "pro-family" movement of evangelical Christians and is founder and president of Focus on the Family.

15. A phrase frequently used by Paul Lehmann.

dicate that Christians are called to take the world seriously. Although God is never bound by what is, there is a physicality to God's presence in the world, i.e., God reveals God's self through physical event. That God became incarnate in Christ, who was born, suffered, and died, reinforces Christian interest in and responsibility for the things of this world. From the beginning the church has discredited tendencies to seek escape from the world. For the discipline of Christian ethics this means that we cannot distance ourselves from specific situations. We cannot hold to abstract norms or principles divorced from what is really going on in the world. We are, rather, called to employ all forms of analysis that are useful for understanding a moral dilemma and its solution: theological, sociological, biological, political, etc. Furthermore, even if we do not give moral priority to consequences as utilitarians do, we cannot discount the concrete consequences of an action, claiming that no matter what harm is done, we are morally right if we follow the law.

4. The Goodness of Creation and Its Need for Redemption

The doctrine of creation also disavows any tendency to ignore or denigrate the physical world. That God created the world and called it good indicates that we cannot hold in disdain the things of the world. Although we recognize that creation stands in need of redemption, we do not for that reason hate what is created. Christians can never overlook this concrete world, for God is radically present in it; Christians also affirm the heavenly world and that God transcends all that is. Hence, we can neither seek to escape the world nor accept the world the way it is.

The church has at times denied the goodness of creation by an inability to affirm the goodness of humanity's sexual nature. Augustine, for instance, believed that there was nothing he should avoid as much as marriage, claiming to know "nothing which brings the manly mind down from the height more than a woman's caress and that joining of bodies without which one cannot have a wife."[16] Jerome believed that the "activities of marriage itself, if

16. Cited by Erich Fuchs, "Christianity and Sexuality: An Ambiguous History," in *Sexual Desire and Love: Origins and History of the Christian Ethic of Sexuality and Marriage* (New York: Seabury Press, 1983), p. 98. Augustine was so disturbed by humanity's sexual nature that he wished the Creator had found another way for procreation to occur: "'Increase and multiply and fill the earth.' Although it seems that this could not happen without the intercourse of a man and woman . . . still we may say that in mortal bodies there could have been another process in which, by the mere emotion of pious charity, with no concupiscence, that sign of corruption, children would be born." Cited by Fuchs, p. 99.

they are not modest and do not take place under the eyes of God as it were, so that the only intention is children, are filth and lust."[17]

At its best, however, the church has celebrated the goodness of human sexuality. Luther, for instance, managed (with some ambiguity) to hold a positive assessment of human sexual activity, believing that one discovers godliness in marriage: "To be sure, when I consider marriage, only the flesh seems to be there. Yet my father must have slept with my mother and made love to her, and they were nevertheless godly people. All the patriarchs and prophets did likewise. The longing of a man for a woman is God's creation, that is to say, when nature is sound, not when it's corrupted as it is among Italians and Turks."[18] In recognizing the goodness of human sexuality, the church has rightly identified two essential functions of intercourse: the unitive and the procreative. The church errs, however, whenever it transforms the celebration of these two functions into commands. Affirming the goodness of sexuality does not, of course, mean that there is a divine command which claims that one *must* be sexually active in order to be fully human. Likewise, affirming the goodness of procreation does not mean that one *must* have children. When the doctrine of vocation and the freedom of God are joined to affirmations regarding the goodness of creation (including the goodness of human sexuality), we celebrate the variety of vocations to which different individuals are called: singleness, marriage, parenthood, etc.

Part II: Homosexuality

1. Theological Shift from Human Freedom to Divine Freedom

The issue of free choice has played a significant but inconsistent role in the argument involving homosexuality. Some proponents of the integrity of homosexual orientation claim that individuals do not choose to be homosexual, but are born into a homosexual orientation. These proponents also affirm the genetic disposition for homosexuality as part of God's good creation. Other proponents assume a nonessentialist position which claims that all of us, homosexuals and heterosexuals alike, determine who we are if given the arena to make a free choice.

17. Cited by Fuchs, p. 98.

18. Martin Luther, *On Married Life* (1522) (German text in Weimar Ausgabe 10/2, pp. 294-96; translated in full in *Luther's Works,* 45:17ff.). Cited in *Luther,* ed. Ian D. Kingston Siggins (New York: Harper & Row, 1972), pp. 148-49.

Opponents of homosexual activity, on the other hand, tend to claim a heterosexual norm for humanity which dictates that human beings remain "faithful in marriage and celibate in singleness." Rejecting any validity to the nonessentialist position, they may or may not agree that a homosexual orientation is determined at birth. Even if the latter is conceded, however, they view such an orientation as inconsistent with divine creation and insist that individuals can exercise the freedom not to act upon such an orientation. Hence, many churches allow celibate homosexuals to be ordained if, of course, they are otherwise qualified for the ministry. Only so-called "practicing" homosexuals are denied ordination outright.

A commonly reported experience among homosexual men finds both support and challenge from the scientific world regarding the genetic origins of sexual orientation: "All my life I have known that I was different. Even in grade school I knew that I wasn't like my friends. All through junior high and high school I tried to be who I was told I was supposed to be. I dated girls. I acted like the other guys. Finally, I have realized that I am gay, and I'm going to accept who I am even if others won't." While we must take this reported experience seriously in our evaluation of the morality of homosexual unions, and encourage science to explore the origins of sexual identity further, uncovering sexual origins does not in itself answer the moral question. Christian faith does not pronounce us moral based on our orientation at birth. Opponents of church-sanctioned homosexual unions correctly point out that while alcoholics and murderers may be born with predispositions toward addiction or rage, this does not validate their behavior.

Nevertheless, supporters of church-sanctioned homosexual unions have equally good reason to point out that homosexual orientation does not by necessity carry the destructive consequences of alcoholism or uncontrollable rage. As Christopher Morse maintains:

> Only those who give no theological heed to consequence as a legitimate test of doctrine can fail to take account of the fact that current church teaching is viewed by increasing numbers of Christians as setting up an intolerable contradiction between their creation as sexual beings and their calling to the Christian life. In what amounts to a tragic cruelty joke, their being human as God has made them and their being faithful as God calls them are presented as antithetical.[19]

19. Christopher Morse, *Not Every Spirit: A Dogmatics of Christian Disbelief* (Valley Forge, Pa.: Trinity Press International, 1994), p. 280. For Morse's insightful discussion of Christian sexual ethics, including the issue of homosexuality, see "Being Human Sexually," pp. 273-83 of his book.

The claim from human experience and from scientific evidence that one is born into a homosexual orientation should be given significant attention, for it raises the question in a particularly powerful way of whether homosexuality represents God's vocation for some individuals. It does not by itself, however, answer the moral question for Christians.

A different argument in favor of homosexual unions discounts the validity of orientation at birth and turns instead to a nonessentialist position which emphasizes free choice. According to Carter Heyward, for instance, the nonessentialist or what she calls "historical" view requires us to frame sexual ethics around actions rather than identity. According to her, the actions of heterosexual or homosexual persons within the context of intimate sexual relations constitute the concern of sexual ethics, not whether heterosexual or homosexual orientation is right or wrong. According to this position, human beings have no fixed and unchanging identity. "All of us, and all of everything, is relative to everything else — changing, becoming, living and dying in relation." Although relationality is our origin, relationality itself "presupposes relativity." According to Heyward, "There is no such thing as a homosexual or a heterosexual if by this we mean to denote a fixed essence, an essential identity. There are rather homosexual and heterosexual people — people who act homosexually or heterosexually."[20]

Rosemary Radford Ruether sets forth a similar argument when she claims that all human beings are born bisexual and are subsequently socialized to be heterosexual by a heterosexist society. The presence of homosexuals reveals that some were able to resist their socialization. Here emphasis on the freedom to choose is paramount. According to Ruether, in the context of a freely chosen, mutual, loving and faithful relationship, we can "appropriate our sexuality not as something biologically necessitated, or as socially coerced, but as a *freely chosen way* of expressing our authentic humanness in relation to the specific others with whom we wish to share our lives."[21] Unlike the position which claims that homosexual orientation is given at birth, this position seeks to protect the freedom to choose one's sexual identity.

Against this nonessentialist position, theological ethics can claim that our identity does not arise solely from who we decide to be but, according to the Christian gospel, from who we are called to be. To act in ways that counter our individual calling constitutes a form of human sin. The argument in support of

20. Carter Heyward, "Notes on Historical Grounding: Beyond Sexual Essentialism," in *Sexuality and the Sacred: Sources for Theological Reflection* (Louisville: Westminster/John Knox, 1994), p. 11.

21. Rosemary Radford Ruether, "Homophobia, Heterosexism, and Pastoral Practice," in *Sexuality and the Sacred,* p. 396, emphasis added.

the integrity of same-sex unions is not dependent on either the nonessentialist position nor on claims regarding a genetically determined sexual orientation. The question to be asked is whether God can call a specific individual into a homosexual orientation through either birth or circumstance.

2. Rejection of Casuistry as the Application of Absolutes to Particular Situations

If neither our orientation at birth nor the freedom to choose entirely determines our vocation, neither do absolute laws (whether gleaned from the Bible or from biology) dictate our vocation in advance. Christians who oppose church-sanctioned homosexual unions usually hold as central to their position that divine commands recorded in the Bible dictate against it. They rightly point out that every passage in the Bible which mentions homosexuality rejects it. While responsible representatives of this view admit that the Bible does not frequently refer to homosexuality, and readily discredit arguments based on erroneous readings (such as appeals to the story of Sodom and Gomorrah),[22] they can still turn to specifically negative texts such as those found in Leviticus, Romans, 1 Corinthians, and 1 Timothy.

In addition to these specific prohibitions against homosexuality, they also rightly point to the biblical celebration of the union between men and women (although in the process they tend to overlook Jesus' marital status and Paul's preference for the single life). Nevertheless, a number of significant claims often arise from those biblical texts which assign great value to the relationship between men and women. Among these claims the following three are especially important for discussions about homosexuality:

- The *imago Dei* is located in our relationship as male and female. Karl Barth has made a powerful argument for interpreting God's words in Genesis, "Let us make humanity in our image," by the clause which completes the verse: "in the image of God he made them, *male and female made he them.*" Although Barth actually writes very little about homosexuality, his interpretation of the essential nature of the male-female relationship is often invoked by Reformed theologians and ethicists who argue against the integrity of homosexual unions.

22. Richard B. Hays proves to be one of the responsible representatives of this view in his discussion of homosexuality in *The Moral Vision of the New Testament: Community, Cross, New Creation: A Contemporary Introduction to New Testament Ethics* (San Francisco: HarperSanFrancisco, 1996).

- The radical otherness of males and females and the resulting need for *complementarity* through relationship with one another mandates the rejection of intimate relationships between people of the same sex. Many Christian theologians and ethicists hold that the essential differences between men and women reflect an otherness in their relationship to one another that prevents idolatry. In contrast, male-to-male or female-to-female relationships represent the idolatry of relating to one like oneself.
- Homosexual activity cannot conform to the biblical injunction to "be fruitful and multiply." Because homosexual activity does not lead to *procreation*, it stands against the divinely appointed purpose for sexual activity.

Typically these claims lead to the conclusion that same-sex unions are idolatrous, self-centered, and devoid of the ability to give life. These same claims, which arise from biblical interpretation, are often reinforced with appeals to nature, apart from any reference to Scripture: "Homosexuality is contrary to the intentions of creation. The structure of sex organs is such that one of their purposes is human reproduction. That is not the only purpose, but it is a real and undeniable purpose — and it is a purpose not capable of being fulfilled homosexually. It is not wrong in this regard, thus, to speak of homosexuality as a terminal sexual behavior. It cannot transmit the gift of life to the next generation."[23] While one can argue that the coincidence between Scripture and nature indicates that creation confirms what revelation teaches in the Bible, one can also argue that the reduction of divine will to absolute commands results in a lessening of the necessity of reference to God. Once the moral code has been extracted from the Bible, one no longer has to discern God's present movement in the world; God's will is always known in advance. Furthermore, once moral imperatives are derived from nature, even reference to Scripture becomes unnecessary; one can discern the morally right path with no reference to God at all.

There is, however, an alternative way to interpret the Bible and in turn to use the Bible for interpreting creation. Claiming that "the Bible says what it means and means what it says," as one Presbyterian leader recently said, lends itself too easily to biblicism and a literalistic interpretation of Scripture.[24] When one reads the Bible through the lens of the freedom of God, one knows

23. Stackhouse, p. 136.

24. For a discussion of the three aspects of biblical interrelation which I believe are important for the present debate, see my "How to Discuss," pp. 152-54.

that the will of God is not captured through individual biblical commands. These individual passages must be set in the context of the entire biblical story, which in turn must be put in conversation with the human story. Only then does the saving story emerge.[25] I contend that the saving story leads to different conclusions than those offered by theologians, ethicists, and biblical scholars who claim that the Bible dictates the church's rejection of the integrity of homosexuality. There are other ways to interpret scriptural references to the *imago Dei,* complementarity between men and women, and the command regarding procreation.

Imago Dei

The *imago Dei* is not located exclusively in our relationship as male and female. Although Barth's interpretation of the image of God as relational continues to be invaluable for today's theological reflection, his insistence that the male-female relationship is the primal expression of the image of God is misguided. While Barth clearly states that his argument does not dictate that an individual *must* be married in order to reflect the image of God, it is a conclusion difficult to avoid. Many theologians and ethicists who hold to this view find it difficult to give full affirmation to those called into the single life.

Complementarity

The insistence on the essential difference between male and female (and therefore their need for one another as complementary) overlooks the fact that two women or two men can be far more radically different from one another than a man and woman may prove to be.[26] The argument based on complementarity rests too heavily on biology. Hence, those who may otherwise denounce natural law actually seem to be dependent upon it; the will of God for individuals is captured within biology. While Scripture certainly shows that men and women are called to be grateful for one another's presence, their appreciation for one another does not rule out the possibility that some individuals can find complementarity through an intimate relationship with another of the same sex.

25. This argument comes from Paul Lehmann. It is most clearly expressed in an unpublished interview by Marvin Brown, "A Conversation with Paul Lehmann on Biblical Hermeneutics."

26. I am grateful to Cindy Rigby for making this point especially clear in a lecture she gave at Princeton Seminary. Cindy now teaches theology at Austin Theological Seminary in Austin, Tex.

Procreation

Surely the world's overpopulation coupled with the existence of thousands of children needing to be adopted demand a reinterpretation of the biblical injunction to "be fruitful and multiply." Because many homosexual couples provide a loving environment for their children (theirs genetically or by adoption), it is incorrect to maintain that homosexual activity is not life-giving. While sexual activity between two people of the same sex cannot result in pregnancy and birth (apart from artificial means of conception), the intimate relationship between them can produce the desire to provide children with a loving home. The tendency to reduce what is "life-giving" to the biological function of conception marks a grave error in this debate.

Same-sex unions are no more idolatrous, self-centered, or devoid of the ability to give life than heterosexual unions are. Just as one would never deny intimate sexual relations between husband and wife who are infertile, claiming that their relationship is not life-giving, the church is not compelled to forbid sexual relations between same-sex partners who are "married" in the eyes of God if not in the eyes of the state.

3. Incarnation Indicates That Consequences Matter

Many arguments which give normative weight to heterosexuality and in turn reject homosexuality as a valid arena of sexual expression for Christians do so with little or no attention to the particular circumstance or consequences of a given homosexual union. Occasionally ethicists who are opposed to the integrity of homosexual activity will give it limited acceptance as an exception (and a less-than-complete human relationship). Perhaps a woman who runs from a violently abusive heterosexual relationship into a caring lesbian one would not be judged harshly, but accepted given the circumstances (though her choice would fall far short of the ideal). Typically, however, persons engaged in homosexual activity are judged guilty of sin regardless of the circumstances under which they live. All homosexuals are described as participating in the same "lifestyle" and are judged equally guilty.

As a result, the homosexual who lives in faithful partnership with another man is as morally culpable as the homosexual who has multiple sexual partners in an evening. The lesbian mother who, along with her partner, seeks to raise her child in Christian faith commits sin equal in weight to the lesbian who makes inappropriate advances toward a heterosexual acquaintance. The actions of homosexual and lesbian couples which look in every way like those of heterosexual couples except that each partner is of the same sex are deemed morally inferior. What does it mean to name something a sin when there are no victims and no negative consequences of the action?

Of course, some homosexual activity creates victims, but the same is true of heterosexual activity. Furthermore, morality is not solely defined by the lack of victims. Nevertheless, when one finds a situation where two adult lives are enhanced by mutual respect and love, where a child is given a home, where the gospel is taught and followed in faithfulness, what does it mean to declare that these two people are living in sin, exhibiting lust and idolatry? Those who oppose the integrity of homosexual activity tend to claim that homosexuals are selfish and idolatrous *apart from any evidence other than the sexual activity itself.* "Homosexual activity is not a complementary union, able to transmit life; and so it thwarts the call to a life of that form of self-giving which the Gospel says is the essence of Christian living. This does not mean that homosexual persons are not often generous and giving of themselves; but when they engage in homosexual activity they confirm within themselves a disordered sexual inclination which is essentially self-indulgent."[27] On what basis is homosexual activity defined as "essentially self-indulgent"? If two homosexual or lesbian partners vow to be faithful to one another, make sacrifices for the sake of the other, and provide an environment of love to a child legally, morally, and spiritually theirs, where does the self-indulgence lie? When one claims that activity is essentially indulgent apart from any visible evidence of it being so, casuistry has lost its moorings and denied the significance of the incarnation for moral thinking. Attention to particular circumstances and consequences — which is demanded by the incarnation — is lost.

When opponents of church-sanctioned homosexual unions do appeal to consequences, the claims are often unconvincing or inappropriate. Some people, for instance, argue that consequences would be grave for society if we claimed that homosexual unions create families equally as valid as families created by heterosexual partners. This argument is no more true than saying that the affirmation of the single life presents grave consequences to society by threatening the American family. Still others who are opposed to homosexuality make highly inappropriate claims regarding consequences. For instance, in a thinly veiled reference to AIDS, a Roman Catholic document claims that "even when the practice of homosexuality may seriously threaten

27. Congregation for the Doctrine of the Faith, "Letter to the Bishops of the Catholic Church on the Pastoral Care of Homosexual Persons," 31 October 1986, printed in *The Vatican and Homosexuality: Reactions to the "Letter to the Bishops of the Catholic Church on the Pastoral Care of Homosexual Persons,"* ed. Jeannine Gramick and Pat Furey (New York: Crossroad, 1988), p. 4.

the lives and well-being of a large number of people, its advocates remain undeterred and refuse to consider the magnitude of the risks involved."[28] Since the church does not condemn all heterosexual relationships even though they, too, can transmit sexual diseases (including AIDS), the link between AIDS and the morality of all homosexual activity seems particularly cruel.

4. The Goodness of Creation and Its Need for Redemption

As stated above, the church has traditionally located the goodness of human sexual intercourse in its two divinely appointed purposes, the unitive and procreative. No argument in favor of church-sanctioned homosexual unions has to disparage these two purposes of sexual activity. In fact, as human beings we can celebrate both the wonder of pleasure and the miracle of conception and birth that can result from sexual intercourse. In affirming the goodness of these two functions of sexual intercourse, we should not, however, transform them from affirmations to prescriptions. Most Protestants and many Roman Catholics feel free to separate the unitive from the procreative functions of sexual intercourse for heterosexuals, recognizing that there is a time when some heterosexual couples are given the gift of children as a result of their sexual activity and there is a time when childbearing is past, or not advisable, or undesirable. When the latter is true, heterosexual couples are not required to refrain from intimate sexual activity. If this is true for heterosexual couples, why can it not be true for homosexuals?

28. Congregation for the Doctrine of the Faith, p. 5.

Concluding Observations by the Editor, Including a Comparison of Christian with Jewish Biblical Interpretation

DAVID L. BALCH

A. Interpretation of Scripture in the Christian Community

The debates in this volume raise the question of how to read the Bible. Several of the contributors assume aspects of a modern discussion which, on the Christian side, has issued largely from Yale Divinity School, from the Old Testament professor Brevard Childs and the theologians George Lindbeck and Hans Frei. Peter Ochs has coupled this Christian discussion with a similar one going on among Orthodox, Conservative, and Reform Jews, that is, between David Halivni, Michael Fishbane, and Steven Fraade.[1] These hermeneutical debates have consequences for how one interprets scriptural statements about the morality of homosexual acts. The hermeneutical and ethical discussions could and should illuminate each other. Some of the essays in this book assume but do not explicitly outline this hermeneutical debate. I will do so briefly in the following paragraphs, hoping that this gives readers easier access to these current discussions of how we might or should read the Bible in relation to ethical questions. I focus on these conservative ways of interpreting Scripture because their advocates appeal to them in our current debates about moral sexual activity.

1. Peter Ochs, introduction to *The Return to Scripture in Judaism and Christianity: Essays in Postcritical Scriptural Interpretation*, ed. Peter Ochs (New York: Paulist, 1993).

For four reasons I will also follow the lead of Childs, Lindbeck, Frei, and Ochs by offering Jewish parallels to our Christian debates. First, these Yale exegetes and theologians want to help our churches deal with questions of communal, not just individual, lifestyle, and so they have turned to Jewish biblical interpreters for insight, since Jews have focused for millennia on how the whole community may be moral. Second, although we are interpreting some of the same biblical texts in Genesis and Leviticus, most Christians remain ignorant of the similar Jewish debates.[2] Third, Jews have given more sophisticated, devoted attention to the "Old Testament" as an important source of contemporary ethics than have Christian biblical interpreters, who move very quickly to the New Testament. Fourth, whether any particular reader of this volume takes a position on the right or the left, I hope that reading similar debates in another group, in which we Christians are not so directly hooked in emotionally and institutionally, may be less threatening.

Many contemporaries have recognized the inadequacy of a lone intellectual attempting to determine the one, original meaning of any text, including biblical texts. Martin Buber criticized the monologic modern self, alone in his or her autonomy, who has often lost a connection to sacrality and further has been dislocated by autonomy from the ability to listen and hear a wider community.[3] Church theologians strongly object to the academic classroom being the only place the Bible is read closely and seriously.[4] Rather than this inadequate, dyadic model of interpretation (one intellectual scholar reading an ancient text), which tends to privatize religious experience,[5] several have proposed a more actual triadic model which realizes that the interpreter of a text does so within a community.[6] With other scholars I want to emphasize the contributions of the historical-critical method employed by

2. Richard B. Hays, *The Moral Vision of the New Testament: Community, Cross, New Creation: A Contemporary Introduction to New Testament Ethics* (San Francisco: Harper, 1996), p. 381, incorrectly says: "This unambiguous legal prohibition [Lev. 18:22; 20:13] stands as the foundation for the subsequent universal rejection of male, same-sex intercourse within Judaism."

3. Ochs, pp. 3, 8, 26, 32, 37, 41. William C. Spohn, *What Are They Saying about Scripture and Ethics?* rev. ed. (New York: Paulist, 1995), pp. 13-14.

4. E.g., Robert W. Jenson, "Hermeneutics and the Life of the Church," in *Reclaiming the Bible for the Church,* ed. Carl E. Braaten and Robert W. Jenson (Grand Rapids: Eerdmans, 1995), pp. 89-105, here p. 94.

5. Ochs, p. 18.

6. Ochs, pp. 13-15, 18, 23, 34-35, 43; Spohn, *Scripture and Ethics,* p. 12. See James A. Sanders, "Canonical Hermeneutics: True and False Prophecy," in *From Sacred Story to Sacred Text* (Philadelphia: Fortress, 1987, 1992), chap. 5.

individual scholars interpreting biblical texts,[7] but recognize that this is always done within a community of some sort.

1. Rules for Reading Scripture

Recent controversies around homosexuality have stimulated interest in the relation between ethics, exegesis, and hermeneutics that has intensely enlivened our exegesis. For example, the theologian Robert Jenson disagreed with a recent, proposed social statement on sexuality, and so was motivated to propose a list of hermeneutical rules for reading Scripture within the Christian community. The crisis in our churches concerning attitudes toward homosexuality provides us the occasion to discuss such proposals. Some excerpts are as follows:

> Rule one. Scripture is a whole. . . . Rule two. Scripture *is* a whole because and only because it is one long *narrative*. . . . Rule three. To be able to *follow* the single story and grasp Scripture whole, we need to know the story's general plot and *dramatis personae*. . . . Rule four. It is the *church* that knows the plot and *dramatis personae* of the scriptural narrative since the church is one continuous community with the story's actors and narrators, as with its tradents, authors, and assemblers. . . .
>
> Rule five. The church's antecedent knowledge of Scripture's plot and *dramatis personae,* without which she could not read the Bible as a whole, is contained in what Irenaeus calls "the rule of faith," . . . something much on the lines of the Apostles' Creed. . . . [Rule six (Irenaeus assumption).] The *unity* of the story told by the Bible is constituted by its having a single hero throughout: the God of Israel. . . . [Rule seven.] Irenaeus's second assumption is that we do indeed know which God it is of whom Scripture speaks, because the "rule of faith" tells us: He is the specifically *Triune* God. . . . There is an exegetical mandate here also.
>
> Historical-critical reading of Scripture has been an affliction for the faith because people have left the *church* out of their self-understanding as they have practiced it.[8]

7. The historical-critical studies in this volume are extraordinary examples of the method. See also Hays, *Moral Vision,* pp. 3, 212, 291-93, and passim; Brevard S. Childs, "On Reclaiming the Bible for Christian Theology," in *Reclaiming the Bible,* pp. 1-17, at pp. 5-9; Karl P. Donfried, "Alien Hermeneutics and the Misappropriation of Scripture," also in *Reclaiming the Bible,* pp. 19-45, at p. 22.

8. Jenson, pp. 97-99, 104, emphasis Jenson's. Compare Hans W. Frei, "The 'Literal Reading' of Biblical Narrative in the Christian Tradition: Does It Stretch or Will It Break?"

In this volume Bird, Seitz, Jewett, and Greene-McCreight emphasize the first rule, the unity of the Old and New Testaments, although Seitz calls Old Testament ritual law only the "[shadow] of . . . Reality."[9] Other participants in this debate enthusiastically agree with the emphasis on narrative in the second and third rules.[10] Richard Hays, for example, writes:

> we may also ask whether it is necessary to ascribe hermeneutical primacy to one of these modes [rules, principles, paradigms (stories), and symbolic worlds]. The shape of the New Testament canon suggests an answer: as Barth, Yoder, and Hauerwas have seen, the New Testament presents itself to us first of all in the form of story. The four Gospels present the figure of Jesus through the medium of narrative. . . . Thus, *narrative texts in the New Testament are fundamental resources for normative ethics.*[11]

Jenson states his rule four radically: "There can be no churchly reading of Scripture that is not activated and guided by the church's teaching. . . . [T]here can be no reading of the Bible that is not churchly. Therefore there can be no reading of the unitary Bible that is not motivated and guided by the church's teaching."[12]

Other interpreters would more clearly include a Jewish reading of Scripture, for example, Brevard Childs, who calls Rabbi Judah Goldin his "revered teacher" at Yale;[13] both Frei and Lindbeck encourage reappraisal of Christian tendencies to de-legitimize Judaism.[14] In a post-Holocaust world, many Christians have insisted that our reading of Scripture has and should be deepened by Jewish teachers, both by Moses, Jesus, and Paul but also, as

---

in *The Return to Scripture,* pp. 75-77; Spohn, *Scripture and Ethics,* chap. 4; Hays, *Moral Vision,* pp. 5-6, 209, 309-10; George Lindbeck, "The Story-Shaped Church: Critical Exegesis and Theological Interpretation," now excerpted in *The Theological Interpretation of Scripture: Classic and Contemporary Readings,* ed. Stephen E. Fowl (Cambridge: Blackwell, 1997), pp. 39-52.

9. Compare also Childs, pp. 12-13.

10. For example, Ochs, p. 8; Frei, pp. 61, 71-72, 78; George Lindbeck, "Toward a Postliberal Theology," in *The Return to Scripture,* pp. 93-95; Spohn, *Scripture and Ethics,* p. 15 and chap. 4; Hays, *Moral Vision,* pp. 193, 292, 295, 310 (#6). Compare Michael Fishbane, "Extra-Biblical Exegesis: The Sense of Not Reading in Rabbinic Midrash," in *The Return to Scripture,* pp. 172-91, at pp. 177-78, quoting, agreeing with, and criticizing Scholem on *aggadah* (narrative) as "a popular mythology of the Jewish universe."

11. Hays, *Moral Vision,* p. 295, emphasis Hays's.

12. Jenson, p. 98.

13. Childs, p. 7.

14. See Ochs, pp. 17, 22-23, 53. Frei, pp. 58, 79, and Lindbeck, "Toward a Postliberal Theology," p. 100.

Childs, Frei, and Lindbeck have seen, by contemporary teachers as wise as Rabbi Judah Goldin.

Jenson's proposed fifth rule perceives Irenaeus's "rule of faith" as the final criterion.[15] The emphasis on narrative typically involves this assumption. Other interpreters choose a different core: Luther insisted on justification by faith as key,[16] and Christian fundamentalists focus on inerrancy and lack of contradiction within Scripture. Ochs outlines several Jewish interpreters' approaches, including Fishbane's kabbalistic (mystical) reading.[17] Methodologically, the choice one makes or the communal consensus formed about the framework within which to read the Bible dramatically influences the interpretation of Scripture, in this debate of Leviticus and Romans.

2. Faithful Reading of Scripture: Continuity and Discontinuity

Tension does exist between exegesis and Christian pastoral teaching. Jenson assumes that the church is a "continuous community with the story's actors and narrators, as with its tradents, authors, and assemblers,"[18] which means that the story is to be interpreted in light of the trinitarian unity of the God whose story our canon narrates. Perhaps surprisingly for many Christians, Orthodox Jews also experience the relative, not the absolute, unity of God; Hasidic Jews perceive ten *sephirot* within the one God,[19] not three "persons" as among Christians. Religious Jews also claim to be in continuity with the Hebrew Bible. But simply for historical reasons, critical exegesis of the biblical books cannot always begin with theological confession of the three "persons" of the Trinity or the ten *sephirot*. Exegesis is a real conversation, recognizing that our conversation partners, Moses and Paul, may not have held exactly the same beliefs as did the fourth-century church or the twelfth-century kabbalistic Jewish mys-

15. Frei, p. 58, agrees.

16. See Spohn, *Scripture and Ethics*, p. 14, on every interpreter having a "canon within the canon." Some liberation theologians ignore Paul, preferring the prophets and the synoptic accounts of Jesus' ministry. Walter Brueggemann criticizes the historians as apologists for the status quo, emphasizing rather the prophets and Job for their outrage and grief that open the people to the transforming action of God. Brueggemann, *The Prophetic Imagination* (Philadelphia: Fortress, 1978), and *Interpretation and Obedience: From Faithful Reading to Faithful Living* (Minneapolis: Fortress, 1991).

17. Ochs, p. 33.

18. Jenson, pp. 97-98, quoted above as part of his rule four.

19. See, e.g., Moshe Idel, *Kabbalah: New Perspectives* (New Haven: Yale University Press, 1988). *Mystical Union and Monotheistic Faith: An Ecumenical Dialogue*, ed. M. Idel and Bernard McGinn (London: Collier Macmillan, 1989).

tics. As confessing Christians, we believe our story is continuous with Moses and Miriam, Jesus, Mary Magdalene, and Paul, but we must also recognize historical development. Might we not also see the possibility that other communities of God's people who are reading (portions of) the same revealed word could also be in continuity with Scripture?

Interpreters raise the question of how we are to be "faithful" in our reading.[20] The assertion of faithful continuity raises the related question of faithful discontinuity,[21] which Käsemann insists is one of the most important questions in theology,[22] a question that is a burning one for those not in power, e.g., for women who in the twentieth century have reinterpreted Scripture and their place in the story with consequences for their functions in the contemporary church. In the present controversy, the question of continuity and discontinuity with Scripture is a burning one for gay or lesbian Jews and Christians.

B. The Plain (Literal) Sense of Scripture

Several chapters in this book assume what the authors describe as the "plain sense" of Leviticus and Romans in order to draw conclusions about the morality of homosexual acts. Clarity about this method and its consequences is crucial for understanding how these authors propose that we read the Bible in making contemporary ethical choices about sexuality. The Jewish editor of *The Return to Scripture,* Peter Ochs, introduces Christian readers who use this method by explaining that they read the text for a normative community, not merely explaining the texts' historical or cognitive sense for any educated reader.[23] The reading for Christians, especially of the Jesus narratives, has

20. Lindbeck, "Toward a Postliberal Theology," pp. 84, 86, 100: "At least in biblical religions, intratextuality cannot be genuine, cannot be faithful, unless it is innovative." Frei, p. 77; Hays, *Moral Vision,* p. 197. Donfried, p. 42 (criticizing Krister Stendahl), differs from Elizabeth A. Castelli, "*Les Belles Infideles*/Fidelity or Feminism? The Meanings of Feminist Biblical Translation," in *Searching the Scriptures: A Feminist Introduction,* ed. Elisabeth Schüssler Fiorenza and Shelly Matthews (New York: Crossroad, 1993), chap. 13. Brueggemann (n. 16 above) is also different from Hays, "Salvation by Trust? Reading the Bible Faithfully," *Christian Century,* 26 February 1997, pp. 218-22.

21. Frei, p. 59.

22. Ernst Käsemann, "Das Problem des historischen Jesus," in *Exegetische Versuche und Besinnungen* (Göttingen: Vandenhoeck & Ruprecht, 1964), pp. 188-214, here p. 213; see Balch, "The Canon: Adaptable and Stable, Oral and Written; Critical Questions for Kelber and Riesner," *Forum* 7, nos. 3-4 (1991 [1993]): 183-205.

23. Ochs, pp. 4 and 27.

"performative force" for the community's code of religious behavior.[24] This literal reading is prescriptive.[25] The community reads Scripture intratextually, interpreting each text within the context of the whole canon, which generates rules of conduct, meaning both the conduct of scriptural reading itself and ethical conduct.[26] The "truth" read has the "strength" to accomplish some change in the world.[27]

Frei also speaks of intratextual reading as the "normative explication of the meaning a religion has for its adherents."[28] Lindbeck's words are still clearer: theology has a normative task and is to be faithful to the sources of the faith, especially Scripture.[29] Practical theology's task is to apply the rules and principles described by dogmatics. Like carpentry, mathematics, and language, intratextual reading is a form of rule-governed human behavior.[30] As one can describe French culture in French terms, American culture in American terms, one can describe Christian culture "reflexively,"[31] which Lindbeck contrasts with the experiential-expressivist and the propositional approaches.[32] These Yale writers typically appeal to Clifford Geertz's anthropological method of "thick description,"[33] so that the theologian is like an ethnographer acquainted with "extremely small matters," who has "detailed familiarity with the imaginative universe in which . . . acts are signs."[34] Lindbeck argues that Christianity is one of the world religions that have "rel-

24. Ochs, pp. 9, 17.

25. Ochs, p. 15.

26. Ochs, pp. 11, 34, 86.

27. Ochs, p. 19.

28. Frei, p. 77 n. 8.

29. Lindbeck, "Toward a Postliberal Theology," p. 84 n. 10.

30. Lindbeck, "Toward a Postliberal Theology," p. 87.

31. Lindbeck, "Toward a Postliberal Theology," p. 87.

32. Lindbeck, "Toward a Postliberal Theology," pp. 83-84.

33. Not only Geertz's anthropological method but, I suggest, Karen Horney's psychology may illumine this debate. When Lindbeck rejects the experiential-expressivist and the propositional approaches to theology and opts instead for a cultural-linguistic one, he employs three options close to Horney's insight that as human beings we function in one of three basic modes, out of our heart, head, or gut, which seems to describe not only psychological but in the present climate also our theological/exegetical options. See Horney, *Our Inner Conflicts: A Constructive Theory of Neurosis* (New York: Norton, 1945), pp. 42, 68-70, 81-85; Horney, *The Neurotic Personality of Our Time* (New York: Norton, 1937); Horney, *Neurosis and Human Growth: The Struggle toward Self-Realization* (New York: Norton, 1950), chaps. 8, 9, 11; Horney, *New Ways in Psychoanalysis* (New York: Norton, 1939).

34. Lindbeck, "Toward a Postliberal Theology," p. 88; see Ochs, pp. 21, 22, 34, and Greene-McCreight, chap. 9 above.

atively fixed canons, . . . normative instantiations of their semiotic codes."[35] The reader is faithful when describing the universe paradigmatically encoded in Holy Writ, a transpersonal authority that oral cultures lack.[36] Canonical texts, then, he concludes, are a condition for the survival of a religion and also for the possibility of normative theological description; Judaism, Christianity, and Islam are religions of the book.[37] The primary focus is on how life is to be lived.[38]

In his discussion of Scripture and ethics, Richard Hays's final criterion is also pragmatic: "the fruits test: How is the vision embodied in a living community? Does the community manifest the fruit of the Spirit (Gal. 5:22-23)?"[39] One of the three primary images shared by all the canonical retellings of the story is "new creation: the church embodies the power of the resurrection in the midst of a not-yet-redeemed world."[40] With other images, this serves as a canon within the canon without replacing the canonical writings. But for Hays, "[t]he slogan of *sola Scriptura* is both conceptually and practically untenable."[41] Needed additional criteria are tradition, reason, and experience.[42]

Despite similar pragmatic goals, however, Lindbeck and Hays offer quite different hermeneutical approaches. Lindbeck suggests the model of an "ethnographer," and then "reflexively" expects those same "extremely small matters" to characterize Christian life expressed in a different language, a different culture, a later century, etc. Hays bridges the gap of time and culture rather by metaphor: the juxtaposition of two unrelated terms provokes new insight.[43] Similarity between diverse items surprises and delights us into see-

35. Lindbeck, "Toward a Postliberal Theology," p. 89.

36. Lindbeck, "Toward a Postliberal Theology," p. 89. Scholars of world religions have recently focused on interpreting scriptures, and their results differ significantly from Lindbeck's. These sacred texts were always read aloud, so that they are both textual *and* oral authorities. Until the eighteenth century all religions were oral phenomena. Only several centuries after the invention of the printing press did readers fall silent, so that Lindbeck's *contrast* between textuality and orality applies only to the post–printing press world, not to early Judaism or Christianity. See Wilfred Cantwell Smith, *What Is Scripture? A Comparative Approach* (Minneapolis: Fortress, 1993), and my article "The Canon" (cited n. 22).

37. Lindbeck, "Toward a Postliberal Theology," p. 90.

38. Lindbeck, "Toward a Postliberal Theology," p. 96.

39. Hays, *Moral Vision*, p. 213.

40. Hays, *Moral Vision*, p. 198; see pp. 213, 304-5, 310 (#10).

41. Hays, *Moral Vision*, p. 209.

42. Hays, *Moral Vision*, pp. 210, 295-97, and passim.

43. See the review of Hays's book by William C. Spohn, "Is There Such a Thing as New Testament Ethics?" *Christian Century*, 21-28 May 1997, pp. 525-31, at pp. 529-30.

ing the world in new ways. Reading Scripture is a metaphor-making activity, imagining our community within the world outlined by the sacred text. These two different hermeneutical strategies potentially, or rather necessarily, have differing performative force, Lindbeck's tending toward reflexive repetition of concrete modes of behavior, toward laws, Hays's toward imaginative connections with new contexts.

Both Lindbeck and Hays insist on a "literal" reading of Scripture, based on the early church's literal reading of the Gospels' stories of Jesus. "The creed . . . which governed the gospels' use in the church asserted the primacy of their literal sense"; Frei notices that this literal or "rule use" of the New Testament presents Christian biblical reading with two enormous problems.[44] First, autonomous Jewish "literal" readings differ from Christian "literal" readings. Second, since Christian literal readings differ from Jewish ones, Frei suggests supposing "that the literal sense of the New Testament prefigures a still newer reading that displaces it in turn. A new set of inside interpreters transcends the now old (i.e. New Testament),"[45] as Muslims claim to have done.

Frei's questions point to the fact that seismic changes have occurred in ways of reading the "plain sense" of the Bible. Frei is obviously correct that the Orthodox Jewish reading of Scripture differs from conservative Christian "literal" readings of the same biblical books; therefore, below I will propose comparing ways Jews and Christians read Levitical texts on sexuality. Comparing interfaith readings of Scripture, specifically of Leviticus, may shed new light on our related debates.

The Jewish author Michael Fishbane asserts that human suffering provides the occasion for biblical exegesis.[46] There are other stimuli to exegesis, "but only suffering gives rise to genuinely symbolic readings, by which I mean readings which engage the revealed word in a mutually transformative dialogue."[47] Fishbane records two such "axial ruptures in the cultural system" which stimulated major hermeneutical innovations: first, Israel's break with the mythic cosmology of the ancient Near East, a change associated with Moses'/Israel's rejection of other gods/goddesses. Related to this change, early Israel also rejected the pervasive ancient Near Eastern practices of kingship and slavery.[48] The theo-

44. Frei, p. 58.

45. Frei, p. 59.

46. Ochs, pp. 35-36, quoting Michael Fishbane, *The Garments of Torah: Essays in Biblical Hermeneutics* (Bloomington: Indiana University Press, 1989), pp. 34, 64-65.

47. Ochs, pp. 35-36.

48. See George Mendenhall, "The Hebrew Conquest of Palestine," in *The Biblical Archaeologist Reader,* ed. E. F. Campbell, Jr., and D. N. Freedman (New York: Doubleday, 1970), 3:100-120, here pp. 110-11.

logical change had practical, ethical consequences that were discontinuous with earlier practices.

Second, beginning in the time of Ezra, Israel moved "from a culture based on direct divine revelations to one based on their study and reinterpretation."[49] The great prophets received oral/aural revelations/visions directly from God, but the rabbis read and debated ancient texts, which also had enormous practical, ethical consequences, some of which were discontinuous with earlier Israelite religion. Religious leadership, for example, became more intellectual, and its center moved away from Jerusalem to schools in the Diaspora, to Babylon, later to western, then eastern, Europe.

To Fishbane's examples I would add a third and perhaps a fourth hermeneutical change in reading Scripture within Judaism, both of which also have had to do with incalculable suffering. In 1492 the Christian emperor and empress of Spain, Ferdinand and Isabella, expelled the Jewish community from the country, and to overstate it, Judaism became Buddhism; religious Jews turned inward, mystically seeking experience of the ten *sephirot* this side of *Ein Sof,* God beyond experience.[50] Again, the ways the Jewish community worships God and interprets Scripture changed dramatically. Genesis 1 and Ezekiel 1, read in ecstasy, displaced Levitical laws as the center of Scripture. Fourth, as a Christian I will not risk describing ways the Holocaust has changed Jewish hermeneutics, but that catastrophe would be one source of Fishbane's emphasis on suffering.

Fishbane helps us see that significant change typically happens in periods of crisis and suffering. North American Christian interpretation of what the Bible has to say about kings changed during our Revolutionary War against the English Crown. Interpretation of what Paul says about slavery changed during and after the American Civil War. In our century hermeneutical debates no longer center around kingship and slavery, but often focus on gender and sexuality, on male/female and gay/straight polarities.[51]

49. Ochs, pp. 35-36.

50. Gershom Scholem interprets the kabbalah in several significant books. See Moshe Idel, *Studies in Ecstatic Kabbalah* (Albany: SUNY Press, 1988), and n. 19 above.

51. Spohn, *Scripture and Ethics,* p. 7. A Roman Catholic ethicist, Spohn assumes that such change in interaction with the text is possible: "because equality in Christ is more central to Pauline theology, it should be taken more seriously than time-bound advice about maintaining an ancient domestic order which kept women and slaves in subordination. . . . Those who are confident that the Spirit of Christ guided the community's tradition can appeal to subsequent developments in order to correct the limitations in Paul's writings."

The Celluloid Closet by Vito Russo,[52] a book made into a movie, sketches the history of gay/lesbian roles in American films. The movie observes that prior to 1970, *all gay characters in American cinema died* before the movie ended,[53] and those images reflect gay and lesbian persons' consciousness of how they have been treated in our society. An ethic which makes a whole class of people inferior and second-rate has actual, lethal consequences in society and produces prejudice and hatred in our churches. "A group of people cast as immoral by religious leaders and illegal by the Supreme Court become natural targets for ridicule in the popular media. . . . Open violence against gay people in America has reached epidemic proportions, fueled by films that encourage young people to believe that such behavior is acceptable. . . ."[54]

Christian disparagement of Jews from the sixteenth into the twentieth century also had lethal consequences. The disparagement of Jews is partially based on interpretations of the Gospels' passion narratives, and we have begun learning to read them differently. The question of homosexuality involves gender issues; the attitude toward Jews involves race and religion. Gender, race, class, and religion cannot be separated; all are related to discussions of hierarchy versus equality, and prejudice versus acceptance of difference in our society and in our churches.

Further, Spohn observes that whether an interpreter emphasizes a theology of creation or redemption has significant practical consequences. "Where the former is stressed, subordination and submission are usually emphasized — sometimes even silence; where the latter is stressed, freedom, mutuality, and equality are usually emphasized."[55] This also means that an emphasis on creation often opposes change, and an emphasis on redemption encourages change. Hays and, in this volume, Jones and Yarhouse, Seitz, Jewett, and Greene-McCreight emphasize creation, and also oppose innovation in how Christians understand the Bible in relation to homosexuality.[56]

52. Vito Russo, *The Celluloid Closet: Homosexuality in the Movies,* rev. ed. (New York: Harper & Row, 1987).

53. Russo, pp. 347-49, lists the necrology of movie characters. The first American film in which the gay characters did not die was *The Boys in the Band* (1970), and even then the characters were not portrayed sympathetically, but as difficult and flamboyant.

54. Russo, p. 249.

55. Spohn, *Scripture and Ethics,* p. 16, quoting Richard N. Longenecker, *New Testament Social Ethics for Today* (Grand Rapids: Eerdmans, 1984), p. 92.

56. Hays, *Moral Vision,* p. 386, on Romans 1 and Genesis 1–3. Donfried, pp. 36-39, appears to abandon attempts to read Genesis into Romans 1 and relies instead on the citations of Genesis in Mark 10:2-12.

In contrast, Gudorf, Bird, Fredrickson, and Duff emphasize redemption, and suggest innovation in the way Christians interpret the Bible with respect to homosexuality.

C. Scripture in Ethics: Description of Texts, Constructive Theology, and Hermeneutics

The discussions at the conference sponsored by the Louisville Institute were purposefully balanced: the scholars whose papers are printed above represent both poles of the debate for and against the morality of gay and lesbian sexual relationships. Giving examples from both poles of the debate, I will arrange some concluding observations related to the interpretive framework suggested by Richard Hays.[57]

1. Descriptive

The first task of interpretation is descriptive: How adequate is the exegesis of related texts? This volume presents polarized options. Phyllis Bird interprets the legal texts, Leviticus 18:22 and 20:13, as prohibiting homosexual humiliation, a threat to male honor, not to marriage or reproductive needs. Further, Genesis 1 is not the historical matrix in which the Levitical prohibitions of homosexual acts arose, since the Genesis story is concerned with relations between male and female as the basis for reproduction of the species. For Chris Seitz, on the contrary, Scripture in both the Old and New Testaments presents the law of God, and its plain literal sense proscribes homosexual behavior.

The three New Testament scholars also offer polarized options. William Schoedel shows that Greco-Roman medical doctors debated whether "passion," understood as a disease because it was insatiable, had its source in the body or the mind. Paul assumes the later opinion in Romans 1, and Schoedel concludes that contemporary medical opinions may have influenced Paul's ethical argument. David Fredrickson attempts to shed new light on Romans 1:24-27. He argues that Paul condemned unnatural "use," insatiable passion, addiction to sex, that Paul assumed current attitudes but expressed no negative argument against homosexuality either in Romans 1

57. Hays, *Moral Vision,* chap. 16. He outlines an interpretive checklist on pp. 212-13; see p. 310.

or in 1 Corinthians 6.[58] In stark contrast, Robert Jewett claims that Paul denounces homoerotic relations in Romans 1, a proof of God's wrath.

At the descriptive level, the discussion has become a debate between professional scholars. In addition, those scholars at this conference who tend to reinterpret texts focus on their ancient Near Eastern or Greco-Roman historical contexts (Bird, Schoedel, and Fredrickson), a historical method disputed by those who understand themselves as traditional (Seitz and Greene-McCreight).

2. *Constructive*

In this volume Greene-McCreight suggests that the debate is essentially about hermeneutics, about how to interpret Scripture. Like Seitz, she emphasizes the two covenants in the Bible, specifically including Old Testament law that has not been replaced in the new, eschatological age. The church does need to repent for allowing and promoting violence toward gays and lesbians, but is not free to bless their relationships that are prohibited by Scripture and tradition.

Nancy Duff, on the contrary, insists that the starting point for constructive theology is not human freedom, whether expressed in heterosexual or homosexual relationships or in celibacy; rather, we must begin with divine freedom. Commandments in the Bible are not prescriptive rules, but descriptive accounts of the world that God has made fit for human beings. God in God's freedom has "called" some to celibacy, others into heterosexual relationships, others into homosexual relationships.

3. *Hermeneutics*

a. Jewish and Christian Tradition

Lindbeck has shown that Luther as pastor and catechist taught Scripture in some ways like the rabbis.[59] Luther, who is usually understood as anti-Jewish

58. On 1 Cor. 6:9, see the important essay by Dale B. Martin, "*Arsenokoites* and *Malakos:* Meanings and Consequences," in *Biblical Ethics and Homosexuality: Listening to Scripture,* ed. Robert L. Brawley (Louisville: Westminster/John Knox, 1996), pp. 117-36.

59. George Lindbeck, "Martin Luther and the Rabbinic Mind," in *Understanding the Rabbinic Mind: Essays on the Hermeneutic of Max Kadushin,* ed. Peter Ochs (Atlanta: Scholars Press, 1990), pp. 141-64, a reference I owe to Prof. Marty Stortz.

or at least un-Jewish in his controversial theology, wrote the Small and Large Catechisms as a pastor, focusing on the Ten Commandments, not as many as the 613 rabbinic laws, but still ten commandments. This is the primary way ordinary folks in congregations knew and still know Luther. And when he explained these catechisms, he interpreted them through scriptural stories, like rabbinic, haggadic midrash. Lindbeck argues that the catechetical Luther is the authoritative one.[60] Like the rabbis, Luther preached the Bible, especially the Decalogue as interpreted by the New Testament, as a practical guide which forms the total life of whole communities.[61]

I suggest that one way forward is to pay attention to some traditions that the church has ignored in our present debates. It may be less threatening for persons on either side of the Christian debate to hear arguments made in Jewish denominations, in which we are not directly involved. As seen above, both Lindbeck and Frei encourage conversations between Jewish and Christian interpretation of Scripture. We worship the same God, or we are at least in ecumenical discussion concerning our different understandings of the God revealed through Moses and the prophets. And we are reading (portions of) the same Scriptures, all of us with serious concern about lifestyle. The conflicts in our communities have similar contours, although Jewish interpreters have paid more serious attention to the Hebrew Bible as a source of ethics than Christians have.

Concerning homosexual practices, however, there is an important difference between Jewish and Christian readings of Scripture: unlike Leviticus, "the New Testament contains no passages that clearly articulate a *rule* against homosexual practices."[62] Paul *assumes* gender differences, but he does not make an *argument* against homosexual acts. With this difference in mind, Christians may benefit by attending to Jewish discussions. I will present selected advocates of both poles of the discussion, for and against the morality of gay and lesbian relationships, beginning with those against.

60. Lindbeck, "Martin Luther," pp. 156, 161.

61. Lindbeck, "Martin Luther," pp. 163-64. On the other hand, Luther supported his colleague Philipp Melanchthon, who composed the foundational Augsburg Confession, which realistically recognizes change: "The apostles directed that one should abstain from blood and from what is strangled. Who observes this prohibition now? . . . Scarcely any of the ancient canons are observed according to the letter, and many of the regulations fall into disuse from day to day even among those who observe such ordinances most jealously. It is impossible to give counsel or help to consciences unless this mitigation is practiced. . . ." *The Book of Concord,* trans. Theodore G. Tappert (Philadelphia: Fortress, 1959), pp. 92-93.

62. Hays, *Moral Vision,* p. 394.

Jewish tradition has unequivocally condemned homosexuality.[63] This has been based on the explicit prohibitions of Leviticus 18:22 and 20:13 as well as on certain narrative passages, including Genesis 9:22; 19:5; and Judges 19. Norman Lamm was an early Orthodox Jewish writer who distinguished four Jewish attitudes: repressive, practical, permissive, and psychological.[64] Lamm chose the "practical" option: laws criminalizing homosexual acts are unenforceable but should remain on the books to indicate societal disapproval; by universal consent, however, they should not be enforced. Psychologically, he thought, homosexuality should be considered an illness. Spero agreed: Halakah (traditional law) is divinely inspired and unchangeable, not relativistic; he advocated therapy to change homosexual orientation.[65] Wurzburger added that Judaism proscribes homosexual practices but does not blame individuals who have pathological preferences.[66] Dresner argued that homosexuality is a violation of the order of creation (Gen. 1:27-28; 2:18-24; 5:2).[67] Traditional law is ultimate for the Orthodox, and modern scientific analysis cannot alter its rejection of homosexual sex.[68]

Dennis Prager, a widely influential Jewish writer, publishes a quarterly journal that devoted a whole issue to the subject.[69] He argues that Judaism has done civilization a service by forcing the (male) sexual genie into the marital bottle. Judaism desexualized God; ethical monotheism was a revolution, including a war on the sexual practices of the world religions. Homosexuality was ubiquitous except in Judaism.[70] Torah's prohibition of same-sex acts began human liberation from unrestrained sexuality and women's liberation from being

63. See the survey by Rabbi Yoel H. Kahn, "Judaism and Homosexuality: The Traditionalist/Progressive Debate," *Journal of Homosexuality* 18, nos. 3-4 (1989-90): 47-82, which begins with the conclusion stated above.

64. Norman Lamm, "Judaism and the Modern Attitude to Homosexuality," in *Encyclopedia Judaica Yearbook 1974* (Jerusalem: Keter, 1974), pp. 194-205, reprinted in *Jewish Bioethics,* ed. Fred Rosner and J. David Bleich (New York: Sanhedrin, 1979), pp. 197-218.

65. Moshe H. Spero, "Homosexuality: Clinical and Ethical Challenges," *Tradition* 17, no. 4 (1979): 53-73.

66. Walter Wurzburger, "Preferences Are Not Practices," *Judaism* 32 (1983): 425.

67. Samuel H. Dresner, "Homosexuality and the Order of Creation," *Judaism* 40, no. 3 (1991): 309-21, referring to the article on "Mixed Species," in *Encyclopedia Judaica* 12 (1971), pp. 169-72. Dresner is cited by Jewett, chap. 8, n. 72 above.

68. An observation by Kahn, "Judaism and Homosexuality," p. 54.

69. Dennis Prager, "Judaism, Homosexuality and Civilization," *Ultimate Issues* 6, no. 2 (1990): 1-24. He approvingly (p. 12) cites Lamm's article (n. 64 above) and calls Reform Judaism's decision to ordain avowed homosexuals a break with the Jewish people, a break not just with Jewish law but with Jewish values (p. 19).

70. He relies on David E. Greenberg, *The Construction of Homosexuality* (Chicago: University of Chicago Press, 1988).

peripheral to men's lives.[71] The essence of Judaism is choosing life, not death (Deut. 30:19); Jewish priests alone among the world's religions are forbidden to come into contact with the dead. Male celibacy, sacred in many religions, is a sin in Judaism. Jews' most distinguishing characteristic has been commitment to family life.[72] Through Abraham, all families of the earth are to be blessed (Gen. 12:3; 28:14). Scripture contains the Song of Songs, a book praising heterosexual sensual love. Judaism's sexual ideal is marital sex; all other forms of sexual behavior deviate from that ideal. There is a continuum of wrong from premarital sex, to celibacy, to adultery, to homosexuality, incest, and bestiality.[73] The millennia-old battle for a family-based, sexually monogamous society has been hard-won; to accept homosexuality would not be new.[74]

Herschel Matt, a Conservative Jewish thinker, moved away from the category of "illness" to speaking of "sexual deviance, malfunctioning, or abnormality — usually unavoidable and often irremediable."[75] Matt recognized traditional reasons for condemning homosexuality, but argued that Halakah (traditional law) recognizes the category of "constraint" *(me'ones)* excusing one in circumstances beyond one's control. Because there is no possibility of change to a heterosexual preference, the homosexual should be considered to be acting under "constraint." A decade later, Matt went further and rejected his own suggestion that homosexuals should be tolerated because they are acting out of uncontrollable compulsion. Homosexuality is rather part of God's creation; therefore, gay men and lesbians may be ordained to the rabbinate.[76] Matt went further than many other Conservative Jews, but virtually all Jewish writers support the decriminalization of private sexual acts.

Another Conservative rabbi, Robert Kirschner, pointed out that "in the interpretation of Jewish tradition, where there is a halachic will, there is a halachic way. In other words, if our understanding of a situation changes, we Jews have always found a way to make the law fit in with our new understanding."[77] In the Talmud the word *heresh* means a deaf person, who was not al-

71. Prager, p. 9.

72. Prager, p. 10.

73. Prager, p. 11.

74. Prager, p. 12.

75. Herschel J. Matt, "Sin, Crime, Sickness or Alternative Life-Style? A Jewish Approach to Homosexuality," *Judaism* 27 (1978): 13-24, at p. 20.

76. H. J. Matt, "Homosexual Rabbis?" *Conservative Judaism* 39, no. 3 (1987): 29-33, at p. 31.

77. Robert Kirschner, "Halakhah and Homosexuality: A Reappraisal," *Judaism* 37, no. 4 (1988): 450-58. "Those who argue for the acceptance of homosexuality assume that halakhah cannot change. . . . [But] Halakhah, like any living thing, must be capable of

lowed to testify in a Jewish court nor to receive other privileges of "unblemished" Jews (see Lev. 21:16-24). But sign language was invented, and doctors have learned more about the abilities of deaf persons, with the result that even in Orthodox Jewish communities, *heresh* is now taken to mean "a mentally incompetent deaf-mute." Since the late nineteenth century, hearing-impaired Jews have been accorded the rights and respect that was their due all along; Jewish law has been changed. Kirschner writes that the Jewish imperative, from within Halakic tradition, is to "rescind the ancient denunciation of homosexuals and to recognize that all persons, in their unique sexual being, are the work of God's hands and the bearers of God's image."[78]

Reconstructionists, one of the four large denominations among American Jews, debated the subject from 1983 to 1985, deciding to admit students to the Reconstructionist Rabbinical College in Philadelphia without discriminating on the basis of sexual orientation. Several years later they published a report.[79] The booklet discusses fifteen values fundamental to Reconstructionism, including human integrity, holiness, equality, caring relationships, stable family life, child rearing, and justice. There are discussions of the Levitical texts and other biblical passages traditionally understood to concern sexual activity between men as well as discussions of contemporary science and its relation to Jewish sources.

> Jewish values that affirm the integrity and equality of human beings have primacy over historically conditioned attitudes based on biblical, rabbinic, and medieval texts that condemn homosexuality. (36) Many who reject Jewish law in other areas assert the binding nature of the biblical condemnation of homosexuality. We bemoan justifying injustice by citing biblical law. (36) Due to contemporary reproductive technologies and the option of adoption, lesbian and gay Jews can and do form stable families with children, contributing to Jewish family life. (37) Same-gender partnerships have the same potential for embodying these qualities [companionship and comfort, holiness, mutual respect, trust, care, and love in committed relationships] as do heterosexual marriages. . . . we support long-term partnerships between gays or lesbians and affirm that *kedushah* [holiness] resides

---

change and growth" (p. 451). Halakic discourse is not a priori, not based on deduction, but is a posteriori, is empirical (p. 451). He refers to David Novak, *Halakhah in a Theological Dimension*, Brown Judaic Studies 68 (Chico, Calif.: Scholars Press, 1985), pp. 1-10.

78. Kirschner, p. 458.

79. *Homosexuality and Judaism: The Reconstructionist Position: The Report of the Reconstructionist Commission on Homosexuality* (Wyncote, Pa.: Federation of Reconstructionist Congregations and Havurot and the Reconstructionist Rabbinical Association, 1993), pp. 1-42.

> in committed relationships between same-gender Jewish couples. (37) Judaism has always insisted upon responsibility in expressing sexuality. This includes concern for both partners' emotional, physical, spiritual, financial, and sexual needs, and a commitment to keeping vows of sexual fidelity. Love and responsibility go hand in hand. (37)
>
> We affirm the 1991 resolution of the Federation of Reconstructionist Congregations and Havurot barring discrimination regarding sexual orientation in the forwarding of resumes for rabbinic positions, as a first step towards ending all discrimination in rabbinic placement. (40) . . . we recognize pluralism within our ranks and acknowledge that the issue of rabbinic officiation at same-gender commitment ceremonies requires sensitive judgments best left to individual rabbis. (40)

The discussion among Reform Jews intensified when Beth Chayim Chadashim (BCC), a gay and lesbian–outreach synagogue of Los Angeles, applied for membership in the Union of American Hebrew Congregations (UAHC).[80] A legal opinion was issued stating that homosexuals are sinners, that they should not organize in separate synagogues, and that all sinners are welcome in existing family-oriented synagogues.[81] Sanford Raggins, rabbi of the synagogue that provided BCC its first home, compared the Jewish experience of intolerance and oppression to the homosexual experience. Calls for justice and liberation must take precedence, Raggins argued, over traditional teaching: "our heritage is not limited to . . . the Book of Leviticus."[82] Against the urging of their rabbis' ad hoc committee on the subject, the lay UAHC accepted Beth Chayim Chadashim's application for membership (1974), and a student rabbi was placed there in 1976.

In 1995 the General Assembly of the UAHC, led by Rabbi Alexander M. Schindler, adopted a resolution "promoting equal employment and leadership opportunities for lesbians and gays in the Reform movement" and commended the use of *Kulanu*,[83] a book with chapters on the history of the de-

80. Reform Judaism is organized into three primary institutions: (1) the rabbinical colleges, (2) the rabbis organized as the Central Conference of American Rabbis (CCAR), and (3) laypeople organized as the Union of American Hebrew Congregations (UAHC). The rabbinical colleges ordain rabbis.

81. See Kahn, "Judaism and Homosexuality," pp. 58-59, which I am summarizing.

82. Sanford Raggins, "An Echo of the Pleas of Our Fathers," *CCAR Journal* 20, no. 3 (1983): 45.

83. *Kulanu (All of Us): A Program for Congregations Implementing Gay and Lesbian Inclusion: A Handbook for UAHC Congregations*, prepared by the UAHC Task Force on Lesbian and Gay Inclusion (New York: Union of American Hebrew Congregations Press, 1996). The 1995 resolution is reproduced in *Kulanu*, p. 138.

bate, on suggesting steps toward inclusivity, on ritually recognizing life cycles, on synagogue leadership training, on (re)defining family and temple membership, and a final one on employment practices. I will conclude my brief survey of attitudes toward "tradition" among contemporary American Jews with some citations from *Kulanu.*

In a sermon of 1993 at Hebrew Union College, Lisa Edwards interpreted the ethics of Leviticus as follows:[84]

> We are the stranger. You must not oppress the stranger. "You shall love the stranger as yourself, for you were strangers in the land of Egypt." (Lev 19:34)
>
> We are your gay brothers and your lesbian sisters: "You shall not hate your brother or sister in your heart." (19:17) We are lesbian and gay victims of gay-bashing and murder. "You may not stand by idly when your neighbor's blood is being shed." (19:16)[85]
>
> We are your gay and lesbian neighbors. "You must not oppress your neighbor," (19:13) "You must judge your neighbor justly." (19:15) "You shall love your neighbor as yourself." (19:18)[86]

Kulanu has an appendix that prints resolutions passed by the lay (UAHC) and rabbinic (CCAR) organizations of Reform Judaism. The Women of Reform Judaism were calling for the decriminalization of homosexuality as early as 1965,[87] followed by UAHC and CCAR in 1977.[88] In 1987 the UAHC General Assembly endorsed a resolution that "[sexual] orientation should not be a criterion for membership or participation in an activity of any synagogue." This resolution was supported by Leviticus 19:18 ("you shall love your neighbor as yourself"), by Isaiah 56:7 ("my house shall be called a house of prayer for all peoples"), and by Genesis 1:26-27 ("Let us make humankind in our image . . ." [NRSV]). Genesis was interpreted in light of Isaiah as follows: "each of us, created in God's image, has a unique talent which can contribute to that high moral purpose *(tikkun olam);* and to exclude any Jew from the community of Israel lessens our chances of achieving that goal."[89] This 1987 UAHC resolution

84. *Kulanu,* p. 8.

85. Also quoted in a similar context by Rabbi Schindler in his Presidential Keynote Address to the UAHC biennial assembly of 1989 (*Kulanu,* p. 5).

86. Also cited by the UAHC in 1987 as support for lesbian and gay participation in Reform Jewish worship and leadership (*Kulanu,* p. 119).

87. *Kulanu,* p. 115.

88. *Kulanu,* pp. 116-17.

89. *Kulanu,* p. 119. See Kahn, "Judaism and Homosexuality," p. 64. Several writers in *Kulanu* appeal to Isa. 56:7 (pp. 77 and 119) and Gen. 1:26-27 (pp. 122 and 138). Contrast Dresner (cited n. 67 above).

recommended that the CCAR committee on liturgy develop liturgically inclusive language. In 1989 the UAHC made clear that membership would be accepted on terms of visibility, not invisibility.[90] In 1990 the CCAR received a committee report on rabbinic placement which discouraged pulpit selection committees from requesting information on the sexual orientation of candidates; the report supported civil rights for gays and lesbians in housing and employment, since all human beings are created in the divine image.[91] The same report commended the rabbinic college for clarifying its admission policy, considering an applicant's sexual orientation only in the context of his or her overall suitability for the rabbinate.[92] In 1991 both Temple Youth and Temple Educators supported the ordination of gay and lesbian rabbis.[93] In the same year the Women of Reform Judaism recommended that "all rabbis, regardless of sexual orientation, be accorded the opportunity to fulfill the sacred vocation which they have chosen."[94] The Commission on Social Action called for the elimination of discrimination in the military.[95] Both the CCAR and the Temple Youth called for the Boy Scouts to open its membership to all men and boys without regard to sexual orientation.[96] In 1993 the UAHC called for the recognition of gay and lesbian partnerships, that partners be included in health programs, receive spousal survivor rights, and be recognized as fit parents.[97]

In June 1998 an ad hoc committee on human sexuality reported to the CCAR, discussing principles such as the created universe, people of the covenant, contemporary knowledge, "in the image of God," justice, family, covenantal relationship, joy, and holiness, concluding: "we believe that the relationship of a Jewish, same-gender couple is worthy of affirmation through appropriate Jewish ritual, and that each rabbi should decide about officiation according to his/her own informed rabbinic conscience."[98]

In conclusion, Orthodox, Conservative, Reconstructionist, and Reform Jews have all engaged in careful and devoted interpretation of the Torah and the prophets. As Toulouse has argued is the case among Christians, all have

90. *Kulanu,* p. 120. Rabbi Schindler argued: "We who were Marranos in Madrid, who clung to the closet of assimilation and conversion in order to live without molestation, cannot deny the demand for gay and lesbian visibility" (*Kulanu,* p. ix).

91. *Kulanu,* p. 122, citing Gen. 1:27-28.

92. *Kulanu,* p. 123.

93. *Kulanu,* pp. 125-26.

94. *Kulanu,* p. 127.

95. *Kulanu,* p. 131.

96. *Kulanu,* pp. 132-33.

97. *Kulanu,* p. 134.

98. The five-page CCAR Ad Hoc Committee Report is available from the Religious Action Center of Reform Judaism, 2027 Massachusetts Ave. NW, Washington, DC 20036.

changed their position, the Orthodox continuing to proscribe homosexual practice while not blaming individuals for their sexual preferences. Some Conservative and many Reform and Reconstructionist Jews have moved beyond most Christian denominations by endorsing gay marriage and ordination. Readers of this volume will have different evaluations of their biblical hermeneutics and of their conclusions concerning moral lifestyles. However one judges their arguments, we might agree that Jews have been more concerned and more insightful about Torah as a source of contemporary ethics than Christians have been.

b. Reason

The essays above have made a significant contribution to this aspect of the discussion. Seitz's first sentence states that "Scripture is the authority that guides the church's reflection on human sexual behavior." For him, reason and experience are not categories that count along with Scripture in arriving at moral values, neither in the priests' Levitical world, in Paul's, or in ours. The wrongfulness of same-sex behavior would best be grounded in the Old Testament, not in rhetorically useful arguments from the (Greco-Roman) "milieu." Seitz's view assumes that the texts were written in response to God's revelation and in relation to each other, isolated from their contemporary historical and cultural milieu. Greene-McCreight also concludes her essay by denying that we can appeal to experience over against Scripture and tradition.

Despite their fascinating review of modern scientific research on homosexuality, Jones's and Yarhouse's position is close to Seitz's. Toward the beginning of their conclusion, they assert that "even if the scientific findings in the four areas we have examined were clear and unequivocal, their relevance to the moral debate would still be less than decisive." In their judgment scientific research does not speak definitively to the ecclesiastical debates of the Christian church. Further, natural science cannot validate moral imperatives. They do modify their position, backing away from completely discounting current, scientific reason: "We would reject, however, the utter independence of science and ethical analysis. Good science should inform ethical analysis." Actually, Nancy Duff agrees that uncovering biological origins of homosexual orientation does not answer the moral question.

As Gudorf observes, the standing of contemporary science within Christian ethical debates is fundamental. Jones, Yarhouse, and Seitz reject any central role for scientific research; Gudorf, however, emphasizes its importance as continuing revelation. Ironically, conservative scholars who appeal to the story of God's creation of the world in Genesis tend to understand that text alone as defining creation, and de-emphasize or often discount scientific research as a source of information and value about the created world.

Both Leviticus and Romans make ancient "scientific" assumptions about nature and gender that neither conservative nor progressive scholars could accept today. Phyllis Bird has argued, agreeing with Nissinen, that the passive sexual role in ancient Near Eastern culture was always defined as feminine, and that homoerotic activity prohibited by Leviticus was a threat to male honor, not to marriage or to reproductive needs, and that Genesis 1, which emphasizes procreation, was not the historical matrix in which homosexual prohibitions arose. The law, then, Bird writes, is a gender-role prescription that defines the male as active, the female as passive. On this "scientific" definition of gender, then, Leviticus and 1 Corinthians 6 agree. As one ancient scientist expresses it:

> All females are less spirited than the males, except the bear and leopard: in these the female is held to be braver. But in the other kinds the females are softer *(malakotera)*, more vicious, less simple, more impetuous, more attentive to the feeding of the young, while the males on the contrary are more spirited, wilder, simpler, less cunning. There are traces of these characters in virtually all animals, but they are all the more evident in those that are more possessed of character and especially in man. For man's nature *(phusin)* is the most complete, so that these dispositions too are more evident in humans. Hence a wife is more compassionate than a husband is and more given to tears, but also more jealous and complaining and more apt to scold and fight. The female is also more dispirited and despondent than the male, more shameless and lying, is readier to deceive and has a longer memory; furthermore she is more wakeful, more afraid of action, and in general is less inclined to move than the male, and takes less nourishment. The male on the other hand, as we have said, is a readier ally and is braver than the female. . . .[99]

In relation to this "biology," Paul condemned any male for being "soft" (1 Cor. 6:9). But since we no longer learn in modern biology classes that all male animals are braver than females, that females are "softer," simpler, less cunning, more jealous and despondent than males, can we still accept the sexual ethic that is correlated with such "biology"? The changes between ancient and modern biology do not put the gospel or the core ethic of loving God and our neighbor in doubt, but the changes do raise serious

99. Aristotle, *History of Animals* 9.1.608a32-608b18 (trans. Balme in Loeb).

questions about particular ethical values that readers of this volume will evaluate differently.

Much remains to be done. Donna Haraway, a biologist trained at Yale, has pointed out that in the ancient and also in the modern world, views of "nature" are a cultural construction.[100] It is obvious to us that Aristotle's ancient patriarchal Greek biology was a cultural product, related to his ethics and politics. Haraway argues the same for modern biology, that scientists have projected cultural systems, including patriarchal ones, onto "nature," which is then used to buttress ethical systems. The essays above on ancient and modern psychological anthropology raise the question of how "nature" and ethics are related.

Schoedel's, Bird's, and Fredrickson's discussions show that our ecclesiastical debates do not concern simply Paul's ethics and ours, but Paul's *science and* ethics and our science and ethics. Schoedel persuasively suggests that Paul's ethical assumptions were related to Greco-Roman science. The pseudo-Aristotelian *Problemata,* dated around the first century C.E., appeals to "nature" to explain why some males continue to play passive sexual roles beyond teenage years, theories that are opposed in the second century C.E. by the doctor Soranus. Some of these theories are reflected in Philo and are close to Romans 1. The biology Paul was taught influenced his ethical assumptions and arguments. The modern psychological observations made above by Jones, Yarhouse, and Gudorf must be part of our discussions. Simply observing that the biblical ethical attitude toward homosexual acts is univocal is not enough. Asking how modern biology and psychology influence Christian ethics is also necessary. Again, readers of this volume will give differing answers to this question.

c. Experience Influencing Scripture Interpretation

As the discussion above illustrates, some Christians but not others are willing to appeal to experience in interpreting the Bible.[101] For example, introducing his

100. Donna J. Haraway, *Simians, Cyborgs, and Women: The Reinvention of Nature* (New York: Routledge, 1991), p. 2; see her bibliography, including her own earlier *Primate Visions: Gender, Race, and Nature in the World of Modern Science* (New York: Routledge, 1989). Also Judith Butler, *Bodies That Matter: The Discursive Limits of "Sex"* (New York: Routledge, 1993), references for which I thank my daughter, Christina Balch.

101. Significant collections of articles are *Gay American History: Lesbians and Gay Men in the USA: A Documentary History,* ed. Jonathan Ned Katz, rev. ed. (New York: Meridian, 1992); *The Lesbian and Gay Studies Reader,* ed. Henry Abelove, Michele Ama Barale, and David M. Halperin (New York: Routledge, 1993); and *We Are Everywhere: A Historical Sourcebook of Gay and Lesbian Politics,* ed. Mark Blasius and Shane Phelan (New

chapter on homosexuality, Richard Hays narrates experiences with his gay friend Gary just before he died of AIDS.[102] In concert with the hermeneutical discussions of Frei and Lindbeck outlined by Ochs, I propose that as Christians we look at the analogous experience of the Jewish community. Janet Marder writes out of her experience as the straight rabbi of the world's first gay and lesbian synagogue, the Beth Chayim Chadashim in Los Angeles, a community she had served for five years by 1989, explaining how living with this group has changed her. Knowing actual people instead of merely theories has changed her understanding of the nature of homosexuality, of Halakah (law) in liberal Judaism, and of the place of lesbians and gays in the Jewish community.

> [After five years of experience:] My attitude toward homosexuality has moved from uncertain tolerance to full acceptance. I see it now as a sexual orientation offering the same opportunities of love, fulfillment, spiritual growth, and ethical action as heterosexuality. I still do not know what "causes" homosexuality, but I must confess that at this point I do not much care — any more than I care about what "causes" some people to have a special aptitude for music and others for baseball. I simply accept with pleasure the diversity of our species.[103]

Rabbi Marder also comments on the place of lesbians and gays in Jewish religious life (similar to ways churches treat them): some official recognition (by Reform and Reconstructionist institutions), denial of the right to marry, refusal to allow them leadership positions, acceptance as long as they remain invisible.

Sheila Shulman, rabbi of Beit Klal Yisrael and lecturer at Leo Baeck College, makes an argument similar to Rabbi Marder's, which we Christians might do well to overhear:

> In the *Sifra*, a collection of midrashim on Leviticus, there is a discussion between Ben Azzai and Akiva about which is the most inclusive com-

York: Routledge, 1997). See also Dennis Altman, *Homosexual Oppression and Liberation* (New York: New York University Press, 1971; revised 1993), chap. 2: "Oppression: The Denial of Identity."

102. Hays, *Moral Vision*, pp. 379-80.

103. Janet R. Marder, "Getting to Know the Gay and Lesbian Shul: A Rabbi Moves from Tolerance to Acceptance," in *Twice Blessed*, ed. Christie Balka and Andy Rose (Boston: Beacon Press, 1989), pp. 209-17, at p. 213. Cp. Rabbi Yoel H. Kahn, "*The Kedushah* of Homosexual Relationships," in *Same-Sex Marriage: Pro and Con: A Reader*, ed. Andrew Sullivan (New York: Vintage, 1997), pp. 71-77, reprinted from *Central Conference of American Rabbis Yearbook* 94 (1989).

> mandment. Ben Azzai says that the verse we have been looking at, "In the image of God made He them" [Gen. 1:27], is more inclusive than "Love your neighbor." (Sifra [Lev.] 19:18) Certainly, as a woman, I share Ben Azzai's preference, for two reasons. . . . How much time, energy, and love has each of us spent with women friends who were depressed, who were caught up in self-hatred . . . ? I have seen those same women, full of self-loathing . . . be courteous and gentle, attentive and caring, to friends, to children, to the most casual acquaintance, to anybody, yet remorseless with themselves. So I began to wonder after a while if it would not make more sense for women, to hear that commandment the other way around — "Love yourself as you love your neighbor. . . ." The second reason I prefer Ben Azzai's position has to do with the degree and extent to which the potentiality and actuality of our bonding with each other has been distorted and often destroyed by the woman-hatred, or at best the obliviousness to our existence as persons, that is embedded in our tradition.[104]

Significant numbers of Christian women, perhaps especially lesbians, may think and feel the same way about our tradition as Rabbi Shulman feels about hers.

From an Orthodox perspective, Alan Unterman writes differently: For Jews sex is pleasurable but above all reproductive.[105] Gays remain Jews, can *daven* (pray) in straight *shuls* (synagogues) and participate in family rituals, as Jewish sinners.[106] The *mitzwoth* (commandments) do not recognize either homosexuals or heterosexuals, because they differentiate males and females, not sexual preferences, but still Maimonides' formulation of the law rules out homosexuality within Orthodox religious space.[107] It is unlikely that the Halakah (traditional law) will ever approve the besetting sins of Anglo-Jewry. The most sympathetic Orthodox response is that Jewish gay people are substantially different and have symptoms of a sickness, an attitude that gays would resent.[108] The divisions

104. Sheila Shulman, "What Is Our Love?" in *Jewish Explorations of Sexuality,* ed. Jonathan Magonet (Providence: Berghahn, 1995), pp. 103-15, at p. 108. See *Sifra: An Analytical Translation,* by Jacob Neusner, Brown Judaic Studies 140 (Atlanta: Scholars Press, 1988), 3:109. Compare n. 113 below.

105. Alan Unterman, "Judaism and Homosexuality: Some Orthodox Perspectives," in *Jewish Explorations of Sexuality,* pp. 67-74, at p. 67.

106. Unterman, p. 69.

107. Unterman, pp. 70-71. Compare Greene-McCreight's remarks above on law and gender.

108. Unterman, pp. 73-74.

these quotations document within Judaism are familiar to Christians engaged in analogous conflicts.[109]

These differences between the ways Reform and Orthodox rabbis read Leviticus are parallel to divisions within the Christian community. As an exegete, it is striking to me that the differences are also parallel to disputes within earliest Judaism and Christianity. Some early Jews understood holiness to mean separation from other peoples (Lev. 20:26), but other Jews were more assimilated, so that Judaism in the Hellenistic age was not uniform.[110] All analogies are faulty, so without intending a precise parallel, I observe that the ancient gap between the Qumran Essenes on the one hand and an Egyptian Jewish text like the letter of Aristeas[111] on the other parallels the modern differences between Orthodox and Reform Judaism. I draw the analogy here because the Essenes and Aristeas drew very different conclusions about lifestyle. Essenes thought most other Jews unclean and avoided them, but Aristeas narrates stories of priestly Jews from Jerusalem eating at a symposium with pagans in Egypt!

The earliest Christians were also divided by similar differences, as we see already in the New Testament. Raymond Brown distinguished four groups, each of which includes both Jews and Gentiles: (1) those who insist on full observance of the Mosaic Law; (2) those who keep some Jewish observances, e.g., James and Peter; (3) those who did not require circumcision or observance of kosher food laws, e.g., Paul; and (4) those who saw no abiding significance in the Jewish cult or feasts, e.g., the Gospel of John.[112] Diversity has characterized both ancient and modern Judaism and Christianity.

109. We can all learn from the striking address by Rabbi Lionel Blue to Christian gays and lesbians, "Godly and Gay," in *Jewish Explorations of Sexuality,* pp. 117-31.

110. Cf. John J. Collins, *Between Athens and Jerusalem: Jewish Identity in the Hellenistic Diaspora* (New York: Crossroad, 1983), pp. 7, 11, 14-15, 244-45, who distinguishes between Judean and Diaspora Judaisms more carefully than most. Compare Alan F. Segal, *Paul the Convert: The Apostolate and Apostasy of Saul the Pharisee* (New Haven: Yale University Press, 1990), pp. 113, 121, 151, 236-40, 264-65, and especially now John M. G. Barclay, *Jews in the Mediterranean Diaspora: From Alexander to Trajan (323 BCE-117 CE)* (Edinburgh: T. & T. Clark, 1996).

111. See V. Tcherikover, "The Ideology of the Letter of Aristeas," *HTR* 51 (1958): 59-85, and Balch, "Attitudes toward Foreigners in 2 Maccabees, Eupolemus, Esther, Aristeas, and Luke-Acts," in *The Early Church in Its Context: Essays in Honor of Everett Ferguson,* ed. Abraham J. Malherbe, Frederick W. Norris, and James W. Thompson, NTSupp 90 (Leiden: Brill, 1998), pp. 22-47, esp. pp. 39-42.

112. Raymond E. Brown, "Not Jewish Christianity and Gentile Christianity, but Types of Jewish/Gentile Christianity," *CBQ* 45 (1983): 74-79; Raymond E. Brown and John P. Meier, *Antioch and Rome: New Testament Cradles of Catholic Christianity* (New York: Paulist, 1983), pp. 2-8.

But the particular type of diversity within *modern* Judaism that we have seen above in debates about homosexuality is strikingly similar to *ancient* debates within Judaism and within (Jewish) Christianity. Both Rabbi Marder and Rabbi Shulman appeal to Leviticus 19:18, "love your neighbor as yourself," as more important than other commandments, as more important than Leviticus 20:13, which commands Israel to kill those who perform homosexual acts.

This interpretation of Torah has a familiar ring to any Christian. We recall Jesus' and Paul's appeal to this same Levitical command to love neighbors (Matt. 5:43-44; 19:19; 22:39; Luke 6:27; 10:27; Rom. 13:9; Gal. 5:14; James 2:8) as the great commandment, as summing up all the others. Paul quotes it in the context of debates about whether to keep kosher or to keep the Sabbath (Rom. 14 interpreting Lev. 11 and Exod. 20), which he calls "quarreling over opinions" (14:1)! Many would judge kosher and the Sabbath more important than the command to kill those who commit homosexual acts. Many commentators parallel Jesus choosing the great commandment with the slightly later debate between ben Azzai (ca. 110 C.E.) and rabbi Akiba (ca. 135 C.E.).[113] This ancient debate is strikingly similar to modern debates between Orthodox and Reform rabbis as well as within Christian denominations, but now over the comparative importance of Leviticus 19:18 and 20:13.

113. H. L. Strack and P. Billerbeck, *Kommentar zum Neuen Testament aus Talmud und Midrasch*, 6 vols. (1926-61), 1:357-58; Ernst Simon, "The Neighbor (Re'a) Whom We Shall Love," in *Modern Jewish Ethics: Theory and Practice*, ed. Marvin Fox (Columbus: Ohio State University Press, 1975), pp. 29-56, pp. 38-39, 53 with n. 17 on the ben Azzai/Akiba debate. Simon quotes Akiba's restrictive interpretation: "Indeed! if he acts as thy people do, thou shalt love him; but if not, thou shalt not love him," from Aboth de R. Nathan 16, trans. Judah Goldin, *The Fathers according to Rabbi Nathan*, Yale Judaica Series X (New Haven: Yale University Press, 1955), p. 86. Jesus' inclusive interpretation of Lev. 19:18 is analogous to ben Azzai's interpretation of Gen. 5:1, both a contrast to Akiba's restrictive interpretation of Lev. 19:18. Hans Dieter Betz, *The Sermon on the Mount*, Hermeneia (Minneapolis: Fortress, 1995), p. 302 with n. 806, p. 309, concludes that Jesus originated the inclusive interpretation of Lev. 19:18.

Index of Contemporary Authors

Adams, J. N., 201n.12, 217n.107
Adkins-Regan, E., 99n.65
Agyei, Y., 91n.36
Albert, Maurice, 61n.26, 62n.28
Albertz, Rainer, 151n.18
Allen, A., 209n.61
Allen, L., 96n.54, 97
Altizer, Thomas J. J., 16
Altman, Dennis, 301n.101
Ames, A., 99n.64, 100n.67, 101n.74
Annas, J., 207n.48
Ard, Roger, 29n.59
Ariès, Philippe, 45

Bailey, J. M., 90, 91, 92, 101n.70, 103n.82, 106, 127
Balch, David L., 5n.1, 53n.12, 278, 283n.22, 285n.36, 303n.111
Barclay, John M. G., 303n.110
Bancroft, J., 98, 104, 119n.124
Barnes, Paul, 26n.54, 27n.55, 28n.56
Barnett, Jeanne, 40
Barr, James, 229n.27, 248n.11
Barrett, C. K., 226n.9
Barth, Karl, 264, 265, 266, 272, 274
Baum, Gregory, 17, 18n.26
Baumrind, D., 105, 106
Baur, Karla, 139n.46
Bayer, Ronald, 243n.1
Bell, Alan P., 85n.25, 111, 124, 127n.17, 128, 129, 130, 131n.29
Benishay, D. S., 127n.17
Bennett, J. C., 31n.65
Berry, Jason, 138n.42
Betz, Hans-Dieter, 304n.113
Beyer, Hermann W., 228n.26
Bieber, Irving, 123, 125
Billerbeck, M., 218n.113
Billerbeck, P., 304n.113
Bird, Phyllis, 2, 3, 142, 145n.3, 160n.47, 167n.54, 170n.58, 172nn.61,62, 173n.67, 281, 289, 290, 299, 300
Bischoff, H., 228n.21
Blair, Ralph, 25, 30
Blanchard, R., 102n.75
Blue, Lionel, 303n.109
Blumstein, P., 85n.24, 111n.107, 114n.114
Bockmuehl, Markus, 188n.6
Bockmuhl, Klaus, 24n.45
Bohlen, J., 91n.40
Boswell, John, 67n.37, 138n.41, 178, 198n.1, 221n.129, 233n.62, 234nn.66,67,71, 236n.77, 257n.22, 258n.25

Bottéro, Jean, 158n.36, 159nn.40,41,42,43, 174n.70, 175nn.77,79, 176nn.80,81,83
Bouchard, T., 91n.40
Boyarin, Daniel, 206n.40, 236n.83
Bradford, J., 109nn.98,100, 110
Bradley, S. J., 102n.75
Braun, Herbert, 237n.90
Brigham, S., 101n.73
Brooten, Bernadette J., 47nn.5,6, 54, 201n.15, 232, 233nn.62,63, 234nn.65,70, 236nn.79,82,83
Brown, D., 200n.6, 201nn.12,14, 207nn.48,49, 209nn.60,61, 210n.67, 211n.77, 212n.79, 213n.86, 215n.96, 217nn.109,110, 219n.123, 221n.130
Brown, Marvin, 274n.25
Brown, Raymond E., 303n.112
Browning, D., 80n.11
Brueggemann, Walter, 282n.16, 283n.20
Bruni, Frank, 138n.42
Brunner, Emil, 266
Brunt, P. A., 218n.112
Bryant, Anita, 22, 29
Buber, Martin, 279
Büchsel, Friedrich, 224n.2
Buffière, Félix, 53n.13
Bugg, F., 117n.121
Burgess, John P., 36n.76
Burkett, Eleanor, 138n.42
Burr, C., 112n.110
Burtoft, L., 83n.19
Butler, Judith, 300n.100
Byne, W., 90n.34, 94n.46, 95n.50, 96nn.55,56,57, 97n.58, 99n.65, 100n.68, 102n.76, 104n.83, 105

Campolo, Peggy, 30
Campolo, Tony, 30
Cantarella, Eva, 232n.53, 239nn.105,106,108,109, 240n.111
Carrier, J., 80n.11
Carroll, Janell L., 123n.4
Castelli, Elizabeth A., 283n.20
Catania, J., 89n.33
Charlesworth, James H., 63n.30
Charlton, Ellie, 40
Cherny, S. S., 93n.45
Childs, Brevard, 5, 248n.11, 278, 279, 280n.7, 281, 282
Christensen, Torben, 227n.21
Clanton, Gordon, 14
Clark, Joan L., 32
Clarkson, Margaret, 25n.52
Coalter, Milton J, 37n.77
Coates, T., 89n.33
Cogley, John, 18
Cohen, D., 198n.2, 221n.130
Cole, S. O., 90n.34
Collins, J. J., 63n.30
Collins, John J., 303n.110
Cook, Jerry, 27, 28n.56
Cornford, Francis MacDonald, 44n.1, 56n.15
Conzelmann, Hans, 227
Corley, R., 106
Countryman, L. William, 69n.41, 136n.38
Cox, Harvey, 13-14, 16, 19, 23
Cranfield, C. E. B., 225n.8, 230n.40
Cranmer, 183
Crewdson, J., 94nn.47,48
Crooks, Robert, 139n.46
Cuneen, Joe, 19n.31
Creech, Jimmy, 39
Curran, Charles, 18

Dabelstein, Rolf, 226n.13
Davies, B., 115n.118
Davies, Margaret, 234n.69
Day, John, 151n.18
Dayton, Donald, 8n.5
De Lacy, P., 204n.29
De Young, J., 198n.1
De Young, James B., 236n.83, 237n.89
Dean-Jones, L., 201n.12, 208n.53, 219n.120
DeCecco, J., 100n.67, 101n.71
Deenen, A. A., 111n.106
Deevy, S., 130n.26
DeFries, J. C., 106n.88
Deiden, Thomas, 235n.74
Dell, Greg, 40
Delling, Gerhard, 229n.27
Deming, W., 210n.63, 218n.115

Diamond, M., 91n.37
Dobson, James, 267n.14
Dodd, C. H., 224n.1
Doll, L. S., 103n.81
Donfried, Karl P., 1, 280n.7, 283n.20
Douglas, Mary, 225n.7
Dover, Kenneth J., 44n.2, 53n.13, 198, 205n.40, 211n.69, 221n.130, 231n.50, 232
Dozeman, Thomas B., 147n.8, 157n.35, 166n.53
Drabkin, I. E., 54n.14
Dresner, Samuel H., 235n.72, 292, 296n.89
Driver, Tom F., 20n.34
Duff, Nancy, 5, 245n.6, 261, 262n.2, 264nn.5,6, 273n.24, 289, 290, 298
Dunn, James D. G., 226n.11, 228n.23, 237n.91, 238n.96

Echegaray, Hugo, 137n.40
Eckert, E., 91n.40
Edgar, J., 22
Edwards, Catherine, 219nn.120,121,123, 235n.76
Edwards, Lisa, 296
Ehrhardt, A. A., 100n.69
Eichel, E., 86n.28
Elliger, Karl, 149n.16, 151n.18, 152n.24
Ellis, L., 99n.64, 100n.67, 101n.74
Erwin, K., 110n.103
Evans, L., 117n.122

Fado, Donald, 39, 40
Falwell, Jerry, 22n.37
Fantham, E., 210n.64, 221n.130
Fascher, Erich, 238n.94
Feder, H., 99n.65
Ferguson, J., 204n.31
Fiorenza, Elisabeth Schüssler, 132n.31
Fishbane, Michael, 278, 281n.10, 282, 286, 287
Fisher, N. R. E., 217n.108, 219n.118
Fitch, Robert, 11
Fitzgerald, J., 215n.98
Fitzmyer Joseph, 194n.10, 198n.3, 227nn.18,20, 234n.67
Fletcher, Joseph, 11, 12
Foerster, Werner, 227nn.20,21
Forster, E. M., 24n.47, 53n.13
Foster, Richard J., 16n.23, 30n.61
Foucault, Michel, 198, 199n.4, 202n.19, 209n.60, 213n.85
Fraade, Steven, 278
Frame, Randy, 25nn.49,51
Fredrickson, David E., 3, 4, 197, 289, 290, 300
Frei, Hans, 5, 179n.1, 278, 279, 280n.8, 281, 282, 283n.21, 284, 286, 301
Freud, Sigmund, 125, 140
Frymer-Kensky, Tikva, 161n.47, 166n.53
Fuchs, Erich, 268n.16, 269n.17
Fulker, D. W., 93n.45, 106n.88
Furnish, Victor Paul, 232n.59, 234n.66

Gaffney, James, 20n.34
Gagnon, J. H., 79n.9, 89n.33
Garrison, D. H., 209n.58, 211n.71
Gebhard, P., 122n.1
Geertz, Clifford, 252, 284
Gerhard, G., 201n.16, 202n.22, 221n.130
Gerstenberger, Erhard S., 151n.20
Gijs, L., 111n.106
Gilbert, Maurice, 236n.83
Gladue, B. A., 96n.56, 100n.68, 102n.76
Gleason, M., 219nn.119,122, 221n.132
Glibert-Thirry, A., 206n.42, 208nn.52,54, 213n.85, 216nn.100,101,102, 220n.125
Godet, Frédric, 226nn.10,14
Golden, Mark, 198
Goldhill, Samuel, 205n.40, 219n.123, 221n.129
Goldin, Judah, 281, 282
Gooren, L. J. G., 96nn.56,57, 102n.76
Gorski, R. A., 96n.54, 97
Graber, B., 96n.56
Graham, Billy, 9, 31n.63
Grant, Robert, 2
Grayson, A. Kirk, 157n.34
Greeley, A., 107n.94
Green, R., 90n.34, 95n.53, 96n.56, 100nn.67,68, 101nn.70,74, 102n.76, 112n.110, 115n.116, 123n.5, 125
Greenberg, David F., 80n.11, 85n.24, 174nn.69,72, 176n.83

Greene-McCreight, Kathryn, 4, 169, 170, 242, 248n.11, 281, 284n.34, 288, 290, 298, 302n.107
Gruber, Mayer I., 171n.59, 172n.63
Grundmann, Walter, 238n.94
Gruuen, R. S., 100n.69
Gudorf, Christine, 2, 3, 121, 139n.44, 289, 298, 300

Hadas, Moses, 48n.7
Haldeman, D. C., 85n.24, 112n.110, 113n.113, 114, 115
Halivni, David, 278
Hallett, Judith P., 231n.51, 235n.76, 239n.108
Halperin, David M., 198n.2, 200n.6, 208n.53, 239nn.106,109,110
Hamer, Dean H., 90n.34, 93, 94, 127
Handy, Robert, 18n.27
Haraway, Donna, 300
Harrison, Paul, 134n.37
Harry, J., 86, 87nn.30,31, 101n.70, 112n.110, 114n.115
Hauck, Friedrich, 225nn.3,4,5
Hays, Richard B., 30n.61, 67n.37, 147, 189, 190n.8, 192, 231n.47, 234nn.64,66,67,71, 272n.22, 279n.2, 280n.7, 281, 283n.20, 285, 286, 288, 289, 291n.62, 301
Heath, A., 117n.122
Heider, George C., 151n.18, 153n.25
Heinemann, I., 209n.60
Heinemann, Uta Ranke, 139n.43
Henderson, J., 198n.2, 200n.7, 210n.64
Henderson, Jeffrey, 235n.76
Hendricks, S., 96n.56
Hengelbrock, J., 229n.31, 230nn.37,39
Henry, Carl F. H., 31n.63
Henshaw, Richard A., 176nn.83,86
Herdt, Gilbert, 126
Hermann, Karl Friedrich, 61n.26
Heston, L., 91n.40
Heyward, Carter, 271
Hofman, M. A., 96n.57, 97, 127n.19
Holmes, David M., 40
Holmgren, Stephen, 258n.24
Holter, K., 235n.73
Hooker, Evelyn, 108, 109, 128
Hoover, J. Edgar, 22
Horn III, Carl, 30n.60
Horney, Karen, 284n.33
Horowitz, Maryanne Cline, 53n.12
Hough, Joseph, 14
Hoult, T., 100n.67
Howe, J., 76n.6
Hu, N., 93n.44
Hu, S., 93nn.44,45, 95, 104n.85
Humbert, Paul, 151n.20
Hume, C. S., 102n.75
Hutcheson, Richard G., Jr., 8, 9n.6

Ide, Arthur Frederick, 233n.62
Idel, Moshe, 282n.19, 287n.50
Inwood, Brad, 206n.42, 213nn.84,87, 214n.94
Isay, R. A., 131n.29

Jacobelli, Luciana, 232
Jacobsen, Thorkild, 167n.56
Janus, C. L., 130n.28
Janus, S. S. S., 130n.28
Jenkins, C., 218n.117
Jenkins, Philip, 138n.42
Jenson, Robert W., 279n.4, 280, 281, 282
Jewett, Paul King, 33
Jewett, Robert, 4, 194n.10, 223, 235n.74, 236n.80, 281, 288, 290, 292n.67
Johnson, Luke Timothy, 253n.17
Johnson, Virginia H., 108n.95
Johnson, Warren, 13n.12
Johnson, William Reagan, 21
Jones, Jim, 36n.76
Jones, S., 116n.120
Jones, Stanton L., 2, 73, 79n.9, 84nn.21,22, 107n.92, 116nn.119,120, 121, 122, 288, 298, 300
Jonsen, Albert R., 265n.9
Joosten, Jan, 149n.16, 166n.53
Jung, Patricia Beattie, 131n.30, 132n.34

Kähler, Else, 233n.62
Kahn, Yoel H., 292nn.63,68, 295n.81, 296n.89, 301n.103
Kallman, F. J., 127

Kant, 48
Kantzer, Kenneth, 21n.36, 25, 29n.58
Käsemann, Ernst, 227n.15, 229n.30, 231n.46, 283
Kendler, H. H., 118
Kendler, K., 117n.122
Kennedy, D. F., 218n.111, 219n.119
Kerford, G. B., 206n.43
Kessler, R., 117n.122
King, M., 91nn.38,39, 92n.43
King, Martin Luther, 7
Kinsey, A., 2, 86, 87, 92, 103n.79, 122
Kirschner, Robert, 293, 294
Koester, Helmut, 232n.57, 234n.68
Kolodny, Robert C., 108n.95, 123n.2
Konstan, D., 199n.5, 208n.50, 221n.131
Kornhardt, Hildegard, 230n.43
Kosnik, Anthony, 19n.29, 20n.33, 123n.6
Kraft, Robert A., 65n.34
Kramer, Samuel Noah, 167n.56
Krenkel, Werner, 239
Krentz, Edgar, 5n.1
Kroll, W., 231n.50
Kruglyak, L., 93n.45
Kühl, Ernst, 230n.40, 238nn.97,98
Kuss, O., 231n.47

L'Hour, Jean, 151n.20
Lagrange, Marie-Joseph, 229n.29
Lambert, Wilfried G., 160n.45, 176n.85
Lamm, Norman, 292
Lampe, Peter, 239n.102
Laney, James T., 11, 12n.9
Laqueur, Thomas, 53n.12
Laumann, E. O., 79nn.9,10, 80n.12, 85nn.23,24, 86, 87n.30, 88, 89, 103n.81, 107n.94, 111n.104
Lausberg, Heinrich, 230nn.43,44
Lee, J. A., 130n.26
Lehmann, Paul, 11, 12, 264n.7, 265, 267nn.13,15, 274n.25
Leick, Gwendolyn, 158n.39, 160n.45, 176n.85
Leigh, B., 129n.24, 131n.29
LeVay, S., 90n.34, 97, 127
Li, L., 93n.45
Lidz, T., 127n.17
Lief, Harold I., 138n.42
Lietzmann, Hans, 237n.86
Lilja, S., 207n.49, 208n.51, 209n.61, 215n.96, 217n.108, 235n.76
Lindbeck, George, 5, 278, 279, 281, 282, 283n.20, 284, 285, 286, 290, 291, 301
Lindesay, J., 95n.52
Lindsell, Harold, 22, 24n.44
Lipman, A., 130n.26
Locher, Clemens, 176n.80
Locke, B. Z., 107n.93
Loewe, Raphael, 248n.11
Lohfink, Norbert, 162n.51
Longenecker, Richard N., 288n.55
Luck, G., 207n.46
Luther, Martin, 183, 269, 290, 291

Magnuson, V. L., 93n.44
Marder, Janet, 301, 304
Markowitz, L., 129n.24
Marshall, I. Howard, 229n.32
Martin, C., 86n.27, 122n.1
Martin, Dale B., 69nn.41,43, 198n.3, 205, 246n.8, 252-53n.15, 257n.22, 290n.58
Martin, J., 91n.37
Marty, Martin E., 9, 10n.7
Masters, William H., 108n.95, 123n.2
Matlovich, Leonard, 32n.65
Matt, Herschel, 293
Mattison, A. M., 85n.25, 111n.105, 130n.26
Mauser, Ulrich W., 166n.53
May, Elaine Tyler, 15n.19
May, Margaret Tallmadge, 51
McCallum, James, 37
McCormick, C. M., 96nn.53,54
McCormick, Patrick, 35n.73
McDonald, E., 91nn.38,39, 92n.43
McKirnan, D. J., 130n.26
McNeill, J. J., 81n.15
McNeill, John J., 33n.67, 140, 141n.48, 233n.62
McWhirter, D. P., 85n.25, 111n.105, 130n.26
Mead, Sidney E., 10n.7, 101n.73
Meehan, Francis X., 20n.34

Meier, John P., 303n.112
Melanchthon, Philipp, 291n.61
Melcher, Sarah, 150n.17
Mendenhall, George, 286n.48
Meyer-Bahlburg, H. F. L., 100n.69
Meyer, Heinrich August Wilhelm, 225, 226nn.9,14
Michael, R., 107n.94
Michael, R. T., 79n.9
Michaelis, Wilhelm, 229n.33, 230nn.38,41
Michaels, S., 79n.9
Michel, O., 226n.12, 229, 236n.78
Miller, James E., 201n.15, 205n.39, 231n.49, 232n.53, 233n.61, 235n.75
Mitchell, Christopher Wright, 228n.25
Money, J., 100n.68
Montgomery, John Warwick, 31n.63
More, P., 213n.88
Morris, Leon, 237n.91
Morrison, Melanie, 30n.61
Morse, Christopher, 270
Muck, Terry, 30n.61
Mulder, John M., 37n.77

Neale, M. C., 91n.36, 117n.122
Nelson, James B., 15, 139n.45, 245n.6
Neusner, Jacob, 302n.104
Neuwalder, N. F., 100n.69
Nicolosi, J., 112n.111
Niebuhr, Reinhold, 13, 16
Niebuhr, H. Richard, 11, 12, 41
Nissinen, Martti, 142n.1, 147nn.6,9, 149, 152n.23, 157n.34, 158nn.36,37,38,39, 159, 160nn.45,46, 161n.48, 171n.59, 174, 175nn.73,75,76,77,79, 176nn.80,81,82,83,85, 299
Nolan, Albert, 137n.39
Noll, Mark, 41n.89
Noonan, John T., Jr., 17n.26
Noth, Martin, 149n.16, 151n.18, 152n.24
Novak, David, 294n.77
Nussbaum, M., 207n.48, 213n.86

Ochs, Peter, 278, 279, 281nn.10,14, 282, 283, 284nn.24,25,26,27,34, 286nn.46,47, 287n.49, 301
O'Day, Gail R., 185n.4
Oden, Robert A., Jr., 172n.61
Odenwald, W. F., 106
Olyan, Saul M., 236n.83
Opelt, I., 66n.35, 67n.38
Osborn, Robert T., 16
Osborne, Wayne, 37
Osiek, Carolyn, 5n.1
Overholser, 23n.42

Pangborn, Cyrus, 12, 13n.11
Parker, R., 217n.107
Parsons, B., 90n.34, 94n.46, 95n.50, 96nn.55,56,57, 99n.65, 100n.68, 102n.76, 104n.83, 105
Paschen, Wilfried, 225n.6
Pattatucci, A. M., 93nn.44,45
Patterson, C., 93n.45
Paul VI, Pope, 18
Paulsen, J., 108n.95
Peplau, L. A., 129
Petersen, W., 221n.129
Peterson, P. L., 130n.26
Petschow, H., 158n.36, 159nn.40,41,42,43, 174n.70, 175nn.77,79, 176nn.80,81,83
Pillard, R. C., 90, 91, 92, 127n.17, 130n.27
Pittenger, Norman, 24n.45
Plomin, R., 106n.88
Pohlenz, M., 207n.46, 230n.42
Pomeroy, S., 202n.21
Pomeroy, W., 86n.27, 122n.1
Pottier, E., 61n.26, 62n.28
Powers, Jeanne Audrey, 32
Prager, Dennis, 292, 293nn.71,72,73,74
Preisker, H., 238n.95
Preston, K., 200n.12, 209nn.56,58, 215n.96, 218n.111, 219n.123, 221n.129
Price, Richard M., 238n.100

Radner, Ephraim, 257n.23
Rado, Sandor, 125n.11
Raggins, Sanford, 295
Reesor, M., 213n.84
Regier, D. A., 107n.93, 110nn.101,102,103

Reisman, J., 86n.27
Rekers, G., 101n.73
Renger, Johannes, 161n.47
Rentzel, L., 115n.118
Richlin, Amy, 198n.2, 219n.119, 221n.130, 235n.76, 236n.77, 237n.88
Ricketts, W., 99n.65, 100n.67, 102n.76
Ricoeur, Paul, 69n.41
Rigby, Cindy, 274n.26
Righter, Walter, 36n.74
Ringgren, Helmer, 225n.3
Risman, B., 79n.9, 101n.72
Robins, Eli, 103n.80, 109n.99, 128
Robins, L. N., 107n.93, 110nn.101,102,103
Rodriguez-Sierra, J., 96n.56
Rohr, Richard, 16n.23
Roscoe, Will, 161n.48
Rosen, A., 101n.73
Rosen, L. R., 100n.69
Ross, M., 108n.95
Rothblum, E. D., 109nn.98,100, 110n.101
Ruether, Rosemary Radford, 19, 20nn.32,34, 271
Russo, Vito, 288
Ryan, C., 109nn.98,100, 110n.101

Saad, Lydia, 35n.73
Sachs, William L., 36n.74
Safrai, S., 237n.85
Saghir, Marcel T., 103n.80, 109n.99, 128
Saglio, E., 61n.26, 62n.28
Sanders, James A., 279n.6
Sarte, Jean-Paul, 264
Sasse, Hermann, 229n.27
Satlow, Michael L., 206n.40, 237n.83
Scanzoni, Letha, 30n.61
Schenk, Wolfgang, 228n.25
Schindler, Alexander M., 295, 296n.85, 297n.90
Schlatter, Adolf, 228n.24, 230n.41
Schlier, H., 225n.8, 238nn.94,100
Schmidt, T., 84n.22
Schneider, Johannes, 236n.78
Schoedel, William R. (Bill), 2, 4, 43, 234n.65, 289, 290, 300
Schofield, M., 208n.54
Scholem, Gershom, 287n.50
Schrage, Wolfgang, 62n.27, 64, 69n.42, 70n.45
Schrijvers, P. H., 46n.4, 54, 57, 63n.31
Schwartz, Howard Eilberg, 132n.33
Schwartz, P., 79n.9, 85n.24, 101n.72, 111n.107, 114n.114
Scroggs, Robin, 63, 218n.117, 235, 236n.80, 237n.87
Searle, G. D., 14
Searle, John, 246n.7
Sedgwick, T., 81, 82
Segal, Alan F., 303n.110
Seitz, Christopher, 3, 144, 177, 281, 288, 289, 290, 298
Sell, R. L., 87n.30, 88
Seow, Choon-Leong, 147n.9, 151n.20, 168n.57
Sheppard, Gerald T., 167n.54
Shinn, Roger, 31n.65
Shulman, Sheila, 301, 302, 304
Siegelman, 103n.79
Siker, Jeffrey, 250n.13, 253, 254, 255, 256, 257
Simon, Ernst, 304n.113
Sindt, David, 35n.71
Sissa, Giulia, 64n.33
Smedes, Lewis, 27, 28n.56, 33
Smith B. L., 22n.36
Smith, C., 208n.51
Smith, Mark D., 231n.50, 235n.75
Smith, Ralph F., 131n.30
Smith, T., 107n.94
Smith, Wilfred Cantwell, 285n.36
Souza, Todd, 26n.53
Spero, Moshe H., 292
Spohn, William C., 279nn.3,6, 281nn.8,10, 282n.16, 285n.43, 287n.51, 288
Spong, John Shelby, 3, 76, 133, 187n.5, 188n.7
Stackhouse, Max, 263, 273n.23
Stafford, W. S., 73n.2
Stager, Larry E., 170n.59
Stall, R., 88, 89n.33
Stalstrom, O., 108n.95
Stegemann, Wolfgang, 230n.45
Steininger, E., 60n.21

Stevenson, M., 139n.46
Storms, M. D., 126
Stott, John, 25n.51, 33n.68
Stowers, Stanley K., 193n.9, 233-34n.63
Strack, H. L., 304n.113
Strathmann, H., 228n.22
Sutker, P. B., 117n.121
Swaab, D. F., 96n.57, 97, 127

Tanner, Kathryn, 248n.11
Taylor, T., 203n.23
Tcherikover, V., 303n.11
Thesleff, H., 203n.23, 219n.123, 220n.125
Thielicke, Helmut, 15, 16n.20
Tomson, Peter J., 231n.48
Toulmin, Stephen, 265n.9
Toulouse, Mark, 1, 6, 245n.6, 297
Trible, Phyllis, 133n.36
Trigg, J. W., 73n.2
Turner, W. J., 88, 94n.46

Unterman, Alan, 302

van de Spijker, A. M. J. M. Herman, 233n.62
van der Horst, P. W., 209n.61, 217nn.107,108
van der Toorn, Karel, 161n.47, 172n.61
van Geytenbeek, A. C., 208n.54, 209n.60
van Naerssen, A. X., 111n.106
Van Wyck, P., 126
Vann, F. H., 100n.69
Veyne, Paul, 44n.2, 239
Veridiano, N. P., 100n.69
Vilbert, Jean-Claude, 230n.45, 235n.76, 238n.101
von der Osten-Sacken, Peter, 235n.75
von Soden, Wolfram, 172n.63

Wacker, Marie-Theres, 172n.61
Walker, A., 211n.12
Ward, Roy Bowen, 232nn.52,56,58, 233nn.60,63
Weeks, Louis B., 37n.77
Weinberg, Martin S., 85n.25, 111, 124, 128, 129, 130, 131n.29
Wellings, 88
Wells, David, 41n.89
Wells, J. A., 87n.30
Wengst, Klaus, 233n.62
West, J. A., 117n.121
Westermann, Claus, 228n.25
Whitaker, Richard E., 167n.54
Whitam, F. L., 91n.37
White, L., 215n.98
Wilckens, Ulrich, 68n.39, 226n.11, 236n.82
Wiley, J., 89n.33
Wilhelm, Gernot, 172n.61
Williams, R., 112n.108
Williams, Rowan, 248n.11
Winkler, John J., 206n.40, 232nn.56,58, 239n.105
Witelson, S. F., 96nn.53,54
Wittgenstein, 247
Wolfson, Harry Austryn, 59n.20
Wolpe, Paul Root, 123n.4
Workman, D., 84n.22, 107n.92, 116n.120
Wright, D., 220n.127, 221n.129
Wright, Elliott, 23n.43
Wurzburger, Walter, 292
Wypij, D., 87n.30

Yancey, Philip, 25
Yarhouse, Mark A., 2, 73, 79n.9, 84n.21, 116nn.119,120, 121, 122, 288, 298, 300

Zahn, Theodor, 225n.8, 236n.78, 237n.92, 238n.97
Zhang, Shang-Ding, 106
Zucker, K. J., 101n.70, 102n.75, 103n.82

Scripture Index

OLD TESTAMENT

Genesis
1–3 167n.54, 245n.5, 288n.56
1–2 166, 191
1 166, 168, 194, 287, 289, 299
1:22 167
1:26-27 296
1:27 302
1:27b 167n.54
1:27-28 151, 167, 292, 297n.91
2:18-24 292
2:24 167
3 167, 256
3:5 194, 227
3:6 194
4:1 147n.11
4:17 147n.11
4:25 147n.11
5:1 304n.113
5:2 292
9:22 292
11 256
12:3 293
16 251
18 189
18:20 195
19 147, 156
19:1-29 147
19:5 147, 195, 292
19:7 148
19:8 148n.13
19:9 147n.10
19:24 195
28:14 293
34:7 148n.12, 152
34:31 148n.14
38 164, 251
38:9-10 158
38:21-22 171
38:26 147n.11

Exodus
14:12 170
20 304
20:26 162n.51, 237
22:19 156
23:17 151n.19

Leviticus
11 304
11:6 [11:5 LXX] 65
17:1–26:46 149
18 150, 152, 153, 154, 156, 157, 163, 164, 166n.53
18:1-16 153
18:2b-5 149
18:6 150
18:6-18 237
18:7-16 150
18:17-18 150
18:17-23 150
18:19 150, 151, 155
18:19-23 150
18:20 150, 151
18:21 151
18:21-22 154
18:22 63n.30, 149, 151, 236, 289, 292
18:23 150, 151, 157n.32
18:24 150
18:24-30 149
18:26 152
18:27 152
18:29 63n.30, 152
18:30 150, 152
19 152, 163
19:2 149, 154
19:13 296
19:15 296

19:16 296
19:17 296
19:18 296, 302, 304
19:26b 250n.13
19:34 296
20 152, 154, 155, 157, 164, 166n.53
20:1-5 153
20:1-16 153
20:6 153
20:9 153
20:10 153, 185
20:10-16 189
20:10-21 153
20:11 153n.27
20:12 153n.27
20:13 63n.30, 152, 153, 156, 178, 186, 250n.14, 289, 292, 304
20:14 153
20:15-16 153
20:16 154
20:17 153n.27
20:17-21 153
20:18 153n.27
20:19 153n.27
20:20 153n.27
20:21 153n.27
20:22-26 153
20:22b 154
20:23-24 154
20:24 154
20:26 154, 303
20:26b 154
21:16-24 294
22:23-24 185
25 162

Numbers
13:30–14:4 170
32 169

Deuteronomy
13:14 152n.21
14:7 65
15:12-18 162n.51
16:11 162n.51
16:14 162n.51
22:5 157
22:23-24 178
23:17-18 152n.21, 170
23:18 172
25:4 66
27:15 152n.21
27:21 156
30:11 48
30:19 293

Judges
19 147, 156, 292
19:22 147
19:22-24 147
19:23 148, 152
19:23-24 148
19:25 148n.13
20:6 148n.12
20:10 148n.12
21:11 151n.19
21:12 151n.19

Ruth
4:11 167n.55

1 Samuel
1:19 147n.11
18:1 146n.6

1 Kings
1:4 147n.11
14:24 172n.62
15:12 172n.62
22:46 172n.62

2 Kings
23:7 172n.62, 173n.67

Ezra
9–10 163n.52

Nehemiah
13:23-30 163n.52

Job
36:14 172n.62

Proverbs
6:26 171

Isaiah
56:7 296
59:13 227

Jeremiah
7:18 173n.67
14:14 227
44:15-19 173n.67

Ezekiel
1 287
8:14 173n.67

Hosea
4:14 171
7:13 227

Habakkuk
2:4 194

APOCRYPHA AND PSEUDEPIGRAPHA

Wisdom of Solomon
13–14 49
14:2 236n.82
14:24-27 226n.11
14:26 49
15:5 236n.82

Sirach
18:30 236n.82
23:6 236n.82

Jubilees
16:5-9 237n.89

Epistle of Aristeas
139 227n.20
151-52 237n.89
152 217n.107

4 Maccabees
2:11 209n.60
3:17 210n.65
5:8 48
5:14-38 48
5:25 48
5:26 48

3 Esdras
8:66 226n.13

Testament of Benjamin
6:5 217n.107
8:2 217n.107

Testament of Joseph
4:5 226n.11
4:6 217n.107

Testament of Judah
16:1 219n.123

Testament of Levi
17:11 221n.132

Testament of Naphtali
3:1-5 216n.103

Testament of Reuben
2:1 215n.97
2:8 215n.97
3:2 215n.97
4:6 215n.97

Assumption of Moses
5:4 227n.16

2 Slavonic Enoch
10:4-5 237n.89
34:1-3 237n.89

NEW TESTAMENT

Matthew
5:17 188
5:17-48 178, 184
5:19 188
5:20 188
5:43-44 304
19:19 304
22:39 304
24:9-14 257n.23

Mark
7 187
7:1-13 187, 188
7:1-23 178, 187
7:9-13 188
7:13 188
7:19 187
7:21 188
10 191
10:2-9 166
10:2-12 288n.56
10:3 191
10:6-8 191

Luke
6:27 304
10:27 304

John
7:53–8:11 185n.4
8:1-11 178, 184
8:5 185
8:12–11:57 186
19:30 178, 186

Acts
10 255n.20, 257

Romans
1–2 191, 193, 196
1 128, 134, 140, 189, 190, 192, 193, 194, 245, 288n.56, 289, 290, 300
1:1-15 223
1:9 228
1:16 193n.9
1:16-17 223, 224
1:17 194
1:18 193, 195, 216, 226, 227
1:18-27 222
1:18-32 48, 49, 67, 198-99n.3, 211, 216, 233n.63
1:18–4:25 223
1:19-21 228
1:20 194, 195
1:21 216, 224
1:22 194
1:23 194, 226
1:24 69, 208, 209, 216, 224, 225, 229
1:24-27 190, 193, 194, 197, 198, 199, 205, 206, 207, 208, 215, 216, 222, 223, 224, 289
1:25 194, 195, 224, 226, 231
1:26 44, 146, 195, 196, 200, 201, 208, 209, 217, 224, 229, 231n.48
1:26-27 47, 48, 53n.12, 67, 68, 134, 154n.29, 204, 236n.79, 238
1:26a 230
1:26b 230, 234, 236
1:27 208, 209n.58, 210, 211, 213, 214, 215, 217, 224, 231nn.47,48, 235, 238
1:27a 234, 236
1:27a-c 238
1:27d 238
1:28-32 190
1:29-30 226
1:29-31 128
2 193, 195, 196
2:1 190, 191, 193, 233n.63
2:9-10 193n.9
2:11 193

2:11-16 68
2:14-15 134
2:17 233n.63
2:23 216n.104
2:29 67
3:2 194, 195
3:31 178, 183
4:1-25 192
5:1–8:39 223
5:15-20 192
6:19 225
7:7-12 183
7:12 187
7:13-25 178, 183
7:18b-20 263
9–10 249n.12, 252
9:1–1:36 223
11:24 68
12:1 67
12:1–15:13 223
13:9 304
14 304
14:1 304
15:14–16:23 223

1 Corinthians
6 290, 299
6:9 29n.58, 63, 136, 190, 198, 199, 218, 220, 222
6:9-10 197, 218, 219
6:12 70, 208n.51
6:12-20 69
6:13 70
6:15 65
6:18 71
6:19 65, 70
7 235n.73
7:1-7 48
7:1-9 166
7:4 233, 234n.63
7:7 233
7:9 48, 140, 210n.63
7:12-16 49
7:19 69
7:29-31 49
7:32-35 49
8–10 69
8:1 69
8:4 69
8:4-6 67
9:9 66
10:1-22 70
10:14-22 70
10:23 69
10:23–11:1 70
11 59, 235n.73
11:2-15 59
11:5 62
11:5-7 62
11:6 62
11:13 62
11:14 68
11:14-15 59, 62
15:25 38n.94
15:53 238n.94

2 Corinthians
5:10 238n.94
12:21 225

Galatians
3:28 62, 258
4:17 208n.51
5:14 304
5:16 190
5:16-24 178, 184
5:19 225
5:24 178, 190

Ephesians
5 245n.5
5:21-33 166

1 Thessalonians
2:3 225, 237n.90
4:1 238n.94
4:3-8 166
4:4 209n.60
4:5 209n.60, 229
4:7 225
4:12 218n.112

2 Thessalonians
2:11 237n.90
3:7 238n.94

1 Timothy
1:8-11 221n.129

Hebrews
47 172n.62
10:1 188
10:1-4 188
10:1-31 178, 187
10:9 188
10:19 188
10:31 189
13:4 166
15 152n.21
18–19 152n.21, 170
18:17 171
19:18 170, 171

James
2:8 304

Revelation
1–3 257n.23

EARLY CHRISTIAN LITERATURE

Epistle of Barnabas
10:6-7 65

Index of Other Ancient Authors

Achilles Tatius, 209n.58, 210n.66, 218n.111, 221n.131
Aeschines, 71
Akiba, 304
Alciphron, 211n.70
Aristeas, 48, 66, 67
Aristippus 200, 201n.16
Aristophanes, 46, 47
Aristotle, 57n.16, 65, 66nn.35,36, 207, 217n.111, 220, 229, 230n.43, 299, 300
Aristoxenus, 204n.34
Artemidoros, 239n.105
Athenaeus, 201n.16, 206n.41, 217n.111
Athenagoras, 200n.11
Augustine, 132, 139, 247, 268
Aurelianus, Caelius, 54, 57
Aurelius, Marcus, 61n.26

ben Azzai, 304

Chariton, 199, 210nn.64,65,66, 211n.76, 212n.80
Chrysippus, 209n.58, 230n.37
Clement of Alexandria, 43, 44, 47, 50, 64, 65, 66, 200nn.10,11, 202n.22, 203, 204nn.31,32,34, 205nn.39,40, 206n.43, 207n.48, 209n.60, 210nn.67,68, 212n.81, 213, 214n.94, 215n.95, 217nn.108,109, 218n.115, 221nn.131,132

Dio Cassius, 201n.13, 202n.17
Dio Chrysostom, 205nn.39,40, 212, 216nn.102,103,105, 217n.107, 217-218n.111, 220n.126, 221n.131
Diodorus Siculus, 202n.18, 219n.122
Diogenes Laertius, 45, 70n.44, 200n.8, 201nn.13,16, 202n.18, 204n.29, 206, 210n.67, 213n.84, 218n.114
Dionysius of Halicarnassus, 221n.130

Epictetus, 46, 60, 61, 200, 201n.13, 202n.18, 203, 204, 205nn.36,37, 206, 207n.46, 212, 213, 214, 215n.98, 217nn.107,110, 218nn.112,113,115, 219n.123, 221n.132
Epicurus, 207
Eusebius, 220n.128, 221n.129

Fronto, 201n.16

Galen, 51, 61, 200n.9, 204n.29, 208n.56, 209n.58, 213n.84, 214n.94

Heliodorus, 211n.75, 215n.95
Hippodamus, 220n.125

Hippolytus, 220n.128

Iamblichus, 202n.22, 203n.25
Irenaeus, 280, 282

Jerome, 268
Josephus, 49, 68
Justin Martyr, 200n.11

Lactantius, 57
Longus, 210n.64
Lucian, 60n.24, 61, 62n.29, 202n.17, 220n.126, 232n.53
Lucretius, 200n.6, 207n.48
Lysis, 219n.123

Macarius, 221n.129
Macrobius, 239n.106
Maximus of Tyre, 210n.66
Musonius Rufus, 48, 60, 61, 200n.9, 204n.32, 205n.39, 206, 218nn.112,115, 220n.126, 221n.129

Ocellus, 204n.34, 205n.39, 213n.85
Origen, 218n.117
Ovid, 210nn.65,66, 211n.70, 215n.96

Parmenides, 55, 57
Philo 2, 43, 44, 45, 46, 47, 48, 49, 50, 51, 52, 53, 54, 55, 56, 57, 58, 59, 60, 61, 63n.30, 67, 68, 71, 200n.10, 203n.24, 205nn.39,40, 209n.60, 210nn.64,67, 212nn.78,81, 214n.94, 216n.105, 217n.109, 218n.115, 219n.123, 221n.132, 230n.45, 300
Philostratus 63, 211n.75, 212n.78
Pindar, 45
Plato, 43, 44, 45, 46, 47, 48, 49, 50, 52, 56, 57, 58, 59, 64, 71, 202n.22, 203n.25, 205n.39, 208n.55, 215n.96, 221n.129, 229, 232, 233
Plautus, 238n.101
Plutarch, 48, 61, 62n.29, 67, 200, 201nn.13,14, 204n.30, 205n.40, 206n.45, 207n.48, 208nn.55,56, 209n.62, 210nn.64,65,66,67, 211nn.73,75,76, 213n.86, 214nn.94,95, 215n.96, 217nn.107,110, 218n.115, 219n.121, 221n.131, 238n.101
Pseudo-Aristotle, 202n.21, 203n.25, 300
Pseudo-Crates, 204n.30, 218n.114, 220n.125
Pseudo-Demosthenes, 221n.129
Pseudo-Diogenes, 205n.39, 220n.125
Pseudo-Heraclitus, 221n.132
Pseudo-Hippocrates, 210n.66, 221n.132
Pseudo-Lucian, 60n.23, 199n.5, 201n.13, 202nn.17,18, 205n.40, 209n.62, 212n.80, 217nn.107,108, 218n.115, 221nn.129,131, 232n.53
Pseudo-Musonius, 218n.115
Pseudo-Phocylides, 209nn.60,61, 218n.115, 221n.132, 232
Pseudo-Plato, 203n.25
Pseudo-Plutarch, 210n.67

Quintilian, 230n.43

Seneca, 201n.12, 203n.26, 204n.35, 205n.40, 206, 207n.46, 212n.78, 215, 217n.110, 239
Sibylline Oracles, 221n.130, 226n.11
Socrates, 45, 229
Soranus, 51, 54, 55, 56, 57, 63
Stobaeus, 200nn.8,9, 203n.25, 204nn.30,32,33,34, 210n.67, 213n.84, 215n.98, 220n.125
Strabo, 218n.111

Theano, 203n.25, 220n.125
Theophilus of Antioch, 221n.129

Virgil, 210n.66, 215n.96

Xenophon, 200n.10, 202nn.17,18, 203n.24, 208n.55, 209n.57, 211n.75

Zeno, 201n.16, 203, 206, 209n.58, 229n.31

261.8357
B174
98640
LINCOLN CHRISTIAN COLLEGE AND SEMINARY
3 4711 00151 9950